Clinical Research in Allied Health and Special Education

Clinical Research in Allied Health and Special Education

Third Edition

Franklin Stein, Ph.D., OTR/L
The University of South Dakota
Vermillion, South Dakota

Susan K. Cutler, Ph.D., NCSP
Morningside College
Souix City, Iowa

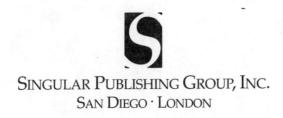

SINGULAR PUBLISHING GROUP, INC.
SAN DIEGO · LONDON

Singular Publishing Group, Inc.
4284 41st Street
San Diego, California 92105-1197

19 Compton Terrace
London, N1, 2UN, UK

Typeset in 10/12 Palatino by So Cal Graphics
Printed in the United States of America by McNaughton & Gunn

Library of Congress Cataloging-in-Publication Data

Stein, Franklin
    Clinical research in allied health and special education / by
Franklin Stein and Susan K. Cutler.—3rd ed.
        p.   cm.
    Rev. ed. of: Anatomy of clinical research / Franklin Stein. c1989.
    Includes bibliographical references and index.
    ISBN 1-56593-631-0
    1. Medical rehabilitation—Research—Methodology.   2. Special
education—Research—Methodology.   I. Cutler, Susan K.   II. Stein,
Franklin. Clinical research in allied health and special education.
III. Title.
    [DNLM: 1. Research.   2. Allied Health Occupations.   3. Research
Design.   4. Education, Special.   W 20.5 S819 1996]
RM930.S74   1996
610'.72—dc20
DNLM/DLC
for Library of Congress   95-46566
                                                                                              CIP

Contents

Chapter 8   Selecting a Test Instrument 315

Preface to the First Edition

This book evolved from questions that arose the first time I worked as an Allied Health student in a clinical facility at the Bronx Veteran's Administration Hospital in New York City. I asked then and I continue to ask:

How can one objectively evaluate and measure the effects of treatment?

Are there causes for patient's improvement other than the direct intervention of the therapist?

If a patient improved as a result of specific therapeutic intervention, can the results be applied to all patients with the same diagnosis?

For fifteen years as a practicing occupational therapist and psychologist, I asked these questions while seeking answers by listening to research papers at conferences, by reading carefully the literature on patient care, by observing therapeutic effects in the clinic, and by following up individual patients over time. As a teacher in a graduate program in the Allied Health Professions at Boston University since 1967, I have continued to raise these questions with students in occupational therapy, physical therapy, nutrition, speech therapy, audiology, rehabilitation counseling, dance therapy, special education, psychology, and health dynamics.

As a clinician in the health field, teacher and social scientist I have found that these questions remain partially unanswered and like many areas of human knowledge generate further questions as we amass evidence and get closer to solutions. The discovery of effective treatment methods and objective measures of patient improvement in many areas of chronic diseases, such as arthritis, psychoses, cardiac insufficiency, multiple sclerosis, cerebral palsy, and cancer, have yet to be found by health researchers.

This book is an attempt to provide the health researcher with a perspective on the history of medical research and the methods of scientific inquiry. The book is directed at the applied scientist who will be carrying out research in such settings as a rehabilitation hospital, residential treatment facility, outpatient clinic, special education classroom, psychiatric hospital, community health center, half-way house, or in the patient's home through outreach programs.

The book is also concerned with research in relation to the health practitioner as a treatment agent. Research in regard to the preparation of the health worker, administration of health care programs and the differential role perceptions are examined. The overall purposes of the book are twofold. One is to assist clinicians and students in the health fields to become effective evaluators and consumers of published research, and two is to facilitate research skills by communicating the process of research and the abilities needed to plan and implement a research project.

The book is organized into eight chapters. The first chapter is a short history of the development of scientific research in medicine, health and rehabilitation. This chapter was included to give the student of research an historical overview that demonstrates the interaction of scientific methods and progress in the treatment of diseases and disabilities. Included in this first chapter is an analysis of medical progress through seven stages of development from the biological description of Galen in the second century to the present concern with development disabilities.

The second chapter relates the scientific method as it applies to the objectivity of the researcher. The relationship between theory, hypothesis and data is diagrammed to describe to the reader the process of arriving at a conclusion. Five fallacies in logic are directly related to health research. These fallacies are directed at the consumer of health research who is many times persuaded to accept a treatment method based on inconclusive evidence. An outline of the research process is presented to give the student an overall view and to suggest questions regarding the validity and adequacy of a researcher's methods and conclusions. The ideal qualities of a researcher are presented in the context of human problem-oriented research. The difference between research that seeks general laws, such as nomothetic, and research that analyzes the underlying dynamics in an individual, such as idiographic, is discussed.

The third chapter describes eight research models that can be applied to health problems—experimental, methodological, evaluation, heuristic, correlational, clinical observation, survey, and historical. The purposes of each model are presented along with examples of application, sequential analysis of the process of research, and the specific methods involved in collecting data. Each research model is treated separately. The problems and limitations of each model are described in detail. By describing eight distinct research models I have attempted to integrate the literature on research methods and to incorporate the most commonly used research models into a comprehensive approach for investigating health problems. The emphasis in this chapter is on how to select and apply a research model to a specific research question.

Chapter four includes strategies for developing and narrowing studies in health and rehabilitation by considering priorities based on incidence of disability, leading causes of death, and human and economic costs of a disability to society, and the significance of a research problem based on the role perceptions and job descriptions of Allied Health professionals. The problems of feasibility in relation to time, cost, instrumentation, and researchability are discussed.

How a student can find previous published studies that are related to an area of research interest is examined in chapter five, Review of the Literature. Sources of bibliographical references in the Allied Health sciences are listed, as well as the use and availability of computer-based information retrieval systems such as Medlars and ERIC.

Research design, which is the title of chapter six, includes the process of planning research and controlling for extraneous variables. The problems of stating a hypothesis, operationally defining terms, and identifying the independent and dependent variables are discussed in relation to the eight research models in health. The need for theoretical explanations for generating a hypothesis is emphasized. The limitations of a study in regard to problems of control, sampling, reliability of instruments and tests, and restrictions involving research with human subjects are examined.

Chapter seven, entitled Methodology, includes the problems of representative sampling, measuring a variable, understanding reliability and validity, and selecting a test instrument.

The relationship between statistics and health research is included in chapter eight entitled Data Analysis and Statistics. Topics in this chapter are: receptivity to statistics, language and design of statistics, application of statistics to health research, descriptive statistics and inferential tests.

The motivation to write a book needs outside energy as well as self-propelled locomotion. The students who have taken HP 701 at Sargent College are as much responsible for this book as I am. They served as the external energy to finish this book. To my colleagues at Sargent College, I am also grateful for their critical examination and scrutiny. To Matt Luzzi, Ruth Jacobson, Dorothy Disher, Don Maietta and Charlotte Renner I express thanks for their editorial support and encouragement. To Dorothy Lundsgaard, an excellent typist who can translate hieroglyphics into English, a public thank you. And to his family, Jennie, David, Jessica and Barbara, an apology for the undue crises that were wrought by writing a book.

In addition to the support from students, colleagues, friends and family, I acknowledge the help from Boston University in awarding me a sabbatical during 1974 that enabled her to study and write in Cambridge, England. I also feel appreciative to the Society of Visiting Scholars in Cambridge, England, who made my adjustment to the world of academia there a pleasant experience.

Preface to the Revised Edition

In working on the revised edition of *Anatomy of Clinical Research*, I became aware of the rapidly changing developments in the delivery of health care in the United States. Consumers of health care—you and I, and everyone else—are demanding quality care at a reasonable cost. National Health Insurance, which seemed so promising ten years ago, now has been pushed further ahead in the future. Medicare and Medicaid, which seemed to be developing lives of their own, have had their progress slowed down. In spite of this, the health care industry has continued to grow, especially in the area of allied health manpower. As this growth continues it represents a larger proportion of the gross national product (GNP) in the United States. Health care expenditures in 1986 were $458.2 billion, an average of $1,837 per person and represented 10.9 percent of the GNP, as compared to $75.0 billion, an average of $399 per person and 7.4 percent of the GNP in 1970.

Technological advances in health care, such as coronary bypass surgery, bionic replacements, and renal dialysis, have had dramatic effects on medical care. These effects on the general health of the populace, however, are comparatively minor compared to the widespread movement toward preventative health care and physical fitness. The epidemic in the incidence of Acquired Immune Deficiency Syndrome (AIDS) and the continuing problem of drug addiction have contributed to changes in the health care system in the last ten years.

Americans are now finding that they have a major responsibility in maintaining their own health through exercise, diet, reduction of stress and control of smoking, and alcohol and drug usage.

It has been substantially documented that lifestyle affects the physical and psychological well-being of the individual. These general findings will continue to influence the direction of research in the next ten years in the Allied Health Professions. Stress and its effects on health will also continue to generate much interest.

In this revision I have sought to update health statistics, references, and sources of information for the health care researcher. I have also expanded upon examples of research models in chapter three so as to help the student researcher better understand the eight research models. In the Appendix I have added a section on the Nobel Prize in Medicine. This was added to give examples in the history of scientific medicine and in the hope that they might perhaps inspire some unknown researcher in the Allied Health professions. I have also revised some parts of the book that needed further elaboration.

I acknowledge the helpful comments from the Allied Health students at the University of Wisconsin-Milwaukee in the classes of 696-423, Writing and Research in Occupational Therapy Practice and 437-207, Data Analysis in Allied Health Sciences.

I also owe much to my present and former colleagues at the University of Wisconsin-Milwaukee for their support and assistance during the period I revised this book.

Introduction

The first edition of this book was published in 1976. At that time it was the first textbook on clinical research in the allied health professions. Since then numerous texts have been published in research from the perspective of clinical practice in occupational therapy, physical therapy, and speech–language pathology and audiology. The current edition, the third, is a collaborative effort where the authors combine their expertise in occupational therapy, counseling psychology, and special education into a textbook on clinical research. In preparing this edition we raised the question: What characterizes a good textbook in clinical research? In reviewing other textbooks and reexamining the strengths and weaknesses of this book we came up with the following points:

- The textbook should be well written and easily understood by undergraduate and graduate students. Complex concepts should be explained carefully and presented in a logical sequence.
- There should be an historical perspective in the text that connects the student to other researchers who laid the foundation for clinical practice. The allied health professions and special education are a continuation of the scientific and medical revolutions that created the helping professions. As clinicians we are dependent upon the early research in anatomy and physiology, testing and measurement, medical instrumentation, clinical medicine, and environmental health. The knowledge gained in the basic sciences impact strongly on the clinical professions. As scholars we know that current practice stands on the shoulders of the giants in basic and clinical research.
- Within the context of the book there should be many examples from the literature as well as hypothetical examples explaining theoretical concepts and research principles. The book should come from a pragmatic perspective that presents feasible ideas.
- The book should be a resource for further study in related areas. References and addresses should be liberally found throughout the book to point the student in the right directions.
- Statistical procedures should be clearly explained in a stepwise procedure. The concept underlying the statistical technique should be emphasized. Although there are a number of software programs and statistical packages it is important for the student to understand how the statistical results are derived. The student should have a strong background in descriptive statistics before learning inferential statistics.
- In the textbook there should be an example of a research proposal that can serve as a model for the student researcher. The research proposal should be feasible and realistically implemented.
- The textbook should be comprehensive and include a number of different research models appropriate for research in occupational therapy, physical therapy, special education, rehabilitation counseling, and other allied health fields.

- Qualitative as well as quantitative research models should be described with examples from the literature. Both models are appropriate and relevant. The research design is judged on its own merits as far as validity and application to clinical practice or health care.
- The emphasis in research is in raising relevant and feasible questions. The student should be encouraged to state many questions that generate intellectual interest and curiosity. The process of doing research and searching the research literature are as important as reporting results. Research should be a process of discovery and intellectual excitement.
- The student who is designing and carrying out a research study should see the relationship between one's research study and one's professional role whether it be as clinician, administrator, educator, or researcher.
- The research text should help the student develop a critical view of research. The student should be able to read the literature with a critical eye and carry over this knowledge to clinical practice especially in clinical reasoning.
- The student should have a strong appreciation of the ethical issues involved with human research. Students should be able to design an informed consent form and to be able to safeguard the research subject from unnecessary psychological or physical risks.

One of the major purposes of this textbook is to link research to clinical practice. It is important within this context that the researcher raise many questions relating to clinical practice in developing a research proposal. As students or clinical researchers work on the preparation of a research design they should keep in mind the practical implications of the research study. The content of the chapters in the book are organized comprehensively to include all the components in research from generating a research topic, carrying out a literature review, designing a research study, selecting a measuring instrument, analyzing statistical data, and writing a scientific paper. The textbook is organized to enable a student to write a research proposal, critically evaluate a published study, and prepare a manuscript for a refereed journal.

In writing this edition, the authors developed a conceptual model that serves as a rationale for the book.

- The medical model underlies the clinical practice in allied health and special education. Historically the medical model includes arriving at a diagnosis that serves as the basis of treatment. Understanding the medical model and its historical perspective is important for clinicians in rehabilitation and special education because we work closely with physicians in a team approach. The development of educational, psychological, and sociological factors in treatment does not negate the medical model. Effective rehabilitation and habilitation depends upon a holistic approach to the patient that includes the medical model and educational–psychological approach.
- Conceptually we emphasize the strengths of individuals with disabilities as the basis of good treatment. In planning treatment interventions, the clinician evaluates both the strengths and weaknesses in the client and then develops with the client a goal-directed plan for achieving functional independence.
- Good treatment means fitting the treatment procedure to the patient and not fitting the patient to a treatment method. The clinician should avoid a

"Procrustean bed" where treatment methods are advocated and generalized to all patients. Good treatment is based on the individual needs of the patient and the consideration of multiple approaches.

- The goal of clinical research is to discover through objective and systematic inquiry the most effective treatment methods that can be applied to the client with a disability. Research should be driven by theory and explanation.
- The relationship between clinical research and clinical practice is based on the premise that good treatment depends upon multiple factors including the therapist's skill, the effectiveness of a treatment methodology, the appropriateness of the client, and environmental factors that affect treatment. Clinical research strives to understand the relationship between these factors in clinical treatment.
- Doing and critically evaluating research findings helps the student to become an effective clinician. Since clinical practice is dependent on clinical reasoning and decision making, the effective clinician applies the scientific method in practice. The research-oriented practitioner is able to evaluate the literature and incorporate current research findings into clinical practice.

Acknowledgments

We are especially grateful for the assistance of many people who read and critiqued chapters in this book and encouraged us to continue with the process. Among them are Jane and Mike Madden, Evelyn Schlenker, Yuhlong Leo, Dorothy Ann Elsberry, Glenna Tevis, Michael Granaas, Mary Ann Kurth, Jacqueline Cunningham, and Karenlee and Floyce Alexander. Especial thanks to Sarah Montgomery for her contribution of an example of a research proposal. We also appreciate the comments from students in the Department of Occupational Therapy at the University of South Dakota on the content of the book. Secretarial and work study support from the Department of Occupational Therapy were extremely timely. Kathy Graff and Cherity Lindgren were helpful in carrying out the detailed tasks that are indispensable in writing a book. We greatly appreciate the support of the faculty and staff at USD (Dean Frank Brady, Denise Rotert, Barbara Brockevelt, Peggy Stoddard, Bob Bing, Cheryl Hovorka) and at Morningside College (President Jerry Israel, Dean Bari Watkins, Tory Marquesen, Carol Phillips, Dick Owens, Sharon Ocker, Aline Bobys).

Frank Stein acknowledges the help from the New York University Occupational Therapy faculty during the summer of 1995 while he was a visiting professor. And to my wife, Jennie, who listened attentively while I struggled to formulate concepts and meet deadlines. Sue Cutler would especially like to acknowledge her father who, as a psychologist, inspired me to ask questions about the world and thus engage in research.

Both of us would also like to thank Marie Linvil and Angie Singh at Singular Publishing for their immense help in the editing of the book and keeping us on track.

CHAPTER
1

A Short History of the Scientific Method in Medicine, Health, Rehabilitation, and Special Education

Medical research on the scale to which it is developed today is a modern invention. A hundred years ago it was limited to the part-time activities of a few dozen individuals working in their private rooms (one could hardly call them laboratories) at home or in a university. Today it provides a life-time's career for thousands of medical scientists working in specially built laboratories in universities and research institutes financed by government or the pharmaceutical industry.—N. Poynter, *Medicine and Man* (p. 6)

Operational Learning Objectives

By the end of this chapter, the reader should be able to

1. describe seven stages in the history of medicine
2. explain the cyclical nature of medical progress
3. recognize the important contributions of medical researchers toward the improvement in environmental health and clinical practice
4. understand the importance of methodological discoveries in diagnosis, prevention, and treatment
5. indicate the reasons for the growth of the allied health professions that are related to the rehabilitation movement
6. explain the important stages in the development of special education
7. identify trends in rehabilitation research

1

Introduction

Before the beginnings of modern science in the latter half of the nineteenth century, relationships between causes and effects still retained explanations that bordered on the supernatural. Vitalism, a recurrent movement in medicine, was typified by the eighteenth century physician who ascribed mysterious substances in the blood to life functions. This theory was an outcome of the prescientific thinking that gave way to the systematic and orderly explanations that we now associate with modern scientific research. The breakthrough in understanding the disease process began with the laboratory experimentation of Pasteur (1822–1895), who served as a model for the medical scientist. The impact of scientific technology in the treatment and rehabilitation of the sick and the disabled has been a remarkable record in human progress. In only a few other areas of knowledge has man made greater strides. How and why did this happen?

The analysis of the progress in medical science, rehabilitation, and special education is divided into seven stages, identified in Figure 1–1. These seven stages are progressive, interactive, and dynamic. For example, basic research in biological and chemical processes in Stage I continues to be important as evidenced by the investigations of

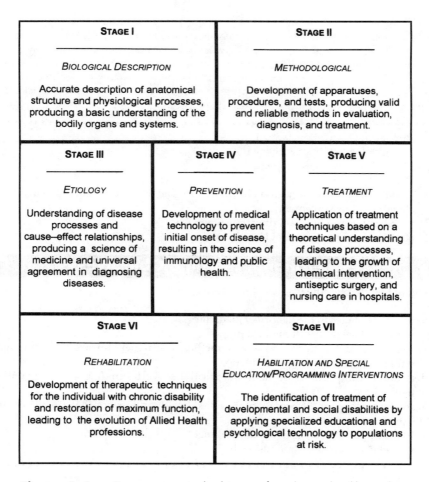

Figure 1–1. Seven stages in the history of medicine, health, and rehabilitation. The seven stages are progressive, interactive, and dynamic.

DNA and RNA as the building blocks in protoplasm. Similarly, methodological research is in the forefront by virtue of the integration of high technology with clinical practice as demonstrated in the areas of prosthetics, transplant operations, kidney dialysis techniques, and artificial replacement of bodily organs. Medical scientists are constantly refining treatment and preventive methodologies. Immunologists who formerly sought chemicals to destroy harmful bacteria and viruses have led the way to present day investigators searching for vaccines to prevent cancerous growths and life-threatening diseases, such as Acquired Immune Deficiency Syndrome (AIDS).

Progress in science is cyclical and cumulative. As knowledge grows, medical scientists refine their methods of research. Stages of development in medicine point to the cumulative process of obtaining knowledge and to the evolutionary process of scientific methodology and its impact on clinical practice.

1.1 Biological Description, Stage I

The Growth of Scientific Anatomy and Physiology

The earliest medical research started with the discovery of the physiological processes and anatomical systems of the body. Biological Description: Stage I, the evolution of medical research, is outlined in Table 1–1. Knowledge of the anatomical structure of animals during the Middle Ages and Renaissance periods was greatly influenced by Galen

Table 1–1   *The Emergence of the Medical Scientist: Stage I*

Medical Events	Discovery Dates	Scientists	Implications
Hippocratic writings	400–500 B.C.	Hippocrates (500 B.C.)	Provided a model for medical practitioners based on ethical and humane treatment
Systematic study of bodily processes	169–180 A.D.	Claudius Galen (129–199 A.D.)	Influenced medical practice for 1300 years, presenting an eclectic synthesis of prior knowledge
"The canon of Medicine"	translated 1187	Avicenna (980–1037)	Significant figure of Arabic medicine whose work was dogma during the Middle Ages
"Paragranum": The four pillars of medicine: philosophy, astronomy, chemistry, and virtue	1530	Paracelsus (1493–1541)	Created the foundation for general medical practice based on a knowledge of pharmaceutical chemistry
Atlas of Anatomy "De humani of corporis fabrica"	1543	Andreas Vesalius (1514–1564)	Made descriptive anatomy the basis of medicine and replaced aspects of Galen's work
Manual of Surgery	1543	Ambroise Pare (1510–1590)	Generated surgical innovations based upon accurate anatomical knowledge
Discovery of the circulation of the blood "Exercitatio"	1628	William Harvey (1578–1657)	Integrated anatomy with physiological knowledge of blood circulation
Digestive system "Experiments and Observations of Gastric Juice and the Physiology of Digestion"	1833	William Beaumont (1785–1853)	Used objective observation in discovering the process of digestion

(138–201 A.D.) who experimented on lower mammals; Leonardo Da Vinci (1452–1519) who made precise drawings of human anatomy; and, later, Vesalius (1514–1564) who, through careful dissection, described human anatomy. Identifying and describing the anatomical structures of the body led to the increased knowledge about relationships between systems and the interrelationships of cardiovascular, respiratory, and genitourinary functions. Harvey's (1578–1657) concept of the circulation of blood, for example, led the way to an understanding of the internal environment of the body. Galen, Da Vinci, and Harvey were among the first scholars to accurately describe the human body. However, it was the ancient Greeks who initially brought rational thought to an evaluation of health and disease. The Hippocratic writings reflect the depth of Greek thought.

The Hippocratic Writings

The first stage in the history of medicine was essentially clinical observation. The healer applying Hippocratic methods used himself as a measuring instrument, carefully noting what he saw, felt, smelled, and heard. He used rational thought regarding the causes and treatments of diseases based on these observations. In the ancient Greek civilization, scholars were allowed the freedom to speculate on all aspects of human life. Thus the model for the Western physician emerged. Hippocrates, who is traditionally called the Father of Medicine, was probably representative of a number of individuals. It is more accurate to speak of the "Hippocratic writings" than to attribute all of ancient Greek medicine to one individual. The Hippocratic writings cover many areas of medicine, including ethics, disease etiology, anatomy, physiology, and treatment. These writings are not a consistent work linking theory to practice, but a compendium of clinical histories and a description of Hellenistic medicine.

We know very little about Hippocrates' life, except that he lived during the fifth century B.C. in Cos, an island off the Greek mainland, and that he was a famous practitioner and teacher of medicine. The following excerpt from the Hippocratic writings, *On the Articulations*, (ca. 400 B.C./1952) translated by Francis Adams, demonstrates the method of clinical observation used to diagnose a dislocation of the shoulder joint and the importance of individual differences in human anatomy:

> A dislocation may be recognized by the following symptoms: Since the parts of a man's body are proportionate to one another, as the arms and the legs, the sound should always be compared with the unsound, the unsound with the sound, not paying regard to the joints of other individuals (for one person's joints are more prominent than another's), but looking to those of the patient, to ascertain whether the sound joint be unlike the unsound. This is a proper rule, and yet it may lead to much error; and on this account it is not sufficient to know this art in theory, but also by actual practice; for many persons from pain, or from any other cause, when their joints are not dislocated, cannot put the parts into the same positions as the sound body can be put into; one ought therefore to know and be acquainted beforehand with such an attitude. But in a dislocated joint the head of the humerus appears lying much more in the armpit than it is in the sound joint; and also, above, at the top of the shoulder, the part appears hollow, and the acromion is prominent, owing to the bone of the joint having sunk into the part below; there is a source of error in this case also, as will be described and also, the elbow of the dislocated arm is farther removed from the ribs than that of the other; but by using force it may be approximated, though with considerable pain; and also they cannot with the elbow extended raise the arm to the ear, as they can the sound arm, nor move it about as formerly in this direction and that. These, then, are the symptoms of dislocation at the shoulder. (Hutchins, 1952, pp. 94–95)

The Hippocratic writings, with their emphasis on dietetics, exercise and natural methods, were the complete holistic guide for the ancient physician.

Galen

Greek medicine provided the foundation for medical practice in the Western World. Galen, a product of the Roman civilization, was the next link in the chain of medicine. He was born in Pergamum, Greece, in the second century A.D. when Roman civilization controlled much of the Western World. Galen was educated in philosophy, mathematics, and natural science. He learned medicine by traveling to places where the great physicians practiced. After acquiring knowledge steeped in the Hippocratic tradition, he became a doctor to the gladiators who performed in the Roman arenas. Galen became an acclaimed practitioner in Rome and later spent his time writing extensively. He is a model for the medical scientist who engages in clinical practice, teaching, and scholarly publication. Galen's genius was in his ability to integrate prior knowledge with his clinical observations of disease. Unfortunately, his writings on medicine became authoritative dogma from the Middle Ages to the time of the rebirth of scientific inquiry in the Renaissance period. The following excerpt from Galen (ca. 192/1971) typifies his skill in teaching anatomy as well as his careful methods of observation.

> Since therefore, the form of the body is assimilated to the bones, to which the nature of the other parts corresponds, I would have you first gain an exact and practical knowledge of human bones. It is not enough to study them casually or read of them in a book; no, not even in mine, which some call Osteologia, others Skeletons, and yet others simply On Bones, though I am persuaded that it excels all earlier works in accuracy, brevity, and lucidity.
>
> Make it rather your serious endeavor not only to acquire accurate book-knowledge of each bone, but also to examine assiduously with your own eyes the human bones themselves. This is quite easy at Alexandria because the physicians there employ ocular demonstration in teaching osteology to students. For this reason, if for no other, try to visit Alexandria. But if you cannot, it is still possible to see something of human bones. I, at least, have done so often on the breaking open of a grave or tomb. Thus once a river, inundating a recent hastily made grave, broke it up, washing away the body. The flesh had putrefied, though the bones still held together in their proper relations. It was carried down a stadium (roughly 200 yards), and reaching marshy ground, drifted ashore. This skeleton was as though deliberately prepared for such elementary teaching.
>
> If you have not the luck to see anything of this sort, dissect an ape and having removed the flesh, observe each bone with care. Choose those apes likest man with short jaws and small canines. You will find other parts also resembling man's, for they can walk and run on two feet. Those, on the other hand, like the dog-faced baboons with long snouts and large canines, far from walking or running on their hindlegs, can hardly stand upright. The more human sort have a nearly erect posture; but firstly the head of the femur fits into the socket at the hipjoint rather transversely, and secondly, of the muscles which extend downward to the knee, some go further (than in man). Both these features check and impede erectness of posture, as do the feet themselves, which have comparatively narrow heels and are deeply cleft between the toes.
>
> I therefore maintain that the bones must be learnt either from man, or ape, or better from both, before dissecting the muscles, for those two (namely bones and muscles) form the ground-work of the other parts, the foundations, as it were, of a building. And next, study arteries, veins, and nerves. Familiarity with dissection of these will bring you to the inward parts and so to a knowledge of the viscera, the fat, and the glands, which also you should examine separately, in detail. Such should be the order of your training. (as cited in Wightman, 1971, pp. 32–33)

Renaissance Medicine in the Sixteenth and Seventeenth Centuries

The history of medicine parallels in many ways the rise of Western civilization. The Middle Ages was a sterile period for the growth of new ideas and experimentation. Medical practice existed then as dogma, closely linked to practices and beliefs of the Church. While Medieval Europe adhered to rigid doctrine, medical practice flourished in the Middle East as represented by the Arab physician, Avicenna (980–1037). With the onset of the Renaissance, scientists carried out experiments on human dissection under great risk of public denouncement and physical punishment. In spite of this, a psychological climate was established in the sixteenth century that allowed medical scholars and scientists to seek the truth by experimentation. Physicians made great strides in integrating laboratory observations with clinical practice.

Renaissance physicians rekindled the torch of medical science that had been stagnant for approximately one thousand years. The scientists of the Renaissance were scholars familiar with Greek and Roman writings who questioned all knowledge and accepted little dogma. Furthermore, they reexamined the anatomical knowledge of Galen, experimented in chemistry, and sought explanations for the life processes in humans, the beginning of the science of physiology.

Andreas Versalius and the Refinement of Human Anatomy

The most important medical anatomist of the Renaissance was Andreas Versalius. He was the first medical specialist in human anatomy. By critically examining the work of Galen, he realized that Galen's observations of anatomy were not based on human dissection but were descriptions of the bodily structures of monkeys, pigs, and goats. From 1537 to 1542, Versalius worked on an anatomical atlas, *De humani corporis fabrica libri septea*, which was published in 1593. The book contained 663 folio pages. Versalius' research on human anatomy became the basis of medical science and provided the necessary knowledge for the surgeon. The interplay between laboratory observations and clinical practice provided scholars with the data they needed for readjusting theory to practice and practice to theory. The model for obtaining anatomical knowledge in the medical sciences was forged in the sixteenth century.

Paracelsus the Medical Chemist

The next great development in medicine was in the area of physiology. Chemistry and physics are the bases of physiology. The understanding of human physiology awaited the great discoveries in these areas. The first physician to apply chemistry to an understanding of biological processes was Paracelsus. He advocated using pharmaceutical agents singly or in combination to treat specific illnesses. He used sulphur, lead, antimony, mercury, iron, and copper as therapeutics. Paracelsus emphasized the relationship between practical clinical experience and scientific experimentation as evidenced in the following quotation from his work *Paragranum* written about 1528 (as cited in Wightman, 1971):

> The doctor must therefore be practised in Experienz; and medicine is nothing but a wide, certain, experienz, namely that every procedure is based in Experienz. And that is experientia which is correctly and truly founded. Anyone who has learnt his stuff without Experienz is a doubtful doctor.

Experientia is like a judge; and whether a procedure is undertaken or not depends on its approval; wherefore Experienz ought to keep pace with science, for without science Experienz is nothing. Similar an Experiment grounded in Experienz is well founded and its further use understood. . . . Experiment divorced from science is but a matter of chance. (pp. 50–51)

William Harvey

The culmination of man's knowledge in physiology during the Renaissance was achieved in the publication by William Harvey in 1628. The publication *Exercitatio* described accurately for the first time the circulation of the blood. Harvey, an English physician, was trained in Padua, Italy, where Versalius had taught human anatomy. After mastering the physiological theories of his time, he proposed questions, such as: What is the pulse? How does breathing affect the actions of the heart? How does the blood move? These questions directed Harvey's experimental procedures. First he systematically stated a testable hypothesis on the circulation of the blood and then he proceeded with rigorous experimental observation. He used precise measurements in recording pulse rate and the volume of blood ejected by the heart over time. He observed the movements of the heart and blood in living animals. He also analyzed the blood circulation of the fetus to support his theory. By using the scientific method, Harvey was able to discover the most vital process in human life. He did this by (a) presenting a researchable question, (b) mastering the published literature on blood flow, (c) using accurate observations, (d) being guided by predictive hypothesis, (e) using rigorous procedures for collecting data, (f) applying measurement to the process of blood flow, and (g) making a deductive analysis and conclusions.

Harvey's achievement in describing the circulation of the blood ranks with Newton's discovery of gravity as one of the greatest scientific accomplishments in the seventeenth century. Harvey's work at first was met with jealousy and suspicion that many times accompanies an important discovery or change of thinking. In the first chapter from *Exercitatio* entitled "The Author's Motives for Writing" (1628/1952), Harvey explained his reasons for publishing his findings and his desire to bring objective criticism to his work.

I have not hesitated to expose my views upon these subjects, not only in private to my friends, but also in public, in my anatomical lectures, after the manner of the Academy of old.

These views as usual, pleased some more, others less; some chide and calumniated me, and laid it to me as a crime that I had dared to depart from the precepts and opinions of all anatomists; others desired further explanations of the novelties, which they said were both worthy of consideration, and might perchance be found of single use. At length, yielding to the requests of my friends, that all might be made participators in my labors, and partly moved by the envy of others, who receiving my views with uncandid minds and understanding them indifferently, have essayed to traduce me publicly. I have moved to commit these things to the press, in order that all may be enabled to form an opinion both of me and my labours. (p. 273–274)

By the end of the seventeenth century the medical scientist had emerged. At this point in history, medical practice was not at all consistent, yet there was a body of knowledge being created that served as the basis for later discoveries and practices. Medical schools were founded in Europe during the seventeenth century, but it was not until the latter half of the nineteenth century that medical education was rigorously evaluated. These discoveries occurred in a comparatively short period of intense activity from the nineteenth century to the present. The early research describing the human organism served as a foundation of scientific knowledge that was later expanded and incorporated into clinical practice.

1.2 Methodological Process, Stage II

Development of Medical Technology in the Eighteenth and Nineteenth Century

The second stage in medical research was the development of precision instruments and test procedures that enabled the medical scientist to examine and measure the internal processes in the body. Typical among early scientific inventors in medicine was Laennec (1781–1826) who, by watching children playing with hollow cylinders, invented the stethoscope. Methodological research over the centuries has brought about technological advances such as the electroencephalogram, electrocardiogram, X-ray, procedures for urine analysis, positron emission tomography (PET), single photon emission computed tomography (SPECT), computed tomographic X-Ray (CT or CAT scan), magnetic resonance imaging (MRI), and other important instruments and procedures that have become basic tools in clinical medicine. Moreover, technology is continually being refined and updated.

Methodological research is unique in its application of industrial technology to the problems of diagnosis and treatment. Initially, the great advances in methodology coincided with the rise of the industrial revolution in the eighteenth century. Medical scientists who were able to apply industrial technology to medical practice found a wealth of ideas. These advances are examples of interdisciplinary research where investigators from diverse disciplines apply their special knowledge to a specific research problem.

Norbert Wiener (1948), who proposed the theory of cybernetics, used interdisciplinary seminars as a means of generating new ideas and stimulating creative thinking. Presently much work is being done by engineers working in conjunction with medical scientists to create artificial materials and devices that can replace organs in the body. Biomedical engineering is a direct application of methodological research to medicine. Prosthetics, self-help devices, and orthotics are examples of methodological research applied to the field of rehabilitation. Table 1–2 summarizes the major methodological inventions that have impacted on medical care.

The Practice of Medicine in the First Half of the Nineteenth Century

The latter half of the nineteenth century was a golden period in the history of medicine. During this time medical schools were given the legal authority to certify physicians. Examinations were required for anyone who practiced medicine in the United States and Europe. In England, for example, a Medical Register was established in 1858. Atwater (1973), in an article documenting the medical profession in Rochester, New York, from 1811–1860, described the current state of medical knowledge available to general practitioners. Table 1–3 contains an abstracted description of the great gains medicine had made in the prior three centuries according to Atwater.

Although medicine had achieved great gains up until this period, most contagious diseases except for smallpox were untreatable. Surgeons worked at a great disadvantage without antiseptic techniques, and hospitals did not provide the care we associate with

Table 1-2 *Methodological Advances: Stage II*

Medical Events	Dates	Scientists	Implications
Clinical Thermometer	1614	Santotio Santorio (1561–1636)	Physical examination in clinical medicine
Microscopical Anatomy	1661	Marcello Malpighi (1628–1694)	Diagnostic studies of the blood
Clinical Microscope	1695	Antony Van Leeuwenhoek (1632–1694)	Refinement of microscope
Technique of Thoracic Percussion	1761	Leopold Auenbrugger (1722–1809)	Diagnosis of respiratory disorders
Stethoscope	1819	Rene Laennec (1781–1826)	Diagnosis of circulatory disorders
Hypodermic Syringe	1853	Alexander Wood (1817–1884)	Blood transfusions
Method for testing for testing the quantity of sugar in urine	1848	Herman von Fehling (1811–1885)	Diagnosis of diabetes mellitus
X-Ray	1895	Wilhelm Roentgen (1845–1923)	Detection of tuberculosis, fractures, and dislocations
Ophthalmoscope	1851	Hermann von Helmholtz (1821–1894)	Detection of morbid changes in the eye
Cystoscope	1890	Max Nitze (1847–1907)	Disease of urinary system
Electrocardiograph (EKG)	1903	Willem Einthoven (1860–1927)	Coronary functioning
Electroencephalograph (EEG)	1929	A. Berger (1873–1941)	Cerebral dysfunction
Computed Axial Tomography (CAT)	1979	A. M. Cormack, G. N. Hounsfield	Diagnostic assistance

Table 1–3   *Progress in Surgery, Clinical Medicine, and Public Health Up Until Pasteur's Formulation of the Germ Theory in 1878*

Surgery	Diagnosis and Treatment	Public Health
Use of ether and chloroform as anesthetics	Use of microscope, auscultation, and stethoscope in diagnosis	Construction of municipal sewers
Setting of broken bones and reduction of dislocated joints	Dynamic understanding of anatomy and physiology	Recording of vital statistics
Removal of superficial diseased tissue and kidney stones	Isolation of patient with contagious diseases	Custodial care of insane, retarded, poor, and homeless
Widespread practice of obstetrics and gynecology	Relief of local pain pharmacologically	Prevention of smallpox through vaccination

excellent nursing. Medical advances would have to wait for Pasteur, Lister, Morton, and Florence Nightingale to provide the revolutionary innovations.

1.3 Etiological Advances, Stage III

Medical Research in the Latter Half of the Nineteenth Century

The third stage in medical research was the integration of physiology and pathology with the use of a reliable methodology to arrive at a diagnosis. The evolution of the *dynamic understanding of the disease process* is described in Table 1–4. During this stage, an understanding of the etiology of a disease through experimental laboratory research was used to verify cause-effect relationships. This breakthrough in treating disease on a scientific basis started with Pasteur's discovery of the germ theory. From Pasteur's work, laboratory scientists were able to investigate disease processes by identifying a specific microorganism. The age of chemotherapy was initiated. For every microorganism causing a disease (that was isolated in the laboratory) a chemical substance harmless to the body was sought to counteract the germ. From 1850 to 1910, the process of identifying the germ responsible for a disease and the discovery of a chemical to eliminate the germ was the basis for the rapid conquest of many communicable diseases. The elimination of many communicable diseases would not have occurred without the microscope and the laboratory techniques of microbiology and biochemistry. The technology for protecting the individual from infectious diseases was a direct result of the understanding of human physiology and cellular theory. Septic techniques for surgery were later developed by Joseph Lister (1827–1912), who was greatly influenced by the work of Louis Pasteur, and by Ignaz Semmelweis (1818–1865), an obstetrician, who recognized the importance of hospital surgeons using prophylactic techniques during childbirth so as to prevent infection.

The knowledge of cellular activity by Rudolf Ludwig Virchow (1821–1902) was another line of evidence verifying the germ theory of disease. According to Virchow, the cause of disease was a result of changes at the cellular level. Virchow's cellular theory of

Table 1–4   *Dynamic Understanding of Disease Processes: Stage III*

Medical Event	Date	Scientist	Implications
Clinical Physiology	1857	Claude Bernard (1813–1878)	Treatment of physiologic and metabolic disorders through pharmacology
Cell Theory	1858	Rudolf Ludwig Virchow (1821–1902)	Cellular pathology as the basis of treatment
Germ Theory	1878	Louis Pasteur (1822–1895)	The role of microorganisms in disease established
Bacteriology	1882	Robert Koch (1843–1910)	Treatment of bacterial infections could be controlled by the physician
Role of Filterable Viruses	1888	Pierre Roux (1853–1933)	Identification of viruses resulted
Immunization Process "Phagocytosis"	1892	Elie Metchnikoff (1845–1916)	Understanding of the body's defense mechanisms against disease recognized
Chemotherapy	1899	Paul Ehrlich (1854–1915)	Specific chemical compounds used to treat communicable diseases

disease compelled pathologists to use microscopes in searching for lesions and abnormalities within the cells. Elie Metchnikoff (1845–1916) discovered phagocytosis, recognizing that white blood corpuscles in the body counteract disease. The understanding of the dynamics of disease led to the science of clinical medicine.

Physicians were then able to diagnose disease through laboratory microscope techniques, thus replacing vitalism and metaphysics as explanations for the onset of communicable disease. Probably the most important work on medical research in the nineteenth century was Claude Bernard's *Introduction to the Study of Experimental Medicine* published in 1895. Pasteur acknowledged Bernard as an important influence in his own work. Bernard's major contributions to understanding disease included physiology of digestion, neurophysiology, pharmacology, and organic chemistry. Bernard's work has had a profound influence in medical science. Concepts such as homeostasis and stress introduced by Cannon (1932) and Selye (1956) are based upon Bernard's experimental findings on the internal gastrointestinal environment. Bernard, through his experimental methodology, established the future direction of medical research based on rigorous observation, repeated replication, and the acceptance or rejection of a hypothesis. "Scientific generalization must proceed from particular facts to principles" (Bernard, 1865/1957, p. 2). This simple statement is the foundation of twentieth century medical research.

With a refined scientific methodology and a comprehensive theory of disease, medical researchers from about 1880 to 1910 made dramatic progress in identifying disease agents. This advance is exemplified by Robert Koch's work in tuberculosis in 1890, Emil von Behring's work in diphtheria in 1900, and Paul Ehrlich's persistent search for a chemical to counteract syphilis, culminating in the discovery of the drug Salvarsan (arsphenamine) in 1910, after 606 experimental trials.

1.4 Prevention, Stage IV

Preventive Medicine in the Twentieth Century

The advances in medical research that had the most dramatic effect in eliminating diseases have been through primary prevention including public health techniques and mass vaccinations. Public health measures such as purification of water, elimination of human waste products, and protection against food spoilage were used by ancient civilizations such as the Egyptians, Greeks, and Romans. However, when superstition prevailed over using prophylactic methods, as during the Middle Ages in Europe, epidemics and widespread disease occurred. Throughout the world, the potential for epidemics still exists in underdeveloped countries or war zones where public health measures have been disregarded. The elimination of typhus, cholera, bubonic plague, polio, and smallpox in areas accessible to modern medicine has been accomplished through the combination of medical advances in preventing diseases and public health technology. Vaccination as a means of preventing diseases has provided the means to control widespread epidemics that in the past have dramatically reduced populations. The first physician to conceive the use of vaccinations to prevent disease was Edward Jenner (1749–1823), who experimented with cowpox infection, a mild disease, as a means of protecting against smallpox, which in the eighteenth century was one of the leading causes of death. Jenner noted that dairymaids who contracted cowpox from milking infected cows developed a natural immunity to smallpox. This observation led him to believe that if people were deliberately infected with cowpox they would escape the dreaded smallpox. In 1798 Jenner published his findings, which included 23 case histories of individuals inoculated with cowpox.

Initially, Jenner's work was not accepted by the medical community in England. He gradually gained recognition after his work was replicated by other physicians. Jenner's original research on vaccinations remained singularly unique until Pasteur's discovery of the germ theory about a hundred years later in 1878. Jenner's method of inoculation to prevent disease was rediscovered by medical researchers who were later able to isolate pathogenic bacteria and viruses. Table 1–5 lists many of the communicable diseases that are now controlled by vaccination.

Presently, the concept of preventive medicine includes the following health procedures:

- Inoculation to prevent communicable diseases
- Environmental health to reduce atmospheric and water pollution
- Prenatal care to prevent birth defects
- Mental health community services to prevent institutionalization
- Family planning and population control
- Supervision of food handling and processing of foods to prevent botulism
- Prevention of industrial accidents through ergonomics
- Sanitary engineering to prevent typhus and cholera.

Until the twentieth century, physicians were able to do very little when a patient became severely ill. The introduction of chemotherapy, aseptic surgery, and efficient hospital care changed the course of medical practice.

Table 1-5   *Control of Communicable Diseases Through Immunization*

Disease	Causative Agent	Medical Researcher	Discovery Date
Bubonic Plague	Bacterium	S. Kitasato, Alexandre Yersin	1893–1894
Cholera	Bacterium	Robert Koch	1884
Diphtheria	Bacterium	Emil Von Behring	1890
Measles	Virus	Francesio Cenci	1901
Poliomyelitis	Virus	Jonas Salk	1954
Rabies	Virus	Louis Pasteur	1885
Rocky Mountain Spotted Fever	Virus	Howard Ricketts	1909
Smallpox	Virus	Edward Jenner	1796
Tuberculosis	Bacterium	Albert Calmette, Camille Guerin	1921
Typhoid Fever	Bacterium	Almroth Wright	1906
Typhus	Virus	Charles Nicolle	1910
Yellow Fever	Virus	Max Thieler	1936

1.5 Chemotherapy, Surgery, and Hospital Care: The Bases of Treatment, Stage V

Chemotherapy

As knowledge about anatomy and physiology progressed, technology was developed to improve the diagnoses of illnesses. The foundations, created to produce a body of knowledge underlying therapeutics, resulted in chemotherapy, surgery, and hospital care as the bases of modern day treatment. Although ancient civilizations, and in primitive cultures existing today, have used various effective treatments, the causes of diseases and the rationale for understanding the processes were veiled in mystery. For example, rauwolfia serpentine was used in India (100 A.D.) as the "medicine of sad men" (Thornwald, 1963, p. 205) without the present understanding of the biochemical process of a tranquilizer. Ancient Egyptian doctors used mud and soil in the treatment of eye diseases. This type of "sewerage pharmacology" was not understood until 1948 when Dr. Benjamin M. Dugger, a professor of plant physiology at the University of Wisconsin, discovered the drug aureomycin, a chemical similar to natural substances found near the Nile River. Aureomycin has been highly effective in the treatment of trachoma. For centuries, practical treatment for many disabilities, diseases, and illnesses has been applied by trial and error without an understanding of the theoretical dynamics of the disease processes. Healers, such as shamans and witch doctors, intersperse treatment with superstition, sometimes attaining positive results. The important difference between applying therapeutics in modern science and in prescientific civilizations is in the explanation of why a specific treatment cures a disease. The search for cures to diseases, beginning with the germ theory of Pasteur and continuing through Alexander Fleming's discovery of penicillin in 1928 and Selman A. Waksman's discovery of streptomycin in 1944, spurred the corporate growth of therapeutic pharmaceutics. Modern medicine is heavily dependent upon the availability of various drugs to control abnormal physical conditions, such as hypertension, arteriosclerosis, blood clotting, edema, and emotional illness. Hormone therapy, the use of vitamins, and dietetics are other common methods akin to chemical therapy as forms of treatment.

Surgery

Surgical intervention, a second form of treatment, along with chemotherapy, accounts for modern medicine's most dramatic successes. Approximately 40,000 to 50,000 major and minor operations are performed everyday in the 6,000 United States hospitals. A list of the fourteen most frequent operations performed in the United States is shown in Table 1–6 (U.S. Dept. Health and Human Services, National Center for Health Statistics, 1993). Like drug therapy, surgery was used by physicians in ancient civilizations. For example, in ancient Rome (ca. 70 B.C.–200 B.C.) up to two hundred different surgical instruments were used in various operations. In addition, ligature of blood vessels was performed; obstetric surgery, specifically Caesarean section, was known; and even anesthesia was used (Marti-Ibanez, 1962).

Modern surgery as an effective and safe method was the result of two important events: the development of antiseptics by Lister in 1867, who tested the capacity of carbolic acid in preventing infection in general surgery, and the discovery of ether anesthesia as a practical method by William Morton, a dentist, in 1846.

Table 1–6   *Fourteen Most Frequent Surgical Procedures in 1991*

Procedure	Number in Thousands	Rate per 100,000 Population
Episiotomy with or without forceps or vacuum extraction	1,684	672.1
Cardiac catherterization	1,000	399.1
Cesarean section	933	372.5
Repair of current obstetric laceration	795	317.3
Artificial rupture of membranes	775	309.3
Cholecystectomy	571	227.8
Hysterectomy	546	218.0
Oophorectomy and salpingo-oophorectomy	458	182.7
Open reduction of fracture, with internal fixation	418	166.7
Coronary artery bypass graft	407	162.6
Bilateral destrctions or occulusion of fallopian tubes	401	160.1
Prostatectomy	363	145.1
Lysis of peritoneal adhesions	339	135.4
Removal of coronary obstruction	331	131.9
Debridement of wound, infection, or burn	326	130.0
Excision or destruction of intervertebral disc	306	122.2
Insertion, replacement, removal, and revision of pacemaker leads or device	300	119.6
Appendectomy, exclusing incidental	255	101.8

Note. The information contained in this table is based on data from the *Vital and Health Statistics, National Hospital Discharge Survey: Annual Summary, 1991,* published by the U. S. Department of Health and Human Services, Public Health Service, Centers for Disease Control and Prevention, National Centers for Health Statistics (1993).

Hospital Care

The third component in the development of modern treatment, parallel to chemotherapy and surgery, was the rise of hospital nursing care. Florence Nightingale's role in developing the nursing profession is legendary. Single-handedly, she was able to arouse world public opinion about the plight of hospital patients, who were often left to die because of neglect. The story of Florence Nightingale's success is well known. During the Crimean War of 1854, she organized a group of nurses to tend wounded British soldiers. Her experience gave her the insight into the need for clean, efficient hospitals. Reform in hospital care became a national issue in England after the Crimean War, and social legislation was enacted to provide governmental support. The first school of nursing was started by Florence Nightingale in St. Thomas' Hospital, London, in 1860. With hospital reform enacted through legislation and a nursing school started, the foundation for progress in the treatment of the hospitalized patient was established.

Below is a short outline of the historical development of hospitals as documented by Rene Sand (1952):

1. Ancient Greece, Sixth Century, B.C.: A large open building was provided for the Greek physician. It comprised a waiting room, consulting room, and theater for operations and dressings.
2. Ancient Rome, First Century, A.D.: Sick bays were attached to the family estates of the wealthy.
3. Early Medieval Europe, Fourth Century, A.D.: Early Christians established "hospitia" for travelers, abandoned children, and the sick who were traveling on their way to pilgrimages. Care was under the direction of monastic and sisterly orders.
4. Middle East, Twelfth Century, A.D.: Moslems in Baghdad founded the first hospitals where physicians cared for the ill. Special wards for mental illness, blindness, and leprosy were established.
5. Later Middle Ages, Europe, Fifth to Fourteenth Centuries: Hostelries under the jurisdiction of the Church provided care for the sick. Brothers and sisters of the Church in attached ecclesiastical hospitals provided treatment remedies, performed simple operations, and attended those with serious illnesses.
6. Renaissance Europe, Fifteenth Century: For the first time in the Western World, physicians and midwives treated the sick in hospitals. Terminal patients were segregated from the acutely ill.
7. Europe, Eighteenth Century: Gradually hospitals began to treat emergency care patients, outpatient departments grew, and hospitals served as training facilities for medical students.
8. Europe, America, Nineteenth Century: Nursing care was established in hospitals. Antiseptic surgery, anesthesia, and improvement in general care of the hospitalized patient were initiated.
9. Worldwide, Twentieth Century: The growth of specialized hospitals, regional planning, and national health services. A world movement exists in extending health care to underdeveloped countries under the auspices of the United Nations, World Health Organization (WHO).

Current medical treatment is based upon the principle of healing—stopping the progression of a disease and promoting natural bodily processes. Chemotherapy, surgery, and nursing care are the three basic methods that have made medical practice effective in treating many communicable diseases and physiological disorders and anatomical defects. The limitations of medical treatment for individuals with severe chronic disabilities, such as schizophrenia, arthritis, cardiovascular disease, and cerebral vascular accident (CVA) are clearly evident. Medical treatment alone is effective only when the disease process can be narrowed down to a specific etiology. Chronic diseases present problems of multiple etiologies and treatment requiring complex solutions and interdisciplinary efforts. The search for solutions to the chronic disabilities led to the rehabilitation movement.

1.6 Rehabilitation Movement, Stage VI

The emergence of rehabilitation as a distinct entity in the health care system began only 75 years ago. The aftermath of the First World War saw the beginnings of the rehabilitation movement, coinciding with the need for restoring function to those who were permanently disabled. One may ask why the rehabilitation field developed at that time and not in prior centuries or periods of recovery from war. The historical factors that led to the rehabilitation movement are outlined in Table 1–7. Until the eighteenth century, chronic illness and permanent disability in general were not always considered medical problems. For instance, psychiatric illness and epilepsy were considered problems of morality and satanic possession. Treatment of psychiatric illness, if any, was stark, brutal, or radical. Before the rise of large institutions providing custodial care for psychiatric patients, the attitude toward chronic mental illness was at best benign neglect and at worst rejection and punishment. In a related area, birth injuries such as cerebral palsy were misunderstood by ancient cultures. Not until 1862, when W. T. Little, an English orthopedic surgeon, described the relationship between birth injury and neurological disorders, was there any dynamic understanding of this disability. Individuals with other chronic disabilities, such as arthritis, emphysema, cerebrovascular stroke, cardiovascular disease, and spinal cord injuries, were left either to the custodial care of the family or were placed into the hands of charlatans who promised miraculous cures.

Social Welfare and Rehabilitation

The change from custodial care to therapeutic treatment of the individual with chronic disabilities occurred at a period of time in history when social welfare had become a worldwide concern. Social Security was the forerunner in public health and medicine for the indigent with chronic disabilities. Germany, in 1883, and England, in 1897, were

Table 1–7   *Historical Factors Leading to the Rehabilitation Movement*

Incorporation of scientific methodology into clinical medicine
- Industrialization and its impact on clinical procedures for diagnosis and treatment
- Large population of veterans with disabilities from the First World War
- The availability of financial resources through Social Security and National Health Insurance schemes
- Medical specialties and the development of allied health professions
- Public acceptability that individuals with disabilities can be restored to independence through rehabilitation
- Public acceptability of individuals with disabilities in social and work situations

the first countries in Europe to enact legislation providing worker's compensation to cover disability and illness resulting from occupational accidents. The progress towards social and occupational health and safety is described in Figure 1–2. Governmental financial support, resulting from national policies on health and welfare, was necessary because of the enormous hospital resources and health personnel required in the rehabilitation of individuals with disabilities. In the United States, social security legislation, first enacted in 1935, has been a major impetus for the development of the rehabilitation movement. Change in societies' attitudes towards the individual with chronic disabilities, as evidenced in the social welfare movement, has encouraged the growth of the allied health professions.

The Evolution of Allied Health Professions, Phase I

Three major phases in the history of rehabilitation have affected the growth of the allied health professions. The first phase occurred shortly after the First World War. During this period, the need for physical and social rehabilitation of the individuals with disabilities was recognized by the medical community. Casualties from the war included individuals with lower extremity amputation, victims of poison gas resulting in neurological disabilities, and soldiers with a psychiatric disabilities due to shell shock. At that time these veterans of the war were seen as needing assistance in readjusting to community living. Reconstruction workers recruited from nursing staffs were the first health personnel in rehabilitation. Immediately after the First World War, the goal of rehabilitation was primarily humane and supportive to the medical treatment. There was no direct effort by the rehabilitation workers to change the course of a disability or to make the individual with disabilities more functional. During the late 1920s, rehabilitation departments were established for the first time in hospitals. The health personnel recruited to work in these departments were, on the whole, dedicated people who applied caring support and activity to facilitate the patient's readjustment to the community.

The Education and Professionalization: Phase II

The second phase of rehabilitation, during the 1930s, 1940s and 1950s, can be identified as the *educational and professionalization* phase. Table 1–8 lists the major landmarks in physical rehabilitation. During this time programs in colleges and universities were initiated, professional associations grew, and rehabilitation services evolved. The training of allied health specialists who had a unique combination of knowledge in the application of activities and rehabilitation techniques, understanding of medical treatment, and a background in the social sciences were considered necessary preparation for working in a hospital setting. The concepts underlying rehabilitation at that time were taken from other clinical and applied disciplines such as anatomy, physiology, nutrition, language development, psychology, clinical medicine, and education.

Physical Medicine and Rehabilitation

The first rehabilitation medical service in a general hospital was created in 1946, in Bellevue Hospital, New York City (Rusk, 1971). This unit served as a model for the interdisciplinary rehabilitation team. In addition, the physiatry specialty in rehabilitation medi-

ANTIQUITY
- Manual labor and tradesmen neglected
- Occupational diseases ignored

PROTECTION OF MINERS (16th Century)
- Ventilating machines for mines

PROTECTION OF VULNERABLE WORKERS IN DANGEROUS TRADES (19th Century)
- Public health legislation to regulate child labor
- Work day reduced to 10 hours

WORKER HEALTH BUREAU (Established 1927)

SCIENTIFIC INVESTIGATIONS OF PREVENTION AND TREATMENT OF OCCUPATIONAL INJURIES & DISEASES (1980s)
- Application of ergonomics and rehabilitation of principles

MEDIEVAL GUILDS
- Voluntary associations formed for mutual aid protection of tradesman
- Assist worker with disabilities
- Assist in funeral expenses

OCCUPATIONAL MEDICINE (Established 17th Century)
- Relationship between occupation & disease investigated medically
- Prevention measures introduced—rest intervals, positioning, cleanliness, protective clothing

WORKMEN'S COMPENSATION (1890–1910)
- Compensate workers for occupational accidents and diseases

SOCIAL SECURITY LEGISLATION (1930s)
- Place safety & health activities within Labor Department

FUTURE TRENDS IN OCCUPATIONAL MEDICINE
- Occupational health teams: ergonomist, occupational therapist, physician, industrial hygienist, physiotherapist, safety officer, and nurse
- Investigation of physical, chemical, biological, and psychological factors in work environment that may cause or aggravate disease in individuals who are vulnerable
- Investigation of long-term effects of exposure to toxic chemicals, repetitive motion, vibration, excessive noise, extreme temperature, radiation, dust, bacteria

SOCIETY OF ARTIFICERS
- Established apprenticeship system
- Workday regulated 12–13 hours

COMPILING OF VITAL STATISTICS ON OCCUPATIONAL DISEASE (18th Century)
- Use of medical inspectors

NATIONAL WOMEN'S TRADE UNION (1920)
- Protection of women from dangerous industries

OCCUPATIONAL SAFETY & HEALTH AGENCIES (Established 1970)
- On site inspections, regulations, & enforcement of laws relating to dangerous and unhealthy conditions in all industries

Figure 1-2. Progress towards social reform in occupational health and safety.

TABLE 1–8   *Rehabilitation Movement: Stage VI*

Rehabilitation Events	Dates	Contributors	Significance
First comprehensive rehabilitation program in a general hospital	1946	Howard Rusk	Served as model for physical medicine rehabilitation team approach
Physical therapy methods	1949	H. O. Kendall and F. P. Kendall	Basis for physical therapy techniques for muscle testing and patient evaluation
Retraining methods of activities of daily living	1956	Edith Buchwald Lawton	Provided functional rehabilitation methods for increasing independence
Vocational rehabilitation	1957	Lloyd H. Lofquist	Established the role of the rehabilitation counselor
Aphasia rehabilitation	1955	Martha L. Taylor and M. Marks	Provided rehabilitation techniques for speech therapy
Prosthetics	1959	M. H. Anderson et al.	Led to cooperative research by physicians, engineers, and prosthetists in the design of artificial limbs
Orthotics	1962	Muriel Zimmerman	Led to the development of self-help devices for the homemaker and worker with physical disabilities

cine was started. Conceptually, rehabilitation was defined as restoring the individual to the highest level of cognitive, physical, economic, social, and emotional independence. This process, involving a team evaluation of the patient's functions, establishment of treatment goals and priorities, and a interdisciplinary approach to treatment, became the model for rehabilitation. This process is listed in Figure 1–3.

Parallel to the evolution of a medical rehabilitation team was the involvement of the federal and state governments in providing vocational rehabilitation services that resulted from the Vocational Rehabilitation Act of 1954. Sheltered workshops, such as Abilities Inc. in New York City, Epi-Hab in Los Angeles, Goodwill Industries, and Community Workshops in Boston, provided the vocational training component and the specialized employment placement that helped reemploy the individual with disabilities.

Allied Health Treatment Technologies

As the training of allied health professionals developed during the 1940s and 1950s, a treatment technology emerged, especially in physical therapy. Methods for objectively assessing muscle function were established (Daniels, Williams & Worthingham, 1956; Kendall & Kendall, 1949). Electrodiagnosis of muscle function, measurement of range of motion, and techniques for improving muscle and joint action through heat, ultraviolet rays, electrical stimulation, whirlpool, and cold packs were developed through trial and error and clinical practice. These techniques were a major part of the physical therapist's treatment procedures (Downer, 1970). The need for retraining patients in activities of daily living was recognized by therapists as an important area for intervention. Lawton (1956), working with Howard Rusk at the Institute of Physical Medicine and Rehabilita-

CHRONIC DISABILITY	EVALUATION OF FUNCTION	TREATMENT
o Amputee	o Activities of daily living	o Chemotherapy
o Arthritis	o Ambulation	o Dietetics
o Cardiovascular	o Diet	o Nursing care
o Degenerative diseases of the CNS	o Leisure activities	o Occupational therapy
o Emphysema and pulmonary disease	o Muscular and joint testing	o Orthotics
o Epilepsy	o Neurological evaluation	o Physical therapy
o Spinal cord injury	o Psychological testing	o Prosthetics
o Stroke	o Speech and language	o Psychological counseling
	o Vocational assessment	o Social work
		o Speech therapy
		o Surgery
		o Vocational rehabilitation

Figure 1–3.   The process of physical medicine and rehabilitation. Rehabilitation is the process of regaining skills after having lost them. After an evaluation of function, treatment can begin.

tion, published a manual for therapists describing methods to retrain patients to become functionally independent in their everyday activities. The need to retrain patients with aphasia to regain their use of language as the result of a stroke or brain injury led to the development of sequentially programmed techniques (Taylor & Marks, 1955).

Another important component of rehabilitation was in the area of vocational rehabilitation. Lofquist (1957), McGowan (1960), and Patterson (1958) were some of the early workers who defined the role of the rehabilitation counselor in prevocational evaluation, special placement, and vocational training. Occupational therapy progressed as an integral part of the rehabilitation movement in a more general direction than physical therapy or speech therapy. The use of activities as treatment modalities in work, leisure, and activities of daily living was applied to a broader spectrum of disabilities. Occupational therapists worked mainly in rehabilitation departments, psychiatric state hospitals, Veteran Administration facilities, and state schools for the physically and mentally handicapped (Willard & Spackman, 1971). As the rehabilitation movement gained momentum in the 1950s, biomedical research in the replacement of limbs and joints led to the field of prosthetics. The design of component parts, fitting of the prosthesis, and gait training gave rise to another member of the physical rehabilitation team, the prosthetist (Anderson, Bechtol, & Sollars, 1959). Specialization in "rehabilitation" also occurred at a rapid rate within the fields of nutrition, social work, psychology, and nursing.

Psychiatric Rehabilitation

In comparison with physical rehabilitation techniques, psychiatric treatment has lagged behind in developing the technology to treat the individual with mental illness. The initial optimism from 1930 to 1950 that was generated by biological interventions, such as electric convulsive therapy, insulin therapy, Metrazol treatment, and psychosurgery, has faded. During the 1960s to the 1990s psychiatric treatment remained in a state of disarray. The onset of neuroleptic drugs and the community mental health movement in the 1960s led to the dismantling of large psychiatric hospitals that served as custodial "warehouses" for the patients who were chronically mentally ill. Since the 1960s, the length of hospitalization for psychiatric patients has been reduced, but the number of individuals with mental illness living in the community and without treatment has increased. Current enlightened psychiatric treatment emphasizes early return to the community in combination with outpatient vocational rehabilitation. In many state hospitals for the mentally ill a large percentage of patients who are elderly form a residual population from the custodial period. This population is mainly rejected, untreated, and provided mainly with maintenance care. Other individuals with mental illness are in nursing homes or left untreated in large cities as members of homeless populations.

Evaluation of psychiatric treatment still remains a fertile area for clinical researchers. Apart from descriptive observations, few comprehensive studies, apart from descriptive observations, have analyzed treatment techniques in depth. Although many clinicians believe that what they are doing is beneficial, there is little evidence or hard data to support their claims.

Why has psychiatric rehabilitation lagged behind other areas of medical progress? First, there has been wide disagreement in identifying, diagnosing, and treating mental illness in spite of the attempt to classify mental illness as exemplified in the *Diagnostic and Statistical Manual of Mental Disorders* (APA, 1994). Theorists have differed widely in their approaches in psychiatry, advocating specific treatment techniques for the broad area of mental illness. Many clinical researchers have failed to recognize the individual needs of patients and the differential effects of treatment. The second reason for the lag in scientific progress in psychiatric rehabilitation is the lack of comprehensive studies. Psychiatric research has been fixed at the nineteenth century two-variable research stage model, which assumed a single factor cause for mental illness. If progress in psychiatric rehabilitation is to occur, multidisciplinary efforts must investigate mental illness on a broad front, using a biopsychosocial model, rather than a narrow, one-dimensional research. The promise in psychiatric rehabilitation lies in a holistic approach, the incorporation of a community mental health model relying on half-way houses, vocational programs, and support groups, with an individualized approach to evaluation, education, psychotherapy, counseling, and drug treatment.

Third Phase of Allied Health 1960–Present

This evolution leads to the present period of rehabilitation, which has been characterized by various treatment theories. Unfortunately, these theories have become so specialized that professionals in allied health fields can no longer change from one disability area to another without familiarizing themselves with a vast amount of knowledge and technology. For example, allied health professionals have specialized in diverse areas such as augmentative communication, computer technology, sensory integration therapy (SI), neurodevelopmental therapy (NDT), robotics, telemetry, cinematography, and biofeedback. These areas of rehabilitation are unique. They are interdisciplinary in nature and incorporate theories and findings from the physical and social sciences. Table 1–9 shows the rapid growth of the allied health professions from 1950 to the present.

The extraordinary growth of the allied health professions in the last fifty years is apparent if one examines the percentage increase in the number of active practitioners and the number of professional schools. In comparison to the United States' population increase from 150,000,000 in 1949 to 210,000,000 in 1972, one would have expected the professions to increase about 40%. We find, however, that professions like occupational therapy and physical therapy increased 300% from 1949 to 1972. The number of radiologic technologists increased 685%, registered nurses increased 149%, and physicians increased 58% during this period. On the other hand, the smallest increases were in the numbers of chiropractic, osteopathy, optometry and pharmacy. The growth of the allied health professions has continued into the 1980s and 1990s, with forecasts of continued growth into the twenty-first century.

Another indication of the rapid expansion of the allied health professions is the emergence of new fields that did not exist forty years ago. *The Occupational Outlook Handbook* (1951) did not include many allied health professions, which appeared in later editions, starting with 1972 (see Table 1–10).

Rehabilitation Research Trends (1950–1975)

Goldberg (1974), in an analysis of rehabilitation research, identified ten areas that are related to clinical practice:

- *Program Evaluation:* the assessment of the effectiveness of a clinical program in reaching stated objectives or meeting a list of criteria
- *Management:* the study of factors related to health manpower, cost effectiveness, and comprehensive planning in providing health care to those in need of services
- *Dissemination:* the process of communicating research findings over a wide area, including to professional and lay persons
- *Involvement of Consumer Groups:* the identification of research problems
- *Chronic Severe Disability:* functional problems as a major focus of research in rehabilitation
- *Social Problems:* alcoholism, adult crime, drug addiction, and juvenile delinquency as areas included under health-related problems instead of correctional
- *Functional Assessment Methods:* targeted to the individuals with severe disabilities who are in supported employment and working at home
- *Need for Follow-Up and Follow-Along Research:* evaluation of the continuity of care
- *Rehabilitation Utilization:* incorporation of rehabilitation research in clinical practices
- *Rehabilitation Engineering:* interdisciplinary research in solving practical rehabilitation problems especially in the fields of prosthetics, orthotics, communication, mobility, and independent living.

These trends continue to have an impact on current rehabilitation research in the 1990s. From the initial emphasis on the physical restoration of the individual, researchers are now turning to the more complex chronic social problems that are associated with poverty, substandard housing, undernourishment, alienation, and addiction. Evidence is present that severe chronic disabilities, such as polio, tuberculosis, stroke, emphysema, and coronary thrombosis, can be alleviated or reduced through public

TABLE 1-9 *The Growth of Health Profession 1950–Present*

Health Specialty	Post-Secondary Training (Years)	Active Practitioners				Increase in Practitioners (%) 1950 to 1972
		1950	1972	1980	1992	
Chiropractor	6–8	14,000	16,000	23,000	46,000	14
Dentist	6–8	75,300	105,000	126,000	183,000	39
Dietitian and Nutritionists	5	15,000	33,000	N.A.	50,000	120
Occupational Therapist	4–5	2,300	7,500	19,000	40,000	226
Optometrist	6	17,000	18,700	23,000	31,000	10
Pharmacist	5–6	100,000	131,000	141,000	163,000	31
Physical Therapist	4–5	4,500	18,000	34,000	90,000	300
Physician	8–15	200,000	316,500	405,000	556,000	58
Physician Assistant[a]	2–5	N.A.	303	9,222	22,305	N.A.
Podiatrist	6–8	6,400	7,300	12,000	14,700	14
Psychologist	5–9	10,000	57,000	106,000	144,000	470
Registered Nurse	3–5	300,500	750,000	1,105,000	1,835,000	150
Respiratory Therapist	2–4	N.A.	17,000	N.A.	74,000	N.A.
Speech Language Pathologist and Audiologist	6	2,000	27,000	40,000	73,000	1250
Social Worker	6	100,000	185,000	345,000	484,000	85

Note. The information contained in this table is based on data from the *Occupational Outlook Handbook* (1951, 1974–1975, 1982–1983, 1992–1993, 1994–1995) published by the United States Department of Labor and from information obtained from professional societies.

[a]Physician Assistant's programs were started in 1967.

TABLE 1-10 *The Growth of Health Professions of Technologists and Assistants, 1972-1990*

Health Field	1972	1986	1990
Dental Hygienist	17,000	87,000	97,000
Electrocardiograph Technician	10,000	18,000	16,000
Electroencephalograph Technician	3,500	5,900	6,700
Medical Record Technician	8,000	40,000	N.A.
Nuclear Medicine Technologist	N.A.	9,700	10,000
Occupational Therapy Assistant	6,000	9,000[a]	9,600
Physical Therapy Assistant	10,000	12,000[a]	45,000
Radiology Technologist	55,000	115,000	149,000
Respiratory Therapist	17,000	56,000	60,000
Surgical Technician	25,000	37,000	38,000

Note. Data in this table are taken from the *Occupational Outlook Handbook*, 1972-1973, 1988-1989, 1992-1993, U.S. Department of Labor.
[a]Projections based on estimates from the professional association

health immunization programs, balanced nutrition, exercise regimes, and self-monitoring of symptoms. The cost of preventing chronic illnesses is much less than the cost of rehabilitation. Primary, secondary, and tertiary prevention have begun to make an impact in the work of allied health professionals. Research has an important part in justifying the efficacy of treatment intervention, either in restoring function or preventing chronic disability. Current trends in rehabilitation research are listed in Table 1-11.

1.7 Habilitation and Special Education, Stage VII

The success of the rehabilitation movement led to the field of habilitation, which goes beyond the medical model (which traditionally relies on etiology, diagnosis, and treatment). Habilitation includes the integration of psychological, sociological, and educational fields of knowledge emphasizing research in developmental theory and educational technology. Rehabilitation is defined traditionally as the restoration of function and the maximization of abilities in individuals with chronic disabilities. In contrast, habilitation is defined as the development of functions and capabilities in individuals with disabilities occurring at birth, during childhood, or during a traumatic incident (e.g., traumatic brain injury, posttraumatic stress). The process of habilitation is presented in Figure 1-4. The child with mental retardation, the individual who is congenitally blind or deaf, the child born with a missing limb or with cerebral palsy, the child with autism, and the child who is extremely disadvantaged have needs that are different from adults who acquired a physical disability. Helping the child develop independence, coping skills, and physical and mental capabilities to adapt to societal demands requires specialized techniques. The child who is developmentally delayed, unlike the adult with a handicap, has not lost a capacity or skill that requires remedial education, sensory retraining, or vocational readjustment. Instead, the child with a disability needs special education, sensorimotor-language training, occupational preparation, and training for activities of daily living basic to the habilitation process. Special education services, available for individuals with special needs, have been developed to provide training

TABLE 1–11 *Current Trends in Rehabilitation Research in 1995*

- Development of standardized outcome measures that have acceptable coefficients of reliability and validity.
- Evaluation of treatment techniques using prospective designs.
- Operational definitions of treatment methods that can be replicated in clinical practice.
- Controlled observation of normal developmental landmarks that serve as reference points for populations with disabilities.
- Fundamental investigations of the biopsychosocial nature of disease and underlying dynamics.
- Survey of the perceptions of patients with chronic disabilities toward their disability and their evaluation of treatment techniques.
- The incorporation of high technology instrumentation in evaluation and treatment, such as microcomputers, cinematography, psychophysiological measures.

DEVELOPMENTAL DISABILITY, GENETIC, EMBRYOLOGIC, OR ENVIRONMENTAL CAUSES	**EVALUATION OF FUNCTION**	**EDUCATIONAL AND TREATMENT TECHNIQUES**
○ Autism	○ Academic	○ Augmentative communication
○ Blindness	○ Activities of Daily Living (ADL)	○ Braille
○ Cerebral palsy	○ Intellectual	○ Computer and robotics assisted treatment
○ Childhood amputee	○ Neuromuscular	○ Individualized learning
○ Dyslexia	○ Psychosocial	○ Medical treatment
○ Fetal alcohol syndrome	○ Sensory	○ Motor therapy
○ Hearing impaired	○ Neuropsychological	○ Psychological counselling
○ Juvenile arthritis	○ Prevocational	○ Self-care skills
○ Learning disabilities	○ Leisure interests	○ Sensorimotor training
○ Mental retardation		○ Sign language
○ Social deprivation		○ Speech and language therapy
		○ Vocational development

Figure 1–4. The process of habilitation, or development of function. Children with special needs are evaluated and then taught using appropriate educational and treatment techniques.

and instruction in functional skills necessary for independent living and self-support. What were the early historical precursors to the field of habilitation?

Initial Concern for Those With Disabilities

Although prior to the twentieth century some services were available for individuals with disabilities, these services were minimal and were generally no more than custodial care and assistance through the efforts of religious orders and voluntary charities. The earliest report of attempts to treat and educate the blind was the establishment of a hospital in 1260 (Hallahan & Kauffman, 1993; Juul, 1981). Rousseau (1712–1779), a philosopher and theorist, petitioned in his treatise "Emile" for the study of children directly rather than using what was known about adults and applying that knowledge to children. "Nature intends that children shall be children before they are men. . . . Treat your pupil as his age demands" (Rousseau, 1762/1883, p. 52, 54).

During the mid 1800s, Jacob Rodreques Pereire (1715–1780), a Spanish medical doctor living in France, developed an oral method to teach individuals with severe hearing loss to read and speak. At the same time, a Frenchman, Abbé de l'Epée (1712–1789) developed a manual sign language for "deaf-mutes." "The natural language of the Deaf and Dumb is the language of signs; nature and their different wants are their only tutors in it: and they have no other language as long as they have no further instructors" (Epée, 1784/1820, as cited in Lane, 1976, p. 79).

Abbé Roche Ambroise Cucurron Sicard (1742–1833), a French medical doctor influential in the education of the "deaf-mutes" expanded Epée's methods, producing a way to teach "deaf-mutes" to read and write:

> [Epée] saw that the deaf-mute expressed his physical needs without instruction; that one could, with the same signs, communicate to him the expression of the same needs and could indicate the things that one wanted to designate: these were the first words of a new language which this great man has enriched, to the astonishment of all of Europe. (Sicard, 1795, as cited in Lane, 1976, p. 79)

Itard's Influence

The earliest reported case of enlightened intervention with children identified as being mentally handicapped was Jean-Marc Gaspard Itard's (1774–1838) work with Victor, "the wild boy of Aveyron" (Lane, 1976). Victor (ca. 1785–1828), who emerged from the forests of Aveyron between 1797 and 1800, was thought to have been abandoned by his parents as an infant or young child. Itard, a young physician, was assigned the responsibility to teach Victor. Itard applied methods developed earlier by Epée and Sicard. These methods included breaking up each task into small segments and using techniques that had been successful for "deaf-mutes." In this way, Itard believed that he could teach Victor to be social and use language (Lane, 1976; Winnie, 1912). After six years, even though Itard considered his work a failure, Victor had developed some social skills and could read a few words. On the other hand, Itard's work with Victor inspired him to further his methods for teaching "deaf-mutes":

> The child, who was called the wild boy of Aveyron, did not receive from my intensive care all the advantages that I had hoped. But the many observations that I could make and the techniques of instruction inspired by the inflexibility of his organs were not entirely fruitless, and I later found a more suitable application for them with some of our

children whose mutism is the result of obstacles that are more easily overcome. (Itard, 1825, as cited in Lane, 1976, p. 185)

Several authors in education (Forness & Kavale, 1984; Hunt & Marshall, 1994) have recognized the significant contribution of Itard's work with Victor to present-day methods used in special education classes. In his effort to teach Victor, Itard developed methods which encompassed multiple senses (auditory, visual, kinesthetic) and demonstrated that individual instruction could be successful. Eduardo Séquin (1812–1880), a student of Itard, advanced these methods. He opened the first school for the intellectually deficient in 1837 and demonstrated that they could be trained and educated. Finally, as a physician involved in the education and treatment of individuals with disabilities, Itard played a significant part in the development of educational and treatment services for the individuals with disabilities (Forness & Kavale, 1984). Initially, the emphasis of special education relied on a medical model using etiology, symptomology, differential diagnosis, and specialized treatment. This resulted in an educational system based on classification and segregation, rather than a system based on community participation and mainstreaming in general education. It is notable that Itard's work using a single case study has lead to the development of general methods for teaching children with disabilities (Kirk & Gallagher, 1989).

Montessori's Contribution to Special Education

The following quote is from Marie Montessori who, as a physician and teacher, established the basis for special education in Italy at the end of the nineteenth century. ". . .In this method the lesson corresponds to an experiment, the more fully the teacher is acquainted with the methods of experimental psychology, the better will she understand how to give the lesson" (Montessori, 1912, p. 107).

Montessori advocated that the special education teacher of the mentally handicapped should use observation and experimentation in sequencing pedagogical activities. Montessori, who acknowledges the influence of Itard and Séquin, was a forerunner in the movement to provide special education methods through perceptual-motor training to the child with disabilities. These materials and methods were based on concrete, three-dimensional manipulatives (hands-on activities) which allowed exploration and learning through discovery. Today these methods are used with populations of typical children and children with special needs (Shea & Bauer, 1994).

Theoretically, Montessori's method changed the direction of treatment from a medical model to a model based on education, psychology, and child development. This approach was not limited to the child with mental retardation. For example, Louis Braille, who was blind, developed a system of reading for the blind over a period from 1825 to 1852 (Illingworth, 1910). This method of teaching was the basis of special education for the blind in the early 1900s. Analogous to Braille, as a method for teaching the blind, was sign language for the deaf devised by Abbé de l'Epée around 1755 (Winnie, 1912). The oral method was later practiced in Germany by Heinicke and Hill, who felt that speech development in the deaf child should parallel normal speech development (Winnie, 1912). Because of the complexity in educating blind and deaf children, special schools that segregated them from the public schools were founded. The significance of the Montessori method for the mentally handicapped, of the Braille system for the blind, and of sign language for the deaf was that these methods compensated for the child's inability to learn in a typical classroom. They are specific, technological advances designed to help the child to learn. As a result of these methods, special education has been effective with the child who is blind, deaf, or mentally handicapped because of these methods.

Services in the United States

Séquin's contribution to the education of individuals with disabilities extended to the United States. Through the efforts of Samuel Gridley Howe, Séquin immigrated to the United States in 1848. Once in the United States, Séquin shared his experiences and knowledge regarding educational methods for teaching individuals with mental retardation. Eventually he was instrumental in founding the American Association on Mental Deficiency (AAMD), an association which continues to further the understanding of mental retardation (Lane, 1976).

In the United States, Reverend Thomas Gallaudet, Horace Mann, and Samuel Gridley Howe were pioneers in the early development of special schools for children with disabilities. In 1817 in Hartford Connecticut, Gallaudet, assisted by Clerc, a "deaf-mute" trained by Sicard, founded the first residential school for the deaf (Lane, 1976). This outstanding school still exists. Gallaudet University, located in Washington, D.C., is the only liberal arts college established for students with hearing impairments. This university was founded by Gallaudet's grandson in 1864 (Lane, 1976). In 1829, Howe opened the Perkins Institute at Watertown, Massachusetts, a residential school for students with visual impairments. This school is well known because Anne Sullivan, teacher of Helen Keller, was trained there. Fernald State School, the first institution for individuals with mental retardation, was opened in 1848, with the Commonwealth of Massachusetts assuming full financial responsibility (Sigmon, 1987). In addition to Séquin in mental retardation, individuals such as Louis Braille and Alexander Graham Bell, who was instrumental in the amplification of sound for the hearing impaired, greatly influenced the teaching methods used in these early institutions (Kirk & Gallagher, 1989).

A major change in educational practices in the United States occurred when individual states mandated compulsory education between 1852 and 1918. While some students with disabilities were taught in the general education program, the degree of severity in these individuals with disabilities resulted in the creation of residential institutions, segregated day schools, and special classes. The first special education day school in the United States, the Horace Mann School, was opened in 1868 in Roxbury, Massachusetts. New Jersey, in 1911, was the first state to mandate programs for students with disabilities (Sigmon, 1987). Individuals confined to wheelchairs or with severe disabilities continued to be excluded from the public schools until the 1960s and 1970s. The right for children with disabilities to be educated in a public school was mandated by court decisions such as Pennsylvania Association of Retarded Citizens (PARC) vs. Pennsylvania (1971) and Mills vs. Board of Education, Washington, D. C. (1971). Decisions from these judicial cases supported the position that individuals with disabilities were entitled to a free and appropriate education (FAPE) regardless of the degree of severity or educational need (Turnbull, 1986).

Special Education and Testing

In 1905, Alfred Binet (1857–1911), a French psychologist, was commissioned by the French Government to provide a useful assessment tool that would identify those children who needed special techniques to learn. Binet began working to develop methods of assessing intelligence in 1886. His first book, published at that time, was entitled *Psychologie du Raissonnement (The Psychology of Reasoning*, 1899/1912). This was the beginning of intelligence testing as we know it today. (More information regarding Binet and the development of intelligence tests can be found in the chapter on testing in the discussion on intelligence testing.) In the United States, Lewis Terman (1877–1956) and Henry Herbert

Goddard (1866–1957), strongly influenced by Binet, continued the development of intelligence tests. Both believed that intelligence was inherited, stable, and did not change over time. A student's failure in the general education curriculum was explained by his/her inadequate intellectual level, not by methods of teaching or environmental factors. As a result, in the first half of the twentieth century, institutionalization and segregation of those individuals with severe intellectual deficits and physical disabilities became the norm. It was not until the 1960s when there was a major push toward normalization (Wolfensberger, 1972) and deinstitutionalization that individuals with mental retardation and physical impairments were returned to the community and local school programs.

Historically, the habilitation of the educable mentally retarded, blind, and deaf has been more successful than the habilitation of individuals with brain damage, autism, or social deprivation. One reason for these differences has been in the specialized educational curricula that have been developed to compensate for the child's disability. Methods for educating students with brain damage, autism, or social deprivation were slower to develop.

During the latter half of the nineteenth century and the beginnings of the twentieth century, physicians such as James Hinshelwood (1917) and Samuel T. Orton (1879–1948) used adult models to understand reasons for learning difficulties in children who were not deaf, blind, or mentally handicapped. Both clinicians developed a multisensory method for teaching reading. Later, their ideas were expanded by special educators. The methods developed are still used today in many classrooms (Mercer, 1983).

The aftermath of the First World War was another turning point in the development of educational programs for individuals with brain injuries. Kurt Goldstein (1878–1965), in his experimental work with soldiers who had sustained head injuries during battle, contributed much to the understanding of the consequences of brain damage. His work inspired Alfred Strauss and Heinz Werner (Strauss & Werner, 1943) to study children with brain damage during the 1930s and 1940s at Wayne County Training School in Michigan. Their findings led to the identification of a group of children with brain damage. Although these children appeared to be mentally retarded, the cause of the retardation was not due to genetic reasons. Moreover, their behavioral characteristics were very much like the symptoms displayed by soldiers with brain injuries, such as perseveration, distractibility, inattention, and memory problems (Mercer, 1983). In their classic book, *Psychopathology and Education of the Brain-Injured Child*, Strauss and Lehtinen (1947) described symptoms and behaviors of the child with brain injury and justified special education methods for teaching this group of children. Prior to the published works by Strauss and collaborators (Strauss & Kephart, 1940; Strauss & Lehtinen, 1947; Strauss & Werner, 1941; Werner & Strauss, 1941), treatment for the child with brain damage was undifferentiated. Strauss and Lehtinen (1947) described the problem as follows: "The response of the brain-injured child to the school situation is frequently inadequate, conspicuously disturbing, and persistently troublesome" (p. 127).

A. R. Luria (1961) and L. Vygotsky (1934/1961), Russian neuropsychologists, were influential in the understanding of brain functioning and language development. Luria believed that the brain was made up of three functional units: the brainstem, involved with arousal and attention; the posterior portion, involved with taking in and processing of sensory information; and the anterior portion, implicated in planning, monitoring, and verifying one's performance. Luria and Vygotsky postulated that the development of language played an important part in one's ability to organize tasks involving planning, self-monitoring, and self-regulating. Individuals with brain damage who no longer use language for organization manifest extreme difficulties in self-regulatory and self-monitoring activities. Likewise, children who do not use language for organization do not develop self-regulation or planning skills. These ideas of Luria and Vygotsky have influenced the way we teach all students in developmentally appropriate early childhood classes.

Until recently, children with autism faced an even more uncertain future because of the lack of effective methods to compensate for their disability. For example, Bettelheim (1967) described the initial reaction to the orthogenic school and the problems of communication in an 11-year-old girl with autism:

> At first what little speech she had consisted of very rare, simple, highly selective and only whispered echolalia. For example, when we asked her if she wanted some candy she would merely echo 'can-dy'. She would say 'no' but never 'yes'. . . . It was not our language she used, but a private one of her own. (p. 162)

Currently programs such as TEACCH (Treatment and Education of Autistic Children and Communication Handicapped Children) at the University of North Carolina in Chapel Hill, NC, provide expertise and technical assistance in diagnosis and treatment to teachers and parents of students with autism (Edwards & Bristol, 1991).

As with the child with brain damage or autism, the socially disadvantaged child has been an enigma in the classroom. Gordon (1968) characterized the child who is socially disadvantaged as unprepared for a normal educational experience. He wrote: "As a consequence, these children show in school disproportionately high rates of social maladjustment, behavioral disturbance, physical disability, academic retardation and mental subnormality" (p. 6). Many of the children formerly characterized as socially disadvantaged are now diagnosed as Attention Deficit-Hyperactivity Disordered (ADHD).

In 1963 at the first national meeting of what later became the Association for Children with Learning Disabilities (now named the Learning Disabilities Association), the term *learning disabilities* was identified by Samuel A. Kirk (1963):

> Recently I have used the term "learning disabilities" to describe a group of children who have disorders in development, in language, speech, reading, and associated communication skills needed for social interaction. In this group I do not include children who have sensory handicaps such as blindness or deafness, because we have methods of managing and training the deaf and the blind. I also exclude from this group children who have generalized mental retardation. (Kirk, 1963, p. 3)

Another impetus for the development of appropriate educational programs for individuals with disabilities was the formation of various organizations, such as the March of Dimes, National Easter Seal Society, and United Cerebral Palsy, designed to provide community-based services. While these organizations originally provided resources for equipment and medical care for children with disabilities, parents of these children became politically proactive in obtaining rehabilitation hospitals and clinics, special education programs, community services, and barrier-free environments. These organizations have been instrumental in the development of support groups for families and in the publication and distribution of educational materials on prevention and treatment of disabilities.

As compared to children with disabilities who have severe problems in communication and learning, children with physical impairment who have normal language and sensory functions present different types of problems in habilitation. Physical barriers present problems in architectural design. Emotional and social adjustment are affected by the self-concept of children with disabilities as well as by their feelings of competence. Other chronic disabilities of childhood such as juvenile arthritis, ulcerative colitis, childhood diabetes, heart defects, and epilepsy profoundly affect the child's development and require adaptive or specialized treatment methods.

Recent Trends in Services for Individuals With Disabilities

Since the passing of Section 504 of the Rehabilitation Act in 1973, the Education for the Handicapped Act (EHA; Public Law 94-142) in 1974, the reauthorization and amendment of EHA as Public Law 99-457, the passing of the Americans with Disabilities Act (1990), and finally the reauthorization and amendment of EHA as Public Law 101-456, also known as Individuals with Disabilities Education Act (IDEA) in 1990, programs for students with special needs have grown by leaps and bounds. Figure 1–5 displays the change in the number of students who receive special education between 1976 and 1992. Table 1–12 describes the need for personnel and allied health professionals in special education. Treatment and educational services are provided by public schools for any student from birth to age 21 who is at risk or disabled. In addition, a continuum of services are available that range from consulting with the general education teacher about a student's need, to providing an intense, restrictive residential setting for these students. Augmentative communication, life-skills training, and assistive technology are provided to the student when needed (Meyen & Skrtic, 1988).

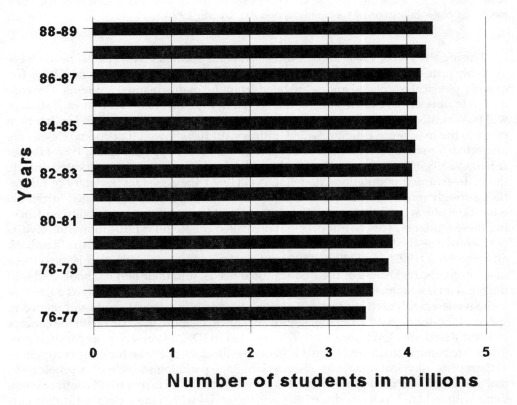

Figure 1–5. The number of students served in special education for specific years. The data are recorded by millions. Thus, in 1976–1977, approximately 3½ million students were being served. Data taken from the Fifteenth Annual Report to Congress on the Implementation of the Individuals with Disabilities Education Act, U.S. Department of Education (1993).

Table 1–12   *Teachers and Allied Therapists Needed to Serve in Special Education for the 1990–1991 School Year*

Personnel Type Needed	Number Employed	Additional Number Needed
Audiologists	837	978
Counselors	7,254	7,608
Diagnostic Staff	7,224	7,899
Local Supervisor/Administrators	16,219	16,891
Occupational Therapists	4,677	4,692
Physical Therapists	3,234	4,082
Physical Education Teachers	5,973	6,338
Psychologists	19,501	20,798
Recreational Therapists	417	506
School Social Workers	9,060	9,794
Special Education Teachers	297,490	324,424
State Supervisors/Administrators	1,154	1,230
Support Staff	52,565	54,023
Teacher Aides	162,043	168,456
Vocational Education Teachers	4,156	4,609
Work-Study Coordinators	1,509	1,829
Total	**557,102**	**634,157**

Note. Data for this table are adapted from the Fifteenth Annual Report to Congress on the Implementation of the Education of the Handicapped Act, USOE, 1994.

During the 1950s, 1960s and 1970s, services for students with special needs were available primarily in residential institutions, special day schools, or special classes frequently physically isolated and segregated from the mainstreamed students. The concept of least restrictive environment, delineated in P. L. 94-142, states that each student will be educated in the program that allows him/her to be educated with his/her own peers to the maximum extent possible. Efficacy studies showed that special classes are ineffective for students with mild disabilities (Dunn, 1968; Epps & Tindall, 1987; Haynes & Jenkins, 1986); however, students with special needs continued to be educated outside the mainstreamed population. Madeline Will (1986), the Assistant Secretary of Education, strongly recommended that students with mild disabilities be returned to general education. She argued that general educators should take more responsibility for teaching these students. This position, originally called the Regular Education Initiative, is now known as the General Education Initiative. Some individuals, such as Stainback and Stainback (1992) and Sailor (1991) have proposed total inclusion, that is, placement of all students, regardless of their educational needs, into their home schools and into the regular classroom. Others (Vergason & Anderegg, 1992) have encouraged a range of inclusiveness, with each student's placement based on individual needs and related to specific long-term goals. This latter stance appears to be more in accord with the concept of Least Restrictive Environment (LRE) as stated in IDEA. Preservice preparation programs are being restructured to enable general educators, special educators, occupational therapists, physical therapists, speech/language pathologists, school psychologists, and audiologists to participate in collaborative efforts. If the current trend continues, students with mild or moderate disabilities will be served within the general education curriculum, with adaptation as needed. Students with severe disabilities may continue to receive educational services in special class placements, especially when the educational needs include self-care skills and independent living skills.

Although much has been accomplished in the development of programs and services for those individuals with special needs, there is much more to be accomplished. We are only beginning to understand how to remediate and improve cognitive deficits. Augmentative communication and use of technology in the education and training of individuals are still in the infancy stage of development. Increased medical technology has made it possible to keep infants and patients with severe disabilities alive. Educational and training needs have just begun to be developed for these individuals.

Habilitation is the latest frontier in health research. Much research remains to be done in developing the knowledge and technology to facilitate growth and learning in the child with disabilities. The progress that already has been made in habilitation is the result of the persistent efforts of investigators devoting a lifetime of work to specific problems.

1.8 Research and the Future of Health Care

What are the future directions and goals of health care? The physician, an individual educated in the arts and science of healing, has been historically the primary health practitioner. At first education of the physician was "at the foot of a master," and later formal training permitted one to legally practice medicine. It is only in the last one hundred years that medicine has become a science with reliable and valid methods. The science of modern medicine began with Claude Bernard and Louis Pasteur, who provided the research methods and theory of disease that underlie clinical practice. Progress has been dramatic from the late 1800s, culminating with the elimination of many major diseases through vaccination, chemotherapy, surgery, and effective hospital care. Preventive medicine is now the cornerstone of health maintenance. Researchers in the present decade are mobilizing their efforts to discover means to prevent premature deaths from heart disease, stroke, cancer, arthritis, emphysema, and AIDS. Ironically, chronic disabilities continue to persist as people live longer and new diseases emerge (e.g., ebola virus) that present new challenges for medical researchers.

A second trend in medical progress is toward self-regulation of health care through education and monitoring of bodily symptoms. The individual's understanding of one's own anatomical, physiological, and psychological make-up through public health education will play an increasingly important role in the future. Why shouldn't compulsory education include an intensive curriculum on health care that includes prevention, diagnosis, and treatment? The recent trend towards self-examination of bodily symptoms in identifying possible cancerous growths is one example of self-regulation. Another example is in the experimental application of biofeedback in controlling migraine headaches, hypertension, and anxiety. The trend toward self-regulation in health will lead to more responsibility for one's own well-being.

Another trend in health care is the growth of specialized health professions. Up until 1920, the doctor and the nurse were the main health care providers. There now exist over one hundred health-related professions. New professions emerging from the advanced technology of medicine will continue to grow. These new professional positions, such as cardiovascular technologist, respiratory therapist, nuclear medicine technologist, sanitarian, and public health educator, are the result of progress made in medical technology and the advancement of public health methods. As research develops in refining the diagnosis and treatment of illness there will be a parallel growth of new specialized health professions.

The medical practice of the future may well be dominated by machines that monitor physiological changes; control the heart rate; stimulate nerves, muscle and skin; replace

TABLE 1–13   *Integrated Physiological Computer Systems*

Bodily Processes	Machine Monitoring	Computer Diagnosis
Circulatory	Electrocardiogram	
Gastrointestinal	Electroencephalogram	Aids heath
Neurophysiological	Chemical Analysis	professionals in
Genitourinary	X-Ray	prescribing treatment
Skeletal-muscular	Thermometer	
Endoscope		

bodily organs; and, in general, receive and transmit information to and from the body (Longmore, 1970). These medical machines will be designed to adapt to the internal organism of the body. Computers connected to the machines will be programmed to interpret accurately the information received. This relationship is shown in Table 1–13.

The merging of medicine with the social sciences to find solutions to the complex problems of mental illness, alcoholism, drug addiction, and criminology is inevitable. Interdisciplinary approaches to prevention and rehabilitation will result in the merging of the physical and social sciences. The relationship of poverty, alienation, malaise, and hopelessness (which are social variables) to the onset of disease, self-destruction, and social aggression will, it is hoped, attract the attention of health researchers who will work closely with social planners. The fear of creating a "1984" or a "Brave New World" where every human need is fulfilled instantly and where the individual foregoes his personal freedom for the security of "Big Brother" should influence social planning and health research. A delicate balance between governmental intervention and the respect for the sanctity and privacy of the individual must be maintained. The right of every individual to the very best health care will hopefully be the most important priority for every nation.

In the following chapters, the methods and procedures intrinsic to scientific health research are presented.

CHAPTER
2

The Scientific Method

Science as a profession, we must remember, is a recent invention. Some of the most important advances in the early development of physics and chemistry were made by amateurs.— J. B. Conant, *Science and Common Sense* (p. 17)

. . . .

.1   Applying Scientific Research to Allied Health, Rehabilitation, and Special Education
2.2   Critical Analysis of the Research Process
2.3   Qualities of a Researcher
2.4   Nomothetic Versus Idiographic Methods

Operational Learning Objectives

By the end of this chapter, the reader should be able to

1. define the terms
    - research
    - theory
    - scientific method
    - intervening variable
    - independent and dependent variable
    - associational or statistical relationship
    - hypothesis.
2. give examples of common fallacies in scientific thinking
3. outline and analyze the components of a research article
4. identify overall objectives of the researcher
5. contrast the nomothetic and idiographic methods of scientific inquiry

. . . .

2.1 Applying Scientific Research to Allied Health, Rehabilitation, and Special Education

The concept of the scientific method was first introduced by the Greeks who proposed that knowledge is enacted by a hypothesis which leads to observation and logical reasoning (Northrop, 1931). The scientific method ensures an empirical view of the world. In general, the scientific method can be summarized in four steps:

1. A hypothesis that is testable is proposed.
2. Objective observations are collected.
3. Results are analyzed in an unbiased manner.

5

4.   Conclusions proposed are based on the results of the study and previous knowledge.

The dictionary definition of *research* is "the diligent and systematic inquiry, or investigation into a subject in order to discuss facts or principles" (American College Dictionary, 1948). *Science* is defined as the "systematic, objective study of empirical phenomena and the resultant bodies of knowledge" (Dictionary of the Social Sciences, 1964). Research and Science are almost identical in definition; both imply systematic objective inquiry resulting in knowledge. Scientific *theory* on the other hand, is a comprehensive explanation of empirical data. Theory predicts what will be observed through research. A theory represents a *deductive* system of understanding the world. It predicts laws in nature that form consistent cause–effect relationships. Theories are developed by considering the underlying processes, linking an observed cause with an effect.

For example, when medical scientists investigated the relationship between a specific bacteria and the cause of a disease, a theory was proposed to explain this relationship. The theory served as the *underlying explanation*, that is, the link between the independent variable (presumed cause) and *dependent variable* (presumed effect). This relationship is schematically diagramed below (Dictionary of the Social Sciences, 1964):

INDEPENDENT VARIABLE	UNDERLYING EXPLANATION	DEPENDENT VARIABLE
Cause	Process	Effect
Germ	Germ Theory	Disease

Theory Building

Theory building is a key part of research. Many assumed cause–effect relationships may be in actuality *associational* or *statistical relationships* where a direct one-to-one ratio between cause and effect does not exist. Instances of associational relationships are those phenomena in nature that may occur together, such as precipitation in India and an increased birth rate, or solar activity and wars. By proposing a theory, a researcher seeks to explain the direct relationship between observed causes and effects. Theory building is a way of distinguishing those relationships that are interdependent. Theories may also be developed by scientists who have systematically collected data. Generally, scientific theories generate research and predict relationships between variables.

Characteristics of a Theory

A theory is defined "as a set of interrelated constructs (concepts), definitions and propositions that present a systematic view of phenomena by specifying relations among variables, with the purpose of explaining and predicting phenomena" (Kerlinger, 1986, p. 9). In general, scientific theories are characterized by certain assumptions:

- *A technical vocabulary, language or terms are generated by a theory*. For example, Piaget, in developing a theory of cognitive development, introduced the terms *assimilation, accommodation, and differentiation*. These terms are now used by theorists in child development to explain how a child thinks. Freud, in introducing the theory of psychoanalysis, gave new meaning to familiar terms such as *ego, id, superego, unconscious, libido,* and *catharsis.* These terms lose their ordinary connotations and take on the precise meanings of the theorist.

- *Natural phenomena or behavior can be explained by a theory.* For example, Darwin's theory of evolution was shaped by his observations of animal behavior and the examination of fossils. He formulated a theory from years of painstaking field observation. The pieces of evidence he amassed on animal and plant evolution were mosaics that he put together like a picture puzzle to form a comprehensive theory. His research expeditions were guided by questions that sought to explain the wide variations in animal behavior that he observed in his travel expeditions to South America.

- *A theory is a tentative set of beliefs that can be verified by scientific research.* Pasteur, in 1863, proposed the germ theory after proving that the processes of putrefaction and fermentation were caused by microorganisms. In 1880, Koch built upon the work of Pasteur by completing scientific laboratory investigation of tuberculosis and cholera, thus demonstrating the validity of the germ theory.

- *A theory predicts events that can be simulated in the laboratory or observed under controlled conditions.* The theory of genetic determinacy predicts that a child born with a chromosomal deficit such as Down Syndrome will become mentally retarded. An infant is diagnosed with Down Syndrome when an extra chromosome 21 is detected through genetic screening.

- *A theory allows a researcher to interpret results and to form conclusions.* Lorenz, who was an ethnologist and who received a Nobel Prize in Medicine, studied instinctive behavior patterns and proposed a theory of aggression. This theory seeks to explain the presence of conflicts and wars throughout human history.

- *A theory generates knowledge and leads to the development of further theory.* Gesell's theory of development predicted that normal human growth is based on sequential, hierarchial stages that unfold at critical ages. Other theorists, such as Erikson (eight stages of psychosocial development), Kohlberg (theory of moral reasoning), and Brofenbrenner (theory of ecological systems), were greatly influenced by Gesell's works in the 1920s.

- *A theory can be completely or partially true, or completely or partially false.* When Freud proposed the psychoanalytic theory at the turn of the nineteenth century, many of his colleagues completely rejected his work as unsubstantiated and based on clinical speculation. Psychoanalysis was later incorporated into psychiatric treatment programs especially in the United States from the beginnings of the twentieth century to about 1960 when criticism started to appear in the professional journals. Many parts of Freud's theory such as the terms he defined are widely used in many studies of psychotherapy. Is psychoanalysis a valid theory of behavior? This question is still unresolved.

For clinical research, theories are a critical component in a study. To paraphrase Kurt Lewin (1939), nothing is so practical as a good theory. A scientific theory implies that phenomena or events in the world can be explained in a logical or rational way. Theories are the engines for scientific research that encompass an inductive system of knowledge. Data, which are collections of facts or information, result from research and in turn can eventually generate scientific laws. The systematic collection of data entails procedures for the review of previous results, the selection of research subjects, and the use of measuring instruments.

The relationship between theories and laws are diagrammed in Figure 2–1. In all scientific research the objectivity of the investigator is the most crucial variable.

Before the development of scientific research at the turn of the century, our knowledge of medicine rested on a combination of trial and error methodology and deductive reasoning based on a priori assumptions. Fallacies growing out of the acceptance of invalid methods of treatment were common during times of superstition, such as in the Dark Ages in Europe and in primitive societies. These fallacies are incorrect arguments that are psychologically persuasive and, in some societies, continue to influence health practices. For example, contemporary practitioners who treat patients with methods that have no theoretical foundation act as if there were data supporting their methods. Some clinicians advocate a particular treatment method or drug based on the fallacious premise that a disease is highly prevalent and, therefore, any treatment is better than no treatment. Also, explanations by "authorities in the field" are used to support therapeutic applications. In the past, experimentation with radical procedures, such as the use of psychosurgery with psychiatric patients, was rationalized as relevant to treatment merely because the patients were severely psychotic and considered hopeless. Or, to cite another fallacy, people refuse to accept data linking smoking to lung cancer and heart disease because they assume it cannot happen to them—only to other persons. A knowledge of the

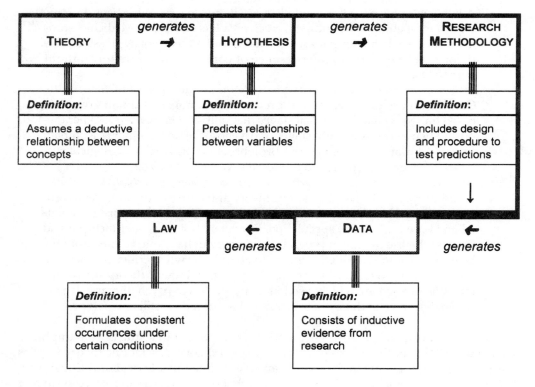

Figure 2–1.   Relationship between theory and law. A theory can become a law only through accurate and systematic research.

more common fallacies is helpful to analyze objectively the validity of published studies. Copi (1953) proposed common fallacies that can occur in scientific research. These fallacies and others applied to health research and clinical practice are listed here.

Irrelevant Conclusion

This fallacy is evident when an investigator intends to establish a particular conclusion by shifting his argument to another conclusion. For example, a clinician seeks support for a treatment method for patients with arthritis by arguing that arthritis is a crippling disease affecting millions of individuals. The fallacy in this argument is that the clinician proposes the acceptance of a treatment method based on the irrelevant fact that a specific disease is widespread. In this case the specific treatment method that is introduced needs objective data to support its use irrespective of the pressing need to help patients with arthritis. Another example of this fallacy in research is the use of unreliable or invalid tests because no other tests for measuring a specific variable exist. For example, a test written in English is given to a speaker whose first language is Navajo because there are no tests written in Navajo. Results obtained are questionable and probably invalid. If a test is invalid or unreliable, it should not be used to measure function.

Appeal to Authority

It is fallacious for a researcher to accept the opinions of a respected scientist on the sole basis of their reputation, without any supporting data. For example, in recognizing an authority's knowledge of nutrition an investigator may use his or her opinions to support a position that megavitamins are an effective treatment for patients with schizophrenia. The authority on nutrition may not have any research data to support or negate this position. A respected authority's personal opinion is not valid scientific evidence. Researchers who appeal to authorities as supporting evidence fail to separate a scientist's previous reputation from his current opinion. In an age of specialization, scientists are no longer encyclopedists who are knowledgeable in all areas. The intensive study required for excellence in one area makes it almost impossible to have expertise even in related areas. When a researcher uses greatly respected scientists' opinions as supporting evidence, especially outside their area of competence, he or she is committing the fallacy of appeal to authority.

False Cause

This fallacy is common in societies where superstition and ignorance of cause and effect exist. Curing diseases through the laying on of hands, special amulets, or magical words are examples of the use of false cause by faith healers. It is also common in nonexperimental research where correlational relationships are observed. For example, it may be noted that a full moon is associated with an increase in admissions to psychiatric hospitals. The relationship between the full moon and insanity is then fallaciously transposed to the conclusion that a full moon causes insanity. A cause and effect relationship is not established by correlational data.

In the absence of valid causes of a disease, simple and reductive explanations are often accepted. For example, a researcher investigating a complex variable, such as a learning disability, may accept prima facie evidence that the learning disability is due to hyperactivity. He bases this conclusion on correlational evidence that children with a learning disability are also hyperactive. The fallaciousness of the argument is illustrated in Figure 2–2.

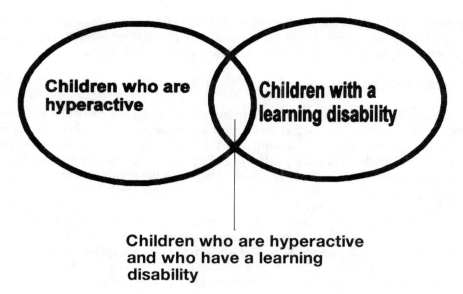

Figure 2–2. The diagram depicts the fallacy of the argument that all children with a learning disablitity are hyperactive. In fact, there are two populations, individuals who are learning disabled and individuals who are hyperactive. A few of the individuals in these populations have both conditions.

In this hypothetical example, not all hyperactive children have a learning disability, although a large number of children who evidence a learning disability are hyperactive. However, there is no evidence to support the conclusion that hyperactivity causes a learning disability or the converse that a learning disability causes hyperactivity. The very nature of a complex variable presupposes multiple causes and interactional effects among variables.

Another example of false cause in clinical practice is observing the effectiveness of a treatment method without adequately explaining the direct effect of treatment on improvement. Even though a treatment method is associated sequentially with improvement, it does not logically follow that it alone changed the condition of the patient. There may be other factors in a patient's experience or in the research conditions that could have contributed to a patient's or subject's improvement. These potential factors, which could affect the result of an experiment, must be controlled before a researcher can conclude that a specific treatment affects improvement. For example, the *placebo effect* (or "dummy treatment") is widely recognized in drug research as a change in a condition brought about seemingly by a drug, but in reality by the power of suggestion that is attached to a drug. The *Hawthorne effect* is another example of a camouflaged relationship between cause and effect. In the Hawthorne effect, the change in behavior is produced by the attention of the researcher or clinician to the subjects or patients rather than solely by the specific treatment method applied. *False cause* is a fallacy based on traditional thinking or superstition and without supporting research evidence.

Ambiguity

The lack of rigor in operationally defining terms and variables used in research produces the fallacy of ambiguity. When researchers compare outcome studies of intelligence, perception, functional capacity, or weight loss, false conclusions may result if their comparisons fail to acknowledge the differences in defining and measuring these variables. Intelligence can be defined in multiple ways and is measured by various group and individual tests and by verbal and performance scales. How the researcher defines and measures intelligence will affect the conclusions and comparisons made. When a researcher states that there is a direct relationship between social class and intelligence, one must denote how these variables were operationally defined. Otherwise one may be operating on a simplistic false basis that fails to take into consideration the various ways of operationally defining intelligence.

For the purpose of explanation let us examine a hypothetical example of ambiguity as shown in Table 2–1. In this example, if the researcher did not state how these two variables—social class and intelligence—are operationally defined, then there is no basis for comparing the results. In actuality there are four different studies measuring the relationship between two abstract variables.

Complex abstract variables that are investigated by researchers must be operationally defined; that is, the measuring instrument or procedure must be clearly identified before studies can be compared and conclusions proposed. Ambiguity is an example of comparing "apples with oranges." For example, an investigator decides to use diet therapy as an *independent variable* (presumed cause) and weight reduction as the *dependent variable* (presumed effect). However, the specific method employed in diet therapy and the method used in measuring weight reduction are the variables in fact being investigated, not diet therapy or weight reduction per se. Clearly operationally defining variables is important in eliminating the fallacy of ambiguity.

Generalization

Much of scientific research involves collecting group data from a representative sample of a target population. Group data represent the average of all individual scores. Also the data imply a range of scores from high to low on specific measured variables. The fallacy of generalization occurs when a researcher applies group data to a specific individual subject. For example, a researcher collects evidence of a statistically significant relationship between the absence of epilepsy and the occurrence of schizophrenia. The researcher concludes this from a study of seizures in which there were fewer individuals with epilepsy among patients with schizophrenia compared to the general population. However, the statistics are based on probability factors and are not based on a one-to-one relationship. The investigator can conclude only that there are fewer individuals with epilepsy in a population of individuals also exhibiting schizophrenia than in the general population—but not that every individual with epilepsy will not become schizophrenic nor that every individual with schizophrenia will not be epileptic. Nor can one conclude that if epilepsy is produced through electric shock, schizophrenia can be pre-

Table 2–1   *Operational Definition of Intelligence*

Presumed Cause: Social Class	**Presumed Effect: Intelligence Operationally Defined in Study**
1. Total family income	1. California Test of Mental Maturity
2. Geographical area	2. Wechsler Intelligence Scale for Children
3. Occupation of father	3. Teacher Reports
4. Valuation of family property	4. Ravens Standard Progressive Matrices

vented or treated. This is a fallacy where group data describing a population is generalized to every individual in the population. Group data cannot be applied to individuals whenever probability statistics do not approach 100%. The error variance in probability makes it impossible to make predictions about the specific individual from group data. One can only describe the general characteristics of groups, not the individual subjects that comprise the group. From probability statistics we can describe groups of patients, students, hospitals, or schools; but we are unable to predict the individual case with any complete certainty.

Another example of generalization fallacy is in the selection of students based on entry examinations, such as the Scholastic Aptitude Test or Graduate Record Examination. For example, a researcher interested in predicting academic success in an allied health program may find a positive correlation of ($r = .73$) between aptitude test scores and grade point averages. However this is not a perfect correlation, and it indicates only that many students with high aptitude test scores will attain relatively high grade point averages. If a program director has to predict a specific individual's success or failure, the data cannot support complete accuracy. In fact, the chances of error in predicting a specific individual's grade point average are very high although there may be accuracy in predicting a group's success in a program.

An example of the fallacy of generalization applied to clinical treatment is the "*Procrustean bed.*" In this case, clinicians who advocate a specific treatment method apply this method as a panacea to all patients regardless of individual differences. The clinician falsely applies the treatment method as a cure-all. Good treatment implies fitting the best available treatment method to the individual based on his or her needs rather than fitting the patient to the treatment.

In spite of the strong arguments used to convince researchers and clinicians to accept the findings of a study or the efficacy of a treatment method, the fallacies of irrelevant conclusion, appeal to authority, false cause, ambiguity, and generalization must be recognized by consumers of research as totally unacceptable means of advancing knowledge. The following discussion includes positive guidelines for analyzing the research process and the qualities of the researcher.

2.2 Critical Analysis of the Research Process

How is a research study judged to be either adequate or valid? How does one analyze the components of research and detect the biases of the investigator, the limitations of the design, and the deficiencies of the sampling procedure? The consumer of research must critically evaluate the methodology of a study before fully accepting the results and conclusions. Many times the results of a study are reported in the media without evaluating the methodology. The results of research can play a prominent role in supporting or negating a particular theory or social action. Governmental policies affecting funding patterns and priorities of social programs are influenced by the results of research studies. For example, continued funding of the children's television program *Sesame Street* is dependent upon data that support the position that the program has educational value. Early childhood programs such as Head Start, manpower retraining, state mental health systems, and graduate training programs in allied health professions are examples where evaluation research is used to justify federal grant support. The unfortunate policy of "benign neglect" toward minority groups during the later half of the 1960s and 1970s was a result of government-sponsored research that supported the discontinuance of many anti-poverty programs. When research is used as evidence to initiate or discontinue social programs, there is an obvious need to evaluate methodology before accepting or rejecting the conclusions. Research is not acceptable merely on the basis of social appeal, no matter how noble the conclusions. Political considerations are one of the abuses of research that confront investigators of controversial social issues, such as community health programs or family planning.

In spite of the diversity in content and the differences in application to treatment, all research has a common methodological format. When a researcher poses a question, the process of research is initiated. The question generates a search of the literature, predictions of results, and a controlled objective procedure for collecting data. Background questions are generated by an investigator to help lead into specific research questions. This is a way of helping students to discover research topics of interest to them and to narrow a research study to feasible dimensions.

Raising background questions is a "brainstorming" tactic to lead one into a review of the literature. The student or clinical investigator is encouraged to list as many basic questions as possible to initiate a study. For example a clinical researcher is interested in the most effective treatment methods of children with traumatic brain injury (TBI). The background questions related to TBI include:

- How is TBI operationally defined?
- What are the diagnostic tests to identify TBI?
- What is the prevalence and incidence rates of TBI?
- What are the most common treatment methods for children with TBI?
- What are the research data supporting treatment interventions for TBI?
- What are outcome measures used to measure treatment effectiveness?
- What is the typical course of the disability?
- What is the prognosis of TBI?
- How can vocational rehabilitation be used to treat individuals with TBI?
- How are functional capacity evaluations applied?

The investigator uses a literature review to answer some of these background questions. This process enables the investigator to become familiar with the research literature and to begin narrowing the study. In general, research is a process of systematically accumulating knowledge. What has been done previously is incorporated into current research. Background questions generate the research process and set in motion the beginning stages of completing a research study. Figure 2–3 describes this process.

The following outline of a research study is based on the scientific method. It is a systematic and objective way to investigate a topic.

    I.   A *Title* includes variables investigated, populations studied, and generalizable settings.

    II.   The *Problem* includes the research questions examined and the stated need and significance of the study.

    III.   A *Literature Review* contains the findings of related studies that are obtained through a systematic search.

    IV.   *Stated Hypotheses* include the operationally defined variables and research predictions.

    V.   A *Methodology* section includes procedures for selecting subjects, screening criteria, measuring instruments, data collection procedures, a plan for statistical analysis, and obtaining of human ethics approval.

    VI.   *Results* include objective findings that are statistically analyzed and organized into tables, charts, and graphs.

    VII.   *Discussion, Conclusions, and Recommendations* include the significance of the findings related to previous research and the implications for further investigations.

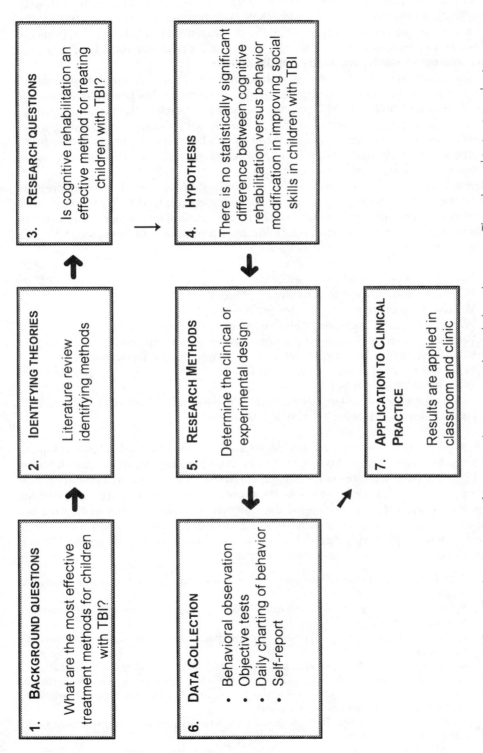

1. **BACKGROUND QUESTIONS**

What are the most effective treatment methods for children with TBI?

2. **IDENTIFYING THEORIES**

Literature review identifying methods

3. **RESEARCH QUESTIONS**

Is cognitive rehabilitation an effective method for treating children with TBI?

4. **HYPOTHESIS**

There is no statistically significant difference between cognitive rehabilitation versus behavior modification in improving social skills in children with TBI

5. **RESEARCH METHODS**

Determine the clinical or experimental design

6. **DATA COLLECTION**

- Behavioral observation
- Objective tests
- Daily charting of behavior
- Self-report

7. **APPLICATION TO CLINICAL PRACTICE**

Results are applied in classroom and clinic

Figure 2–3. Relationship between scientific inquiry, theory, research, and clinical practice. This relationship is pictured using an example of research in traumatic brain injury (TBI).

Each of the subsections can be analyzed by posing specific questions relating to the objectivity of the investigator and the validity of the methods. For example:

I. Title

1. Does the title of the study clearly define what was actually done by the investigator or does it refer only to a segment of the study?
2. Can the results of the study be generalized to the population identified by the title?
3. Are the variables stated in the title identifiable and unambiguous?

II. The Problem

1. Are the research problems clearly identified?
2. Is the study justified in relation to social need, significance, or potential contribution to health care?
3. Are statistics used to support the incidence and prevalence of the problem and its social significance?
4. What is the relationship of the study to medicine, allied health, rehabilitation or special education?
5. Does the study have a potential significant contribution to evaluation methods, treatment techniques, student training, or program administration?
6. Can results of the study be realistically implemented?
7. Is the researcher being objective in selecting a specific problem for investigation, or is there evidence that personal biases will affect the results?

III. Literature Review

1. What data collection methods did the investigator use in systematically reviewing the literature?
2. Are there theoretical assumptions that are unstated but are tacitly accepted?
3. What major areas were reviewed?
4. Was the literature search exhaustive in regard to the research problem?
5. Did the investigator separate subjective opinions and untested theories from research findings?
6. Was the investigator objective in listing results from studies that refute the stated hypotheses as well as those studies that support the hypotheses?
7. How were previous studies reported? Did the investigator describe the number and characteristics of subjects and tests used when reporting the results of studies?
8. Are references up to date?
9. Did the researcher review a wide range of journals related to the research topic?

IV. Stated Hypotheses

1. Are independent and dependent variables identifiable?
2. Are variables operationally defined?
3. Did the investigator present guiding questions?
4. Were hypotheses generated from a review of the literature, and did the investigator cite previous findings?
5. Were the hypotheses stated in null form or directionally?

V. Research Methodology

1. How were the subjects selected for the study: randomly, convenient sample, or volunteers?
2. Were screening criteria used in selecting a representative sample?

3. Were subjects a representative sample for a specified target population?
4. How were the measuring instruments selected?
5. Did the investigator state the reliability and validity of measuring instruments?
6. Do the measuring instruments have a test manual including standardized procedures for data collection and scoring?
7. How did researcher inform subjects of risks and benefits of study?
8. Can the research study be replicated?
9. Did the investigator carefully outline the procedure for data collection?

VI. Results

1. What statistical techniques were used in analyzing the data?
2. How were the results reported?
3. At what level of statistical significance were results accepted?
4. Were limitations of the study presented?

VII. Discussion, Conclusions, and Recommendations

1. Were the findings incorporated with previous literature?
2. Were conclusions justified from reported results?
3. Is researcher bias evident in interpreting results or "rationalizing away" results?
4. Were there unforeseen events that influenced results?
5. Are results omitted that contradict the hypothesis?
6. Is further research indicated?

2.3 Qualities of a Researcher

What are the qualities of a researcher? Scholars analyzing the process of research consider that the attitudes and integrity of the researcher are sometimes more important than the rigor of the methodology and the veneer of scientism. The following has been enlarged from Gee's (1950) discussion of the qualities of a researcher.

Dissonance

The researcher feels uncomfortable with an aspect of the world and the problem serves as the energizer for action. Research is perceived as problem oriented. Semmelweis's concern over the large number of maternal deaths after pregnancy and Salk's experimenting with a vaccine to prevent polio are two examples of medical researchers who were motivated by dissonance. Investigators starting with a problem such as delinquency, malnutrition, AIDS, cancer, or homelessness are energized and moved to action by the amount of pain, anxiety, and degradation that a problem produces in society and arouses public empathy.

Objectivity

This quality enables an investigator to follow the data where it takes one instead of arriving at a conclusion first and then collecting data to support personal biases. Objectivity many times leads to accidental discoveries made through serendipity and happenstance. The researcher is open to accepting whatever the data reveal. Accidental discoveries of major significance are numerous in the history of science and technology: Bell's discovery of the telephone; Edison's stumbling upon the phonograph; Goodyear's accidentally inventing a process to vulcanize rubber; Roentgen's noticing chemical changes on paper, which led to the invention of the X-ray; and Fleming's discovery of penicillin.

Perseverance

The scientist's persistence and dedication to an area of research is prominent in medicine. The history of medical research is filled with researchers like the Curies, who devoted their entire professional lives to uncovering the properties of radium. Perseverance and persistence are necessary qualities if a researcher wants to provide oneself with ample evidence before publishing one's findings. The pressure on the contemporary researcher to rush to publish results discourages persistent and painstaking efforts to accumulate overwhelming evidence. The tendency to release findings prematurely, such as in pharmaceutics, has led to medical calamities like the effects of the drug Thalidomide on fetal development. The need still remains for the researcher to persevere in the face of the pressure to publish.

Intellectual Curiosity

The scientist pursues a topic not only for the practical benefits that may result from the study, but because of the desire to know. Basic research is ordinarily carried out because of the intellectual curiosity of the investigator. The basic research that produced the breakthrough in understanding the anatomy and physiology of humans came about because of Renaissance scientists' need to know. How does the body function? What are the basic processes in cell division? What is the basic chemistry of living protoplasm? Questions regarding the essential nature of the universe and matter can be answered by only such research as is undertaken by individuals with intellectual curiosity. The researcher who earnestly seeks knowledge is likely to be diligent and persevere in attaining some significant goal.

Self-Criticism

The investigator pursuing an area of interest needs to evaluate work critically, by redesigning problems, reworking hypotheses, and initiating new methods for collecting data. The ability to examine one's work critically is important in preventing one from stagnating. Research involves a continual process of questioning, of obtaining evidence, and requestioning. The data from research serve as feedback for the reformulation of hypotheses only if the researcher is able to criticize oneself objectively.

Creativity

Being creative does not necessarily mean being novel or different. The creative researcher juxtaposes different ideas and integrates previous knowledge with contemporary issues. The qualities of risk, innovation, and independence are aspects of creativity. In contrast to creativity is conformity and the need to please others while denying one's own ideas. Creativity may be a necessary quality in the researcher who desires more than fulfilling the needs of a corporate body or serving as a data collector for someone else's mission. Formulation and planning a research design is a creative act. The process of identifying a research problem and designing an objective method to test a hypothesis demands a creative quality.

Integrity

The researcher represents an attitude of mind. In applied health and educational fields, the researcher must be guided by ethical principles that involve a respect for the rights of partipants and the honesty to bide by one's own research design and report data as found. The researcher who is engaging in human research is ethically bound not to abuse partipants. The demand by social action groups and consumer advocates for formalized regulations in regard to the use of human subjects—especially in institutional environments such as prisons, psychiatric centers, chronic disease hospitals, and state schools for individuals with retardation—reflects the past abuses in human research. An informed consent contract between researcher and subject must be included in every research design. The contract shall include the following considerations:

1. The exact procedure to be carried out must be explained in language that is understandable by the participants. Jargon and technical terms should be avoided.
2. The possible physical and psychological side effects in the study and the steps taken by the researcher to prevent harm to the participants should be stated.
3. The participant's time commitment in the study, procedures involved, and place of study should be clearly stated.
4. If the participants are mentally or physically incompetent or under age, then legal guardians or parents should be asked to provide written consent for the participants' inclusion in a study.
5. If the researcher requires that the purposes of the study not be revealed to the participants, then the researcher should explain this openly to the participants.
6. The researcher should not use coercion through any means that imply social disapproval or by penalizing the participants for not participating in the study.
7. If participants are paid for participation in an experiment, it should be based on work and time considerations, not as a camouflaged attempt to disguise the risks involved in being a participant or as an inducement to vulnerable individuals.
8. The findings of the research are to be treated as confidential; an individual participant's data should not be identified. Ongoing research data should be stored in a locked cabinet.

No research is so important that it disregards the rights of participants. The practices during the Second World War by the Nazis who engaged in human research without any regard for human rights is an extreme example of the abuse of research done with fanaticism and conformity to political goals. A researcher's integrity should be within the confines of an ethical code that must go beyond the mere search for data. Research with human subjects is not a pure or amoral theoretical activity.

Integrity in research also involves honesty in abiding by a research design and in reporting data accurately. Many times overzealous researchers are eager to present a theory of treatment or technological advance without having conclusive evidence. The pressure to present significant or dramatic findings sometimes is a result of the ego needs of the researcher. Unfortunately, it may become more important for the researcher to gain personal distinction than to report one's data honestly. Within recent years the scientific community witnessed the personality struggles in which rival researchers engaged competitively while climbing for national recognition (Watson, 1968). The research in heart transplants, cancer, and DNA have been marked by personality conflicts.

Replication

Scientific research does not exist in a vacuum, nor is it usually the product of a single individual. When a researcher investigates an area he or she typically builds upon the work of others. Even the giants of science, such as Newton, Einstein, Pasteur, and Edison, were vitally aware of previous research findings in the literature. Replication means that the researcher is able to repeat an experiment that was reported previously. The researcher who initially carries through an experiment must be able to describe the methodology in sufficient detail, so that other researchers can repeat the experiment. Research is not a mysterious activity carefully guarded and left to mystics. It is an open activity engaged in by a scientific community of scholars. Without replication, knowledge would be stagnant, as in the Dark Ages when researchers carefully hid their methods of alchemy and magic. In clinical research it is vital that investigators share their findings with the clinical community and also receive feedback from clinicians who undertake pilot studies of new practices and treatments.

2.4 Nomothetic Versus Idiographic Methods

One of the most important goals in scientific research is prediction. Whether it is the prediction that a drug will cause certain beneficial effects in the body or that a surgical operation will improve the functioning of a bodily organ, the scientific investigator seeks to discover relationships that may be universally true. The search for general laws in nature is defined as a *nomothetic* approach to science. However, the individual is affected by numerous idiosyncratic factors, such as physiological, emotional, and social influences, that are complex, unique, and sometimes unpredictable. The *idiographic* approach to science pertains to the intensive study of individuals within their own particular genetic milieu and environment.

Nomothetic Approach to Science

If we assume that every individual's behavior can be predicted, then we ascribe to a nomothetic approach; and as scientists we seek general laws that can predict behavior. Behavior modification and operant conditioning assume that individuals are operating under general laws of nature, especially defined as reward and punishment (Skinner, 1953). The precursors of behaviorism were the logical positivists who theorized that all meaningful scientific propositions are derived from experience and can be expressed in physicalistic language that can be quantified (Spence, 1948). This concept of physicalism has tried to incorporate empirical methods of collecting data into the social sciences. The technology of the logical positivists in social science is based on empirical methods of experimental control and objective observation. The major limitation of a nomothetic approach to social science is in the inability to operationally define and measure social variables such as motivation, interests, attitudes, emotions, and thinking. Behaviorism and scientific empiricism apply a psycho-physiological model; historically, the major contributions of behaviorism to social science has been by investigators, such as Pavlov (1927) in classical conditioning, Wolpe (1969) in desensitization experiments, and in the research on biofeedback and conditioning experiments of the autonomic nervous systems of the body by Miller (1969).

Idiographic Approach to Science

Psychoanalysis, phenomenology, Gestalt psychology, and the humanistic movement in the social sciences are examples of idiographic approaches. The subjective nature of experience and the uniqueness of the individual are, in these approaches, the vantage points for investigations. Psychoanalysts use the case study approach in trying to understand the dynamic forces that influence an individual's behavior. The individual is perceived as an active agent interacting with the world continuously and always in the process of change. Gestalt investigations are concerned with the perceptual processes and individual differences among people and within a humanistic framework (Perls, 1969). These idiographic approaches to scientific knowledge assume that prediction in human beings is limited to the single individual, as no two individuals share the same genetic background, physiological make-up, or psychological experiences.

How does an understanding of these two approaches, nomothetic and idiographic, affect our understanding of health research? In the nomothetic approach we assume that general laws control human behavior and physiological responses. For example, in medicine, when an individual is treated for a specific illness with a drug, the physician assumes that the individual patient will react as other individuals do to the same drug. Treatment is presented in relation to the illness, not in relation to the specific individual. Researchers investigating cause and effect relationships frequently assume a nomothetic approach. By contrast, with the idiographic approach the clinician evaluates the patient by considering individual differences and idiosyncratic traits and treats by prescribing a specific regimen. Case studies, single-subject design, and naturalistic observations are the methods used in idiographic approaches.

The history of medicine, rehabilitation, and special education contains many examples of both approaches. In analyzing a research study or in designing an experiment, either a nomothetic or idiographic approach may be appropriate.

CHAPTER
3

Eight Research Models

This fusion of art and science has pushed medical knowledge to the point where persons doing research are aware that human beings should be studied in their day-to-day environments as well as in the laboratory and the clinic, and in psychosocial as well as biophysical perspective, if we are to understand fully the conditions and processes of both health and disease.—L. W. Simmons and H. G. Wolff, *Social Science in Medicine* (p. 5)

• •

3.1   Experimental Research
3.2   Methodological Research
3.3   Evaluation Research
3.4   Heuristic Research
3.5   Correlational Research
3.6   Clinical Observation and Qualitative Research Methods
3.7   Survey Research
3.8   Historical Research

Operational Learning Objectives

By the end of this chapter, the reader should be able to

1.   compare and contrast the eight research models
2.   critically analyze examples of research from the allied health literature

• •

Research is defined as objective systematic investigation. The process of designing a research plan is one of the most creative acts in science. In this process the researcher can generate new knowledge by applying the most modern technology to an existing problem. The research design is an outline of the systematic work of collecting data. From this outline, the investigator develops a plan of action. The diversity of research designs in allied health, rehabilitation, and special education is exemplified by problems, such as evaluating the specific effectiveness of a treatment method in physical therapy, surveying the attitudes of a population of individuals with paraplegia, analyzing systematically a sheltered workshop, constructing a rating scale for speech-language interns, or correlating a relationship between perceptual ability and academic ability. In each of these research examples, a method of data collection serves as the "skeleton" for the study. The research model chosen, experimental or correlational, for example, is a decision based on the purposes of the study and the data collection methods available to the investigator.

Eight research models appropriate to problems in health, rehabilitation and special education are summarized in Table 3–1. These models were identified by analyzing the methods used in the important landmark studies in the biological and social sciences and in the allied health and rehabilitation literature. The authors are aware that some of

Table 3-1   *Eight Research Models*

Research Models	Tasks of Researcher	Significance
1. Experimental (Prospective Design)	Direct manipulation of causes and examination of effects in highly controlled settings	Ability to observe empirically, interactional effects of variables
2. Methodological	Construction of a measuring instrument, curriculum or therapeutic procedures/ approaches	Innovation of technology in allied health, rehabilitation, and special education
3. Evaluation	Critical analysis of health care delivery systems and educational programs	Objective assessment of the effectiveness of systems and treatment programs
4. Heuristic	Discovery of possible causative factors in chronic disabilities, analysis of time, space, and cost factors	Generate further research by identifying significant variables
5. Correlational (Retrospective Design)	Test of the relationships between nonmanipulated variables	Knowledge of factors that assume an associational relationship
6. Clinical or Qualitative	In-depth study of individuals, groups, or systems	Understanding of the underlying dynamics affecting individuals, groups, or systems
7. Survey	Study of the characteristics of populations (homogeneous) groups	Description of general factors that characterize groups
8. Historical	Investigation of past events through primary sources	Reconstruction of events in the past that lead to an understanding of contemporary problems

the research models described in this chapter are not universally recognized by writers on research methodology. Some writers consider the experimental model as the only research model; this point of view wrongly equates research with experimental design. The image of the laboratory investigator injecting chemicals into animals to investigate a disease is a stereotype of scientific research methodology. On the other hand, the task of a researcher interviewing a patient with arthritis, as in the qualitative research model, is lightly dismissed by some writers as *nonresearch*. Research is not limited to one methodology. The investigator who carries out an unbiased research plan and collects objective data is engaging in research whether he/she wears a white coat in a laboratory or does historical research in a library.

In practice, investigators combine research models. For example, the same experiment may involve constructing an instrument for measuring clinical effectiveness and then carrying out an experimental design. Another frequently used research methodology is to survey two populations (survey research models) and then compare differences between the two samples (correlational research model).

The diversity of research models available for the multiple problems of a disability is illustrated by the varied approaches in investigating the aging process. For example, amyloid has been identified hypothetically as a protein that, when accumulating in the body, may be a factor in accelerating the general process of aging. The relationship between amyloid and aging can be analyzed from many perspectives by using more than one research model. For instance, an experimental design using animal research is one possibility. Here the investigator can form two animal groups, one receiving amyloid injections and the other as a control. The results of this hypothetical design could yield empirical data regarding the direct relationship between amyloid and aging in mammals.

Another design applying a correlational model could be created by testing, retrospectively, the relationship between the presence of amyloid in individuals with dementia as compared to normals. A methodologist may be interested in devising an instrument for detecting the presence of amyloid in the bloodstream. A clinical case study of dementia and the examination of dynamic factors is another research possibility. A survey of the diets of older subjects analyzing for the presence of precursors to amyloid would add another dimension to data collection.

The research models employed by investigators imply certain assumptions in the data collection procedures and the interpretation of the data. Research investigations into specific problems can take place from many perspectives. A knowledge of specific research models enables the investigator to attack problems from more than one dimension. Table 3–2 demonstrates how the eight research models can be applied to a multifaceted investigation of the aging process.

The eight research models described in detail in the following pages are objective, systematic methods for collecting data. Each model has specific qualities and limitations that affect its application to a research problem.

These eight research models are not the only methods of organizing knowledge. A theoretical paper in which a scientist integrates and synthesizes knowledge by creating a conceptual schemata and predicting relationships between variables, and a position paper in which a health practitioner advocates a governmental policy are both examples of nonresearch that are scholarly and original. The important difference between research and a scholarly essay or exposition is that in research the investigator formulates a problem first and then objectively collects data related to the problem. In nonresearch or scholarship the investigator presents a position or theory and then cites evidence in its support.

Table 3–2 *Relationship Between Research Models: Aging Example*

Experimental or Prospective:	Use of laboratory animals (induce aging or retard aging) and study of physiological variables
Methodological:	Construct tests and instruments to measure aging
Evaluation:	Evaluate the effectiveness of an institution for individuals who are older to provide a therapeutic environment
Heuristic:	Discover deductively the underlying factors related to aging
Correlational or Retrospective:	Compare a self–actualizing group of individuals who are older with a passive-dependent group
Clinical or Qualitative:	Use a case study analysis of an individual who is older expressing feelings of hopelessness
Survey:	Identify the life-styles of a homogeneous group of individuals who are older living in an independent living environment
Historical:	Document through a study of federal legislation a society's changing attitudes toward individuals who have dementia

The following factors are the <u>sine qua non</u> of applied scientific research. Scholarly models that do not fulfill these requisites of research are described in Table 3–3.

1. A justification and rationale for the research
2. An extensive review of previous literature
3. Operational definitions of research variables
4. Statement of hypothesis or guiding question
5. An objective, unbiased method for collecting data
6. Separate sections for results and discussion.

3.1 Experimental Research

Purposes of Experimental Research

The experimental researcher seeks to collect empirical data by manipulating independent variables and observing their effects. Maximum control of the data collection procedure and environmental conditions is sought in the investigation. An experimenter achieves *internal validity* when he or she is able to control extraneous factors that could possibly affect the results. The degree of experimental rigor depends upon these controls. In general, the purposes of experimental research (see Figure 3–1) are to:

1. compare the effectiveness of clinical treatment methods
2. observe cause-effect relationships established in a laboratory
3. discover general laws of human responses.

Comparison of Treatment Methods

Is treatment method "A" more effective than treatment method "B"? This question is a clinical problem affecting every patient treated by a therapist in a hospital or clinic. Yet the impact of clinical research remains limited. Many therapists continue to cling to traditional methods of treatment without searching the literature to determine whether their effectiveness has been established experimentally. The classical research design employed in testing the relative effectiveness of clinical treatment methods is the following paradigm:

PRETEST OF PATIENT		EXPERIMENTAL INTERVENTION		POSTTEST OF PATIENT
function before	→	of treatment method with	→	function dependent on
treatment		control group		treatment method

In this example the experimental intervention represents the independent or manipulated variable while the degree of improvement represents the dependent variable. A cause-effect relationship is observed directly by the experimenter.

Clinical Research

The clinician's major concern is the effectiveness of a specific treatment method for a specific patient. He or she evaluates the patient, defines behavioral objectives of treat-

Table 3–3 *Scholarly Nonresearch Articles*

Scholarly Article	Tasks of Writer	Significance
Position paper	Advocate reforms of health care systems, legislation, ethics of research, standards of practice	Presentation of policy statements and editorials
Theoretical exposition	Explain relationships between variables and predict outcomes	Logical explanation in science using deductive reasoning
Case study presentation[a]	Present chronological history of patient's illness	Sequential description of disease process in one patient
Literature review	Integrate and synthesize published research	Exploration of current state of knowledge in specified field

[a]*Note.* A case study that is used as a research model is discussed in the section on clinical observational methods.

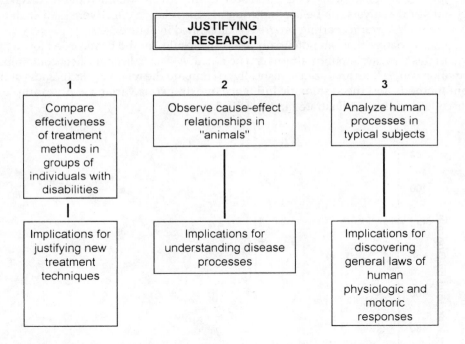

Figure 3–1. Purposes of experimental research. Note that there are three purposes for research, all of which lead to implications for treatment or intervention.

ment, applies the best treatment methods available, and then reevaluates the improvement the patient has made by the time of discharge, concluding that if the patient improved, then the treatment intervention was successful. If the treatment method is successful the clinician assumes that the treatment method should be used for other similar patients (*external validity*). However, before one can generalize the results, further data must be obtained to corroborate the conclusions. The therapist may also postulate that the treatment method selected is better than other comparable methods. Again this must be confirmed by comparing the effectiveness of various treatment methods. Another assumption is that the evaluation of treatment outcome is objective. The technique of measuring the effectiveness of a treatment method can make the difference between labeling it successful or worthless. The test for an adequate measure or evaluation of treatment effectiveness is its replicability by other clinicians. General application to other patients, relative effectiveness compared to other methods of treatment, and objective measurement of improvement are factors that clinicians must examine if their results are to be considered valid and generalizable.

Clinical research provides an experimental method for clinicians to compare the relative effectiveness of treatment methods. In clinical research, the therapist carefully documents the effects of treatment over time. Comparable treatment methods are allocated randomly, and the patient's improvement is correlated with the specific treatment method employed. One method for carrying out clinical research, without setting up experimental and control groups beforehand, is to alternate treatment methods randomly for patients as they are admitted in succession for therapy. For example, if patients with arthritis are referred to physical therapy for treatment, the clinician can employ heat packs, diathermy, exercise, and hydrotherapy methods randomly. Range of motion in the shoulder joint can be used as a measure of improvement. Each patient is charted, and statistical analysis can be used to compare the relative effectiveness of each treatment method. A graph charting progress is illustrated in Figure 3–2.

Other variables that can potentially affect the results should be recorded for each patient. In this way, systematic patterns can be noted. A data collection sheet containing information can be later analyzed statistically to compare the relative effectiveness of treatment methods and the systematic influence of extraneous variables. An example of a data collection sheet is illustrated in Figure 3–3.

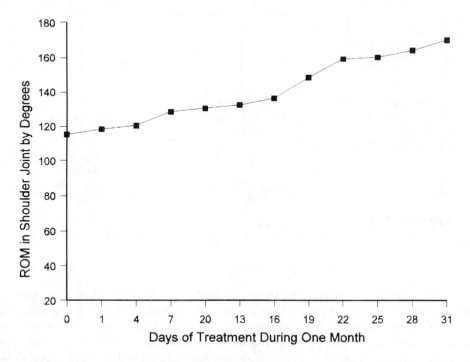

Figure 3–2.   Example of progress chart. The range of motion (ROM) in the shoulder is charted by degree along the vertical axis (Y). The day of measurement is located along the horizontal axis (X). By finding the intersection of X and Y, one can identify the ROM for a particular day.

Reliable —
Valid — R

Designing Experimental Grou

The advantage of using clinical resea
numbers of subjects to initiate resea
the lack of control by the experim
perimental research with matc

In experimental research
or more independent va
compare treatment me
equal groups and en
lustrated below:

DATA COLLECTION SHEET

Background Data

1. Patient code number (based on treatment group)

2. Sex   3. Date of Birth   4. Handedness

5. Diagnosis

6. Date of onset of illness

7. Occupation

8. Years of formal education

9. Marital status

10. Date of data collection

Test Data

11. Pretest scores on dependent variable

12. Posttest scores

    a. 1 week ___   c. 3 weeks

    b. 2 weeks ___   d. 4 weeks

                  e. 3 months

13. Treatment method

14. Other test data, including psychological tests, physiological me

Figure 3–3. Example of a data collection sheet. The information cont
the researcher.

ps

rch is that the experimenter does not need large
arch. The major disadvantage in clinical research is
enter in matching the groups on specific variables. Ex-
ed groups increases the internal validity.
with groups, the investigator compares the effects of two
iables in a patient population. If the experimenter wants to
thod X_1 with treatment method X_2, one must create relatively
ploy a reliable and valid test to measure outcome. The design is il-

DEPENDENT VARIABLE MEASURE	GROUPS	DEPENDENT VARIABLE MEASURE
PRETEST BASE STATE	TREATMENT INTERVENTION	POSTTEST OUTCOME
Y_1 before -----------------	X_1 ------------------	Y_1 after
Y_2 before -----------------	X_2 ------------------	Y_2 after

Experimental research with two or more groups can potentially eliminate the Hawthorne effect. Each group is given equal attention by the researcher. The procedure for guarding against the Hawthorne effect is described in Figure 3–4.

The foregoing sequential analysis illustrates the many controls necessary in isolating the experimental effect and in controlling for extraneous variables. In designing experimental research with human subjects and a control group, it is important for the researcher to match the groups on variables that could potentially affect the results of the study, such as age, sex, socioeconomic status, intelligence, and education. For instance, how can an investigator design an experiment applying biofeedback techniques in reducing hypertension in patients with postcardiac disease? The first step in this hypothetical design is to select a population of patients with postcardiac disease by establishing a screening criteria for inclusion based on age, sex, diagnosis, length of hospitalization, and vital capacities. The number of subjects to be included in the study is determined by statistical and practical considerations. (See Chapter 6 for discussion of these considerations.) Subjects are then randomly assigned to an experimental (e.g., biofeedback) group and a control (e.g., exercise) group. A check is done to determine if the groups are evenly matched on the relevant variables that are being considered. After two matched groups have been established, a pretest of blood pressure is taken in various conditions, such as at rest and at several stages of exertion. A check is made to determine if both groups have approximately equal mean scores of blood pressure. If not, the groups are re-formed until the researcher is satisfied that the two groups are comparable.

The two groups then undergo the experiment within a specified time period of, for example, two 2-hour sessions per week over a 3-month time period. To avoid researcher bias, the test administrator would not know whether a subject was in the biofeedback group or exercise group. Research assistants, who would not be told the purpose of the study, would be responsible for implementing the design. This method, called *double-blind control*, eliminates experimenter bias. Subject motivation, fatigue, anxiety, and dis-

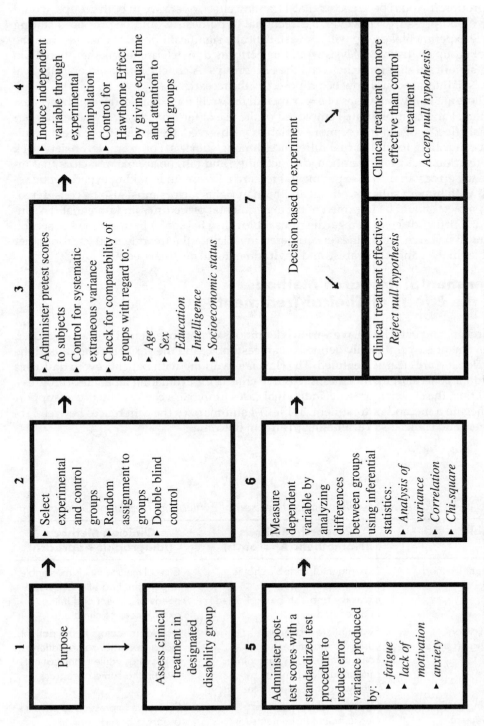

1
Purpose

Assess clinical treatment in designated disability group

2
- Select experimental and control groups
- Random assignment to groups
- Double blind control

3
- Administer pretest scores to subjects
- Control for systematic extraneous variance
- Check for comparability of groups with regard to:
  - *Age*
  - *Sex*
  - *Education*
  - *Intelligence*
  - *Socioeconomic status*

4
- Induce independent variable through experimental manipulation
- Control for Hawthorne Effect by giving equal time and attention to both groups

5
Administer post-test scores with a standardized test procedure to reduce error variance produced by:
- *fatigue*
- *lack of motivation*
- *anxiety*

6
Measure dependent variable by analyzing differences between groups using inferential statistics:
- *Analysis of variance*
- *Correlation*
- *Chi-square*

7
Decision based on experiment

Clinical treatment effective:
Reject null hypothesis

Clinical treatment no more effective than control treatment
Accept null hypothesis

Figure 3–4. Sequential analysis of control factors in experimental research. Controlling for each of these factors helps prevent possible error due to the Hawthorne effect.

tractibility should be carefully monitored because these variables could affect the results. After the 3-month time period a posttest of blood pressures would be obtained from both groups. It would be expected that a training effect, operative in both groups, would lower blood pressure. However, a directional hypothesis would be proposed stating that the experimental group will show statistically significant positive changes than the control group. Statistical analysis would be performed to determine whether there is, in fact, a significant difference between the two groups. A conclusion based on statistical analysis of the data could now be proposed by the researcher.

There are many variations of experimental research, for example, the numbers of experimental and control groups employed or the use of factorial designs where an interactional effect between two or more variables is observed. Generally, there are difficulties in controlling for individual differences among subjects. For example, anxiety, lack of motivation, lack of cooperation, distractibility, and fatigue are major factors that increase the error variance in experimental research. Before undertaking experimental research with human subjects, ethical and human rights factors must also be considered. Every subject should be informed of the experimental procedures and potential risks involved. (Further discussion regarding this topic is in Chapter 5.) In the following section on clinical research, difficulties encountered in isolating the treatment effect from other variables in the patient, therapist, and environment will be discussed.

Experimental Research Methods and the Effects of Clinical Treatment

Researchers and clinicians have various definitions of improvement. For the researcher, improvement is operationally defined and measurable, and the variables that caused the improvement are clearly identified. The clinician, working with patients every day, uses individual goals and, many times, subjective criteria for evaluating a patient's progress. In addition, the clinician presents individual cases from one's clinical practice to support or to negate a method of treatment. Table 3–4 summarizes the differences between researchers and clinicians in evaluating treatment outcome.

Table 3–4   *Researcher–Clinician Comparison of Evaluating Treatment Outcome*

Variable	Research Methods (Nomothetic Approach)	Clinician Methods (Idiographic Approach)
Treatment Method	Experimental variable that is independent, mutually exclusive and can be replicated in other studies	Clinical method that is modifiable, dependent upon the observed needs of patient and the experiences of clinician
Other Factors Affecting Treatment	Systematic extraneous variables that must be controlled (e.g., by matching, random assignment, or by narrowing the scope of the study)	Individual factors in the patient that account for some patients improving, while other patients remain the same or regress
Assessing Improvement	Operational definition of measurement instruments for improvement and control for the Hawthorne effect	Subjective impression of patient's progress based upon the clinician's initial evaluation and subsequent observed changes

The problem of investigating the effectiveness of a treatment method is a complex issue. What criteria are used in evaluating improvement? How can other variables in a patient's life space, such as family, friends, diet, activities, and work, be separated from the treatment procedure in the evaluation of improvement? How can the therapist's relationship be separated from the treatment method or process in determining its effect on treatment outcome?

The interactional effects between the therapist and patient, treatment method and patient, and external environment and patient make it difficult for the experimenter to isolate the specific variables causing specific results. These interrelationships are schematically shown in Figure 3–5.

Before the experimenter can determine if one treatment method is more effective than another method, he or she must identify and control possible extraneous variables that could influence the results. These four areas of influence as shown in Figure 3–5 are variables within the patient, therapist, and environment as well as the treatment method. All of these factors can potentially affect outcome. Knowing this, the researcher must reword the question to be: What specific *treatment* method by what specific *therapist* for what specific *patient* in what specific *environment* is effective as measured by what specific *test instrument*? The interactional effects of these variables are shown in Figure 3–6.

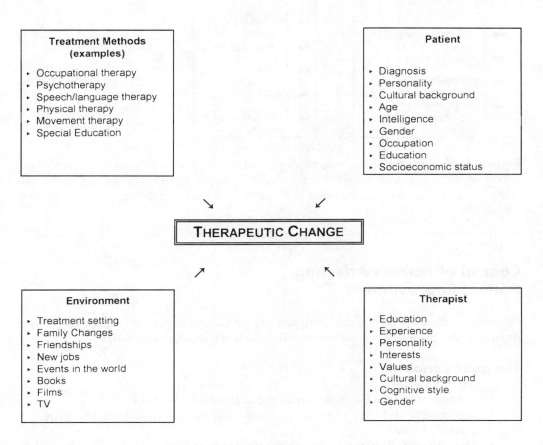

Figure 3–5. Potential factors affecting change in a patient. Each of these factors (i.e., treatment method, patient, treatment settting, and therapist) are multifaceted.

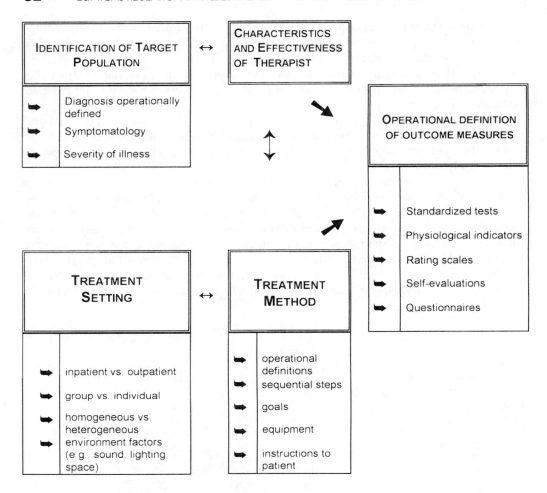

Figure 3–6.   Interactional effects of treatment method, therapist, patient, and treatment setting. While the operational definition remains the same, the results obtained on the outcome measures are dependent upon the interactional effects of method, therapist, patient, and setting.

Control of Factors Affecting Patient Improvement

When controlling for factors that may account for patient improvement, the researcher must consider the following questions within each of the variables listed.

Therapist Variables

- Is age or sex of the therapist significant in affecting outcome?
- Is cognitive style (the characteristic way that the individual perceives the world) a factor?
- How does the therapist's personality affect change?
- Is the level of education or expertise obtained by the therapist a factor in improvement?

- What part does the experience of the therapist play in patient improvement?
- Are there cultural or ethnic factors in the therapist that facilitate or retard patient progress?
- What other qualities of the therapist can potentially affect patient improvement?

Patient Variables

- Do specific demographic factors such as age, sex, or marital status affect treatment outcome?
- What are the effects of diagnosis and severity of illness on treatment?
- How does the patient's intelligence, education, occupation, and social class affect the treatment process?
- Does the congruence or conflict between the personality of the patient and therapist affect outcome?
- Is the patient's environment a factor?

Treatment Method Variables

- Is special training needed in applying the treatment method?
- Is the treatment method reliable; that is, has a standard operational procedure been applied to patients?
- Is there an underlying theoretical explanation for treatment effect on patient improvement?

Environmental Variables

- Does the setting where treatment takes place affect outcome? (Hospital, clinic, patient's home, classroom, special school, and sheltered workshop are examples.)
- How does the timing (the length of individual treatment sessions and frequency of treatments during a week) affect outcome?
- Does group versus individual treatment affect outcome?
- What are the effects of interactions of co-therapists who are simultaneously treating the same patients?
- Do physical variables in the treatment setting such as lighting, background, sound, color, temperature, atmospheric pressure, and visual distractions affect treatment outcome?

In addition to these four variables (therapist, patient, treatment method, and environment) the researcher must pose the following questions regarding the measurement of outcome.

Measurement of Treatment

What criteria are used for measuring outcome? These criteria include the following:

- Change in physical capacity, such as range of motion, ambulation, lowering blood sugar level, fine motor dexterity, aerobic capacity, lowering of heart rate
- Increase in psychosocial functioning, such as ability to work, self-esteem, interpersonal relationships (e.g., family, peers, authority figures), and ability to cope with stress

- Increase in health knowledge, such as in diet, methods to deal with stress, use of activity, family relationships, and knowledge of pharmaceutical drugs.

Interactional Effects on Treatment Outcome

The researcher must also account for the interactional effects among variables. For example, a therapist with a penchant for order may be more effective using a behavioral modification treatment method than a therapist who has a personality characterized by a strong need for nurturing others. A treatment method that is effectively employed with one therapist may not be as effective with another therapist. The importance of therapist characteristics is recognized by clinicians in the practice of assigning patients to therapists based on the clinician's preferences, such as working with children or adults, males or females, or with certain diagnostic categories. Therapists' preferences for working with specific patients are usually indicative of personality variables. However, the self-selecting process of the therapists' preference for a specific treatment method, in a specific treatment setting with a designated diagnostic group may be limited by the therapist's education and experience. As therapists gain insight into their own skills and perceived effectiveness in working with patients, they develop specified preferences. For the researcher evaluating the effectiveness of a treatment procedure, a sensitivity to and awareness of the interactional effects of variables on treatment outcome is a necessity.

An example of a hypothetical research study examining the interaction between treatment methods in speech-language therapy and therapists' characteristics is shown in Figure 3–7. In this example, four treatment methods are compared: behavior management, developmental, direct language training, and nondirective counseling. The therapist's characteristics in working with patients are typified as:

1. Laissez-faire: The therapist is permissive in approaching patients
2. Authoritarian: The therapist is directive in instruction to patients
3. Democratic: The therapist allows the patients' input into their treatment.

The hypothetical results show that behavior management is most effective with therapists who are authoritarian and that a developmental approach is most effective with a therapist who is laissez-faire. A nondirective counseling approach may be most effective with a therapist who is democratic.

Experimental Case Study: Prospective Case

Analysis of Human Processes in Normal Subject

Experimental research models have been used to investigate physiological and psychological responses to various stimuli with normal human subjects. In general, experimental research with normal subjects tends to be *nomothetic* in that the researcher seeks general laws of nature that govern kinesthetic, physiological, neurological, or psychological processes. Potential relationships that can be studied with experimental research are the following:

- Exercise and oxygen uptake
- Food ingestion and traces of minerals in the blood
- Cognitive style and choice of leisure activities
- Exercise and emotional state
- Body alignment and mechanical stress on joints

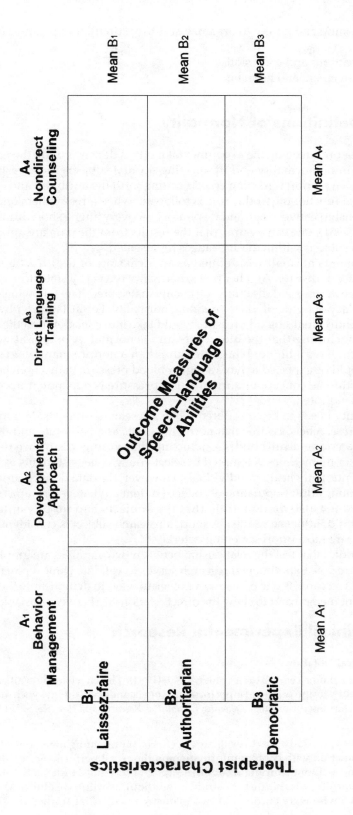

Figure 3-7. Interaction between treatment methods and therapist characteristics of speech-language therapists.

- Dichotic listening and ability to organize auditory stimuli into meaningful patterns
- Movement patterns and sport skills
- Verbal reinforcement and learning

Operational Definitions of Normality

Interpretation of data produced by the experimental method depends upon the concept of normality. In defining normality and in selecting normal subjects the investigator should be guided by an a priori screening criteria setting forth the attributes and continuous range of normal functioning. If this rule is followed, when a researcher concludes that there is a relationship between age and respiratory recovery after a short duration of exercise (Anderson, 1961), one can assume that the results from the data are applicable to all normal human subjects within the age ranges represented.

In some experiments normality is defined as an ideal state of health without the presence of a disability or disease. At other times, normality refers to a statistical average of a population where disease and disability are evenly distributed. The following examples illustrate the fallacy of rigid criteria for defining normality. For instance, a physician evaluating an older individual's blood pressure would take into consideration the age of the individual in concluding that the blood pressure is normal. A pregnant woman would be expected to have a higher blood pressure than a nonpregnant woman. An obese individual would be expected to have a higher blood pressure than a nonobese individual, and so forth. The concept of normal blood pressure is dependent upon age, sex, and weight as is indicated.

Relative normality needs to be considered when a researcher reports data for normal subjects. Many researchers assume that normality exists as an absolute and that the most healthy age is young adulthood. Concluding that young adults are usually healthy, the researcher many times is tempted to select young college students as representative samples of normally healthy individuals. However, the data derived are representative only of a young adult population of college students. Whatever group is selected, the researcher must also demonstrate that the subjects had no physiological abnormalities that could influence results. In short, a research subject is considered normal only when compared to a priori screening criteria.

Experimental studies that test the relationship between two variables are graphically diagrammed in Figure 3–8. Experimental research serves to validate clinical practice. In general, experimental research is one of the most powerful ways to demonstrate the effectiveness of a treatment method and to show the direct relationship between variables.

Example of Clinical Experimental Research

1. **Bibliographical Notation**

   Bulgren, J. A., Schumaker, J. B., & Deshler, D. D. (1994). The effects of a recall enhancement routine on the test performance of secondary students with and without learning disabilities. *Learning Disabilities Research and Practice, 9*, 2–11.

2. **Abstract**

   "The purpose of this study was to evaluate the effects of presenting mnemonic devices in conjunction with content information on the recall performance of students with and without learning disabilities" (p. 2). Forty-one students (18 students with learning disabilities, 23 students without learning disabilities) in grades 7 and 8 who were enrolled in two mainstreamed social studies classes

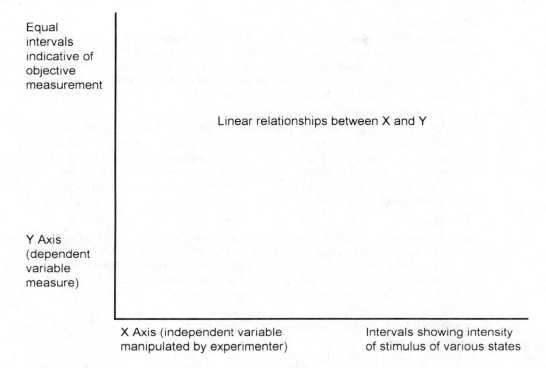

Figure 3–8. The relationship between the independent and dependent variables in experimental research.

were randomly placed in a control group and an experimental group. The two classes were team taught by a special educator and social studies teacher. After a class lecture in which important material had been verbally and visually cued (e.g., "This is important, write this down"), and a period of systematic review of some of the material, the students were given a multiple-choice test covering material from the class lecture. The systematic review differed for each group. The experimental group reviewed material through an enhanced memory routine designed to relate memory of information to specific mnemonic procedures. The control group was drilled repeatedly on the facts. Results of the data analysis indicated that students in the experimental group showed statistically significantly greater recall of information than the control group. In addition, more of the students in the experimental group received passing grades than did students in the control group. The researchers hypothesized that use of the memory enhancement system was beneficial in increasing recall of factual information for students with and without learning disabilities.

3. **Justification and Need for Study**

   The investigators stated that the purpose of the study was to investigate ways in which students with learning disabilities could learn content material presented in lectures in the general classroom and the ways in which general educators could structure classroom lectures to facilitate and enhance learning for all students. The theoretical basis for the study was previous findings that when students with learning disabilities are taught mnemonic techniques, their ability to recall factual information increases. The study extended findings from previous research at the University of Kansas Center for Research on Learning (KU-CRL) regarding the needs of students with learning disabilities who are enrolled in general education classes.

4. **Literature Review**

   Twenty-six references were cited in this article. Articles came from several different journals, including *American School Board Journal, Learning Disability Quarterly,
   Journal of Learning Disabilities,* and *Remedial and Special Education.* The authors
   cited in the references were well known in the field of learning disabilities, memory training, and strategy instruction.

5. **Research Hypothesis or Guiding Question**

   Implicit in the investigator's research design were the following nondirectional
   hypotheses: (a) There is no statistically significant difference between the experimental and the control group in the recall of reviewed facts; and (b) There is no
   statistically significantly difference between the experimental and the control
   group in the recall of unreviewed facts. The latter hypothesis was raised to ensure
   that the two groups were similar.

6. **Methodology**

   Statistical analysis was carried out through a two by two ANOVA design comparing diagnosed and undiagnosed students in experimental and control groups.
   The experimental group reviewed factual material through an enhanced memory
   system, whereas the control group reviewed the same material through repeated
   questioning. Both groups were tested on nonreviewed material to determine similarities between the groups.

7. **Operational Definition of Variables**

   Independent variables
   • control and experimental groups
   • students with and without learning diabilities

   Dependent variables
   • score obtained on reviewed facts
   • score obtained on nonreviewed facts: used to determine similarity between
     groups

8. **Analysis of Results**

   The authors used an analysis of variance (ANOVA) to test their hypothesis. Results confirmed the first null hypothesis (there was no statistically significant difference between the two groups) and led to rejection of the second null hypothesis (there was no statistically significant difference between the two groups in
   recall of reviewed material).

   A significant main effect for exceptionality was seen with nonreviewed and
   reviewed facts ($F = 12.197, p = .001; F = 10.173, p = .003$). This was expected, as there
   was a statistically significant difference between students with learning disability
   and students without learning disabilities. There was no statistical significance between group 1 and group 2 for nonreviewed facts, both of which contained students with and without learning disabilities. However, there was a statically significant difference between groups for reviewed facts ($F = 18.900, p = 000$).

9. **Stated Limitations of Study**

   a. ". . .The practicality of incorporating the Recall Enhancement Routine into
       secondary lessons on an ongoing basis. . . " (p. 10) was not addressed.
   b. The ability of students to "generate their own mnemonic devices within
       mainstream setting" (p. 10) was not addressed. The students in this study
       were taught a mnemonic device and instructional modifications were made
       within the classroom setting.
   c. ". . .the levels at which LD students can perform in the mainstream secondary
       classroom" (p. 10) is a third limitation. Although more students with learning
       disabilities showed passing scores, approximately 25% of the students still
       failed, even when given extra accommodation and instruction.

10. **Major References in Study**

Bulgren, J., Deshler, D. D., & Schumaker, J.B. (1993). *Teacher use of a recall enhancement routine in secondary content classrooms.* Unpublished manuscript, University of Kansas, Center for Research on Learning, Lawrence.

King-Sears, M. E., Mercer, C. D., & Sindelar, P. T. (1992). Toward independence with keyword mnemonics: A strategy for science vocabulary instruction. *Remedial and Special Education, 13,* 22–33.

Mastropieri, M. A., Scruggs, T. E., McLoone, B., & Levin, J. R. (1985). Facilitating learning disabled students' acquisition of science classifications. *Learning Disability Quarterly, 8,* 299–309.

Scruggs, T.E., & Mastropieri, M.A. (1990). Mnemonic instruction for students with learning disabilities: What it is and what it does. *Learning Disability Quarterly, 13,* 271–280.

3.2 Methodological Research

Purposes of Methodological Research

Rehabilitation workers have for many years seen the need to develop devices and apparati to help individuals with disabilities maximize their independence and functional activities. The growth of the fields of orthotics (braces and splints), self-help devices, and prosthetics (design of artificial limbs) is a direct result of this vision. Methodological research in health care is an example of interdisciplinary cooperation between scientists. Biomedical engineering, which emerged as a complex multidisciplinary field incorporating medicine, engineering, psychology, economics, computer technology, law, sociology, and the environmental sciences has grown rapidly in the last 30 years. R. Rushmer, a researcher at the Center for Bioengineering, University of Washington, Seattle, was one of the first to describe the interaction of these multidisciplines. Table 3–5 is adapted from his description.

Table 3–5   *The Current Scope of Biomedical Engineering: Potential Areas of Interaction Between Life Sciences and Engineering*

Applied Bioengineering			
Technological Development	**Therapeutic Techniques**	**Health Care System**	**Environmental Engineering**
Research Tools	Occupational Therapy	Organization	*Pollution*
• Physical measure	Physical Therapy	Medical economics	• Air
• Chemical	Radiation Therapy	Long-range planning	• Water
composition	Respiratory Treatments		• Noise
• Microscopy	Special Education		• Solid waste
• Isotope	Speech/Language Therapy		• Food
	Surgical instruments		
Clinical Interventions	*Monitoring*	*Methods*	Human fertility
• Audiology	• Intensive care	*Improvements*	Population control
• Cardiology	• Surgical, postop	• Support functions	
• Gastrointestinal	• Coronary care	• Service functions	
• Genitourinal	• Ward supervision	• Nursing	

(continued)

Table 3–5   *(continued)*

	Applied Bioengineering		
Technological Development	**Therapeutic Techniques**	**Health Care System**	**Environmental Engineering**
• Musculoskeletal • Neurology • Respiratory		• Facilities design • Medical care • Community care • Independent Living	
Diagnostic data • Automation • Chemistry • Microbiology • Pathology • Multiphasic screening	*Artificial organs* • Sensory aids • Heart–lung machine • Artificial kidneys • Artificial extremities: arms, legs	*Operations research* • Optimization of laboratories • Support functions • Personnel • Processing • Scheduling	*Aerospace* • Environment control • Closed ecological systems • Physiological adaptation
Computer Applications • Data processing • Analysis • Retrieval • Diagnosis	*Transplants* • Liver • Heart • Blood vessels • Kidneys	*Cost Benefit Analysis* • Cost accounting • Evaluation of results • Beneficial economy	Underwater compression effects Heat conservation Communication

Note. Adapted from "Medical Engineering: Projections for Health Care Delivery," by R. F. Rushmer, 1972, p. 13.

The main purposes of methodological research in rehabilitation and special education are the construction of therapeutic hardware, the development of objective tests, the design of physical facilities, and the planning of curriculum and treatment interventions. Figure 3–9 outlines specific areas of applying methodological research to allied health, rehabilitation, and special education.

As seen in Chapter 1, significant advances in medicine and rehabilitation occurred because of technological inventions via the microscope, X-Ray machine, electrocardiogram, otoadmittance bridge in audiology, electroencephalogram, and the numerous diagnostic scopes, all of which are results of methodological research. The introduction of psychophysiological measures and functional capacity evaluation procedures are examples of the ongoing importance of methodological research and its relationship to clinical practice.

Strategies

In devising an instrument or method of treatment, the researcher poses the question: What are the relevant factors that must be considered in devising a device or test instrument? Questions regarding the applicability of an instrument to a specific age group; intellectual, motor, perceptual, and educational factors; and the minimal level of functioning required to use a device must be considered. The content of the instrument or test should be devised after a systematic review of related literature.

An example of methodological research involves developing a practical method of independent feeding for a population of individuals with severe disabilities. What aspects of feeding, such as use of utensils, eye–hand coordination, psychological factors of motivation, instructional methods, and attention should be considered? Or, if a re-

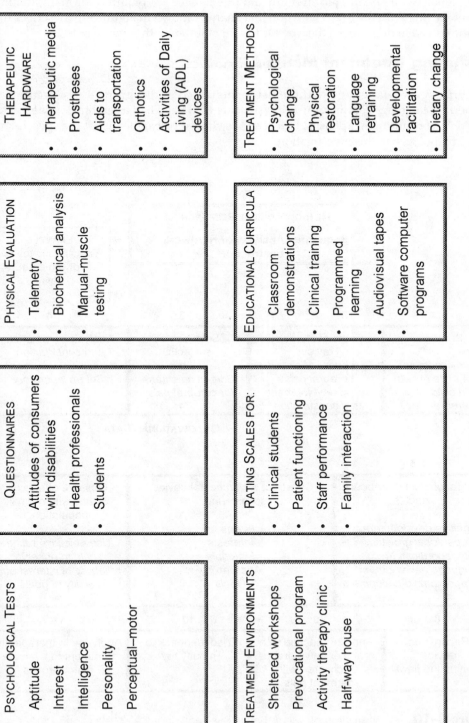

PSYCHOLOGICAL TESTS	QUESTIONNAIRES	PHYSICAL EVALUATION	THERAPEUTIC HARDWARE
• Aptitude • Interest • Intelligence • Personality • Perceptual–motor	• Attitudes of consumers with disabilities • Health professionals • Students	• Telemetry • Biochemical analysis • Manual-muscle testing	• Therapeutic media • Prostheses • Aids to transportation • Orthotics • Activities of Daily Living (ADL) devices

TREATMENT ENVIRONMENTS	RATING SCALES FOR:	EDUCATIONAL CURRICULA	TREATMENT METHODS
• Sheltered workshops • Prevocational program • Activity therapy clinic • Half-way house	• Clinical students • Patient functioning • Staff performance • Family interaction	• Classroom demonstrations • Clinical training • Programmed learning • Audiovisual tapes • Software computer programs	• Psychological change • Physical restoration • Language retraining • Developmental facilitation • Dietary change

Figure 3-9. Methodological research: Purposes and content examples. The application of methodological research to allied health, rehabilitation, and special education.

searcher is interested in devising therapeutic toys for children disabled by cerebral palsy, what factors relating to strength and intelligence are required for manipulating and interacting with the toy? The sequential analysis shown in Figure 3–10 describes the steps involved in designing a therapeutic toy for children with cerebral palsy.

Designing Treatment Method

What if a speech-language pathologist is interested in designing a new treatment method for language retraining in adult patients who have had a cerebral vascular accident (CVA) resulting in aphasia? How can the clinical researcher assist the speech-language pathologist in this investigation?

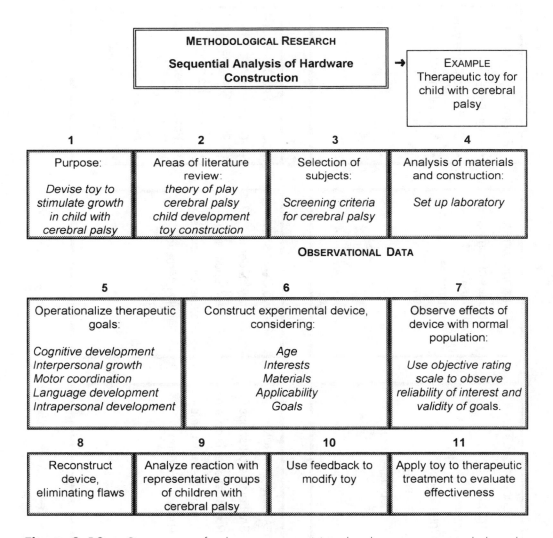

Figure 3–10.   Construction of a therapeutic toy. Note that the construction includes a literature review, operationalized goals, pilot testing on students with and without disabilities, and evaluation of effectiveness.

The overall design of the research is organized into five phases. Phase I is an examination of the need for developing a new language retraining method for adults with aphasia that take into account the incidence of aphasia in the population and its human and economic costs.

Phase II includes a search of the literature reviewing the etiology, incidence and prevalence rates, and treatment methods of aphasia. The specific speech therapy methods currently used for treating aphasia would be included.

Phase III considers the variables that enter into the design of a specific treatment method. The research plan is described in Table 3–6. In this phase, the clinical researcher's goal is to design the treatment method so that it can be used by trained speech-language pathologists in working with individuals with aphasia.

Phase IV includes the experimental pilot testing of the treatment method. Are the instructions clear in presenting the treatment method to patients? Are there areas for further theoretical development in considering aspects of the method? Should the treatment be shortened or lengthened in time? Are there limitations within the treatment procedure? During this phase the researcher is concerned with the refinement of the procedure and initial evaluation by speech-language pathologists working with patients with aphasia. A rating scale for assessing the clarity and relevancy of the treatment method is developed by the researcher and completed by clinicians. The actual testing of the effectiveness of the treatment method cannot be accomplished until the method has been refined.

Phase V includes the discussion of the treatment method, its applicability to patients with aphasia, and the level of skill necessary in administering the treatment. Consideration of the potential effectiveness of the treatment method compared to other procedures as identified in the literature review should also be discussed.

Psychological Tests

The design of psychological tests is a traditional role for psychologists who are trained in measurement theory and test construction. Recently clinicians of diverse disciplines in rehabilitation and special education have also become involved in developing new assessment measures that are directly related to clinical evaluation. For example, interest among occupational therapists in perceptual-motor functions and child development has led to the construction of new tests designed for specific treatment populations. Application and use of standardized tests is becoming an increasingly important task of the clinician who routinely evaluates the level of patient function. Even so, this area has not yet generally been incorporated into most undergraduate curriculums in the allied health professions. The construction of reliable and valid instruments for measuring human capacities is a relatively fertile area of methodological research in the allied health professions. A more in depth discussion of testing and measurement is in Chapter 8. Figure 3–11 analyzes the steps involved in test construction.

Table 3–6 *Variables in Devising a Treatment Model*

Patient	Therapist	Method
• diagnosis	• educational level	• operationalized treatment goals
• severity of illness	• experience	• time factors
• gender	• specific training	• manual of directions
• intelligence	• personality	• individual vs. group factors
• education		
• socioeconomic status		

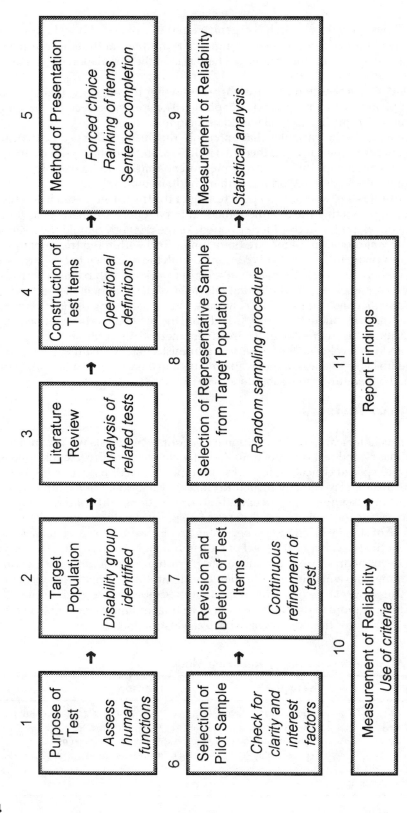

Figure 3-11. Test construction. Note that there is a sequential order to the construction, with many validity checks on the task.

Rating Scales

Rating scales are employed most frequently in evaluating the performance of students, patients, and staff. Typically, the evaluator checks off the description most indicative of performance from a list of adjective phrases. Rating scales are of three types: numerical, dichotomous, and descriptive. In a numerical scale, ratings are distributed along a continuum, such as in the following example:

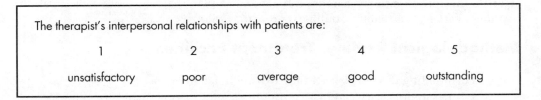

The therapist's interpersonal relationships with patients are:

1	2	3	4	5
unsatisfactory	poor	average	good	outstanding

In a dichotomous scale, the extremes, along a continuum, are identified and the rater places a line indicative of performance anywhere between these two points. For example:

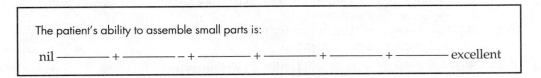

The patient's ability to assemble small parts is:

nil ———— + ———— – + ———— + ———— + ———— + ———— excellent

In a descriptive scale, the rater chooses a phrase from a presented list. For example:

Consistently passive	Shows restraint in acting	Mostly independent	Shows originality	Consistently highly creative in in planning treatment

Questionnaires

The need to gather information regarding the characteristics and attitudes of populations has led to the wide abuse of questionnaires, especially in marketing research. Individuals are deluged by questionnaires asking whether they use a certain brand of toothpaste or deodorant, ad infinitum. Despite abuses, questionnaires can be useful tools in obtaining information about a homogeneous population. In constructing a questionnaire, the researcher must resolve the following questions:

- Was there an overall theoretical framework or rationale for selecting questionnaire items?
- Do the items in the questionnaire measure accurately what the researcher purports to measure? (Validity)
- Are the items clear, unambiguous, and consistent? (Reliability)
- Was a representative pilot sample selected for testing reliability?

For a further discussion of questionnaires see Chapter 8.

Treatment Facilities

How can an investigator contribute in the design of an effective treatment environment for patients with disabilities? The tasks of designing sheltered workshops, outpatient clinics, and "halfway houses" are a joint effort by architects, administrators, therapists, and other rehabilitation personnel. The investigator applying methodological research to the construction of a treatment environment should first pose the question: What factors must be considered in providing a therapeutic environment for patients? From answers to this question the researcher can generate a plan that takes into consideration treatment variables. A tentative outline for research follows.

Methodological Review: Treatment Facilities

1. Formulating the purposes for the treatment facility
   a. Disabilities serviced (e.g., individuals with mental disorders, retardation, or physical impairments)
   b. Treatment goals (e.g., mental and physical development, prevocational, independent living)
   c. Demographic considerations for screening clients (e.g., age, gender, socioeconomic variables)
   d. Location of treatment facility (e.g., urban, suburban, or rural area) and impact on neighborhood.

2. Surveying need for treatment facility by documenting
   a. Number of potential clients to be serviced
   b. Number of other treatment facilities in service area
   c. Attitudes toward facility's location by potential clients, community residents, and health care providers.

3. Reviewing literature describing similar programs
   a. Architectural descriptions of physical layouts
   b. Analysis of staff functions and patient ratios
   c. Policies regarding patient admissions, discharges, and follow-up
   d. Evaluation research of treatment effectiveness
   e. Administrative considerations (e.g., budgeting, departmental responsibilities).

4. Stating guiding assumptions and rationale for
   a. Setting screening criteria for patient admission and discharges
   b. Designing physical layout and geographical location
   c. Proposing staff positions
   d. Setting criteria for evaluating effectiveness.

5. Surveying resources of community
   a. Potential source of staff
   b. Transportation facilities
   c. Consultative services
   d. Community support.

6. Survey cost effectiveness factors
   a. Construction cost
   b. Cost of providing patient care and treatment

c. Cost of providing supportive and maintenance services
d. Sources of potential income
   (1) Fees
   (2) Government grants
   (3) Private contributions.

Designing Education Curricula in Rehabilitation and Special Education

The training of occupational therapists, dietitians, rehabilitation counselors, speech-language pathologists, audiologists, physical therapists, special educators, school psychologists, and other related professional groups involves interdisciplinary approaches. What knowledge in the areas of physiology, anatomy, psychology, and sociology are necessary? What interpersonal skills in working with clients with disabilities must be developed? What evaluation and treatment procedures should be taught? These questions regarding the content of educational curricula are continually being reevaluated in light of the rapid growth of the allied health and special education fields. Parallel to the growth of the curricula content areas is the interest in designing methods for effectively communicating knowledge to health students. How do students learn most effectively? What should be the role of programmed instruction, computer programs, audiovisual techniques, clinical supervision, and lecture demonstrations in the educational curricula? These questions lend themselves to methodological research. The researcher objectively designs a curriculum after an extensive review of the literature and by identifying the relevant factors related to the student, teacher, behavioral objectives of the curriculum, content, and teaching methods.

Physical Evaluation Techniques and Treatment Hardware

Another area of methodological research that is appropriate to allied health and rehabilitation pertains to the use of machines and hardware for evaluating a patient's functional capacity. Electromyography (EMG), electrodiagnostic recording, perceptual-motor tests, visual, auditory and kinesthesis testing, and manual muscle testing are examples of the broad areas for potential research.

Of all the allied health professionals, physical therapists make the maximum use of mechanical methods in clinical treatment. These methods include ultrasound, diathermy, infrared light, ultraviolet rays, whirlpool, electrical stimulation, hot packs, and paraffin. New methods of treatment, especially in muscle retraining are now relying on electrophysiological methods involving oscilloscopes, telemetry, and computers.

The growth in the area of prosthetics has been the result of the combined talents of researchers coming from backgrounds in engineering, neurophysiology, and rehabilitation. Orthotics, the development of splints and braces for individuals with physical disabilities, is another area for research development.

Example of Methodological Research

1. **Bibliographical Notation**
   Kluge, J. B. (1972). The Walldius prosthesis: A total treatment program. *Physical Therapy 52*, 26–33.

2. **Abstract**

Kluge describes the Walldius prosthesis (surgical and postoperative treatment aspects of concern to the physical therapist) and the advantages and disadvantages of prosthesis replacement of the knee joint. The results of a review of 24 cases of total replacement with the Walldius prosthesis performed at North Carolina Memorial Hospital are presented, and a suggested physical therapy program for these patients is described.

3. **Justification and Need for Study**

The Walldius prosthesis, first developed in Sweden, in 1951, is a total replacement endoprosthesis for the knee for those individuals with disabilities who have severe pain and extensive destructive changes in the knee joints. It is one of five major surgical treatment procedures that include arthroplasty, fusion, synovectomy, and osteotomy.

Results of the investigation imply that the follow-up physical rehabilitation "is critical for a successful surgical result" (p. 28). However "little material is available to aid the physical therapist in designing and executing an effective rehabilitation program for the postoperative period" (p. 26).

4. **Literature Review**

Kluge examined the literature and surgical procedures of the knee and cites articles from the following journals; *Journal of American Medical Association; Surgery, Gynecology, and Obstetrics; Journal of Bone Joint Surgery; Acta Orthopedic Scandinavia;* and *Acta Chair Scandinavia.* Her conclusion from the literature was "that the Walldius prostheus provides satisfactory results more consistently than any previous methods of knee arthroplasty" (p. 33).

5. **Research Hypothesis or Guiding Questions**

What factors must be considered in designing a physical therapy postoperative program for patients who have received a Walldius prosthesis knee replacement? This question is implied in the methodological investigation.

6. **Methodology**

The medical records of 16 patients with rheumatoid arthritis who had a surgical implantation of the Walldius prosthesis were reviewed for the purpose of determining the specific physical therapy program prescribed. The following variables were analyzed: age, days in hospital, and passive and active range of motion at discharge and after 1 year.

After analyzing the preliminary results the investigator established the following criteria for successful physical therapy follow-up:

a. "Motivational goals should be included with the basic treatment goals, as progression toward optimal function is slow, often taking a year or longer" (p. 30).

b. ". . . a good result should demonstrate freedom from pain, active mobility from full knee extension through at least 70 degrees of flexion. . ." (p. 31).

c. ". . . complete lateral stability of the knee joint" (p. 31).

d. "Full extension is required for utilization of the internal locking mechanism of the prosthesis" (p. 31).

e. "At least 70 degrees of flexing is desirable for ease in sitting, standing, and elevation activities " (p. 31).

f. "Ideally the patient should progress to independent ambulation" (pp. 31–32).

Based on these criteria the investigator developed a preoperative and postoperative physical therapy program.

7. **Operational Definition of Variables**

The Walldius prosthesis and surgical procedure were described in detail (photograph included), and the investigator identifies the specific model analyzed in the study.

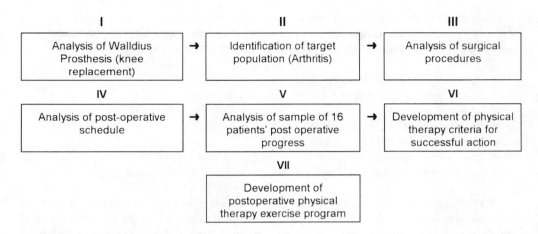

Figure 3–12. Flow plan in methodological research. This example uses the plan from the Walldius Prosthesis. Other flow plans would include the same steps but use different data.

8. **Flow Plan in Methodological Research (see Figure 3–12).**

9. **Analysis of Results**

Based on the analysis of the postsurgical progress of the 16 patients, the investigator developed the following five guidelines or recommendations for physical therapists in the preoperative and postoperative management:

 a. Document preoperative evaluations of functions on film.

 b. On the first postoperative day, describe exercise program.

 c. After the fifth postoperative day, detail exercise program.

 d. When the orthopedist discontinues the balance suspension, detail ambulation exercises. Recommend home program.

 e. Conduct follow-up evaluations and recommend exercise programs.

10. **Limitations of the Study**

 a. The guidelines for establishing a treatment program should be evaluated by physical therapists who work with postoperative patients with a Walldius prosthesis knee replacement. As a follow-up to the study the investigator should develop a rating scale for evaluating the treatment program.

 b. The treatment program should be further developed so that it can serve as a prototype to be replicated in the clinical environment.

11. **Major References in Study**

Walldius, B. (1957). Arthroplasty of the knee using an endoprosthesis. *Acta Orthopaedica Scandinavica Supplementum* XXIV:1–112.

Walldius, B. (1970). Arthroplasty of the knee using an endoprosthesis: 8 years experience. *Acta Orthopaedica Scandinavica, 30 (20)*, 137–148.

3.3 Evaluation Research

Purposes of Evaluation Research

Evaluation research relates to the assessment of programs that provide direct health care, prepare health personnel, and administer services to private and governmental agencies. When engaged in evaluation research, the investigator considers a total corporate unit and the components that comprise it. Program effectiveness, quality of service, productivity, organizational communication, cost effectiveness, stated objectives, and personnel practices are areas considered in evaluation research. Evaluation research is commonly applied in the following programs, services, and agencies:

- Certification of treatment program
- Accreditation of college or educational program
- Agency evaluation
- Analysis of cost-per-patient treatment
- Follow-up studies of patients
- Study of community's health needs and resources available
- Evaluation of program effectiveness.

An historical example of the impact of evaluation research on changing an institution was Abraham Flexner's (1910) report on *Medical Education in the United States and Canada*, which was made to the Carnegie Foundation for the Advancement of Training. Flexner personally toured the 155 medical schools that existed in the United States and Canada. Although he did not use a standardized questionnaire or test instrument for evaluation, he did apply specific criteria in evaluating the quality and effectiveness of schools in preparing physicians. These criteria were the following:

1. The entrance requirements for gaining admission to the medical school (whether they were nominal, high school graduation or equivalent, or college training)
2. The number of students in attendance
3. The size of the faculty, including number of full-time professors and part-time instructors
4. The financial resources available to the college for endowments, tuition, and other income
5. The quality and adequacy of the physical plant, including laboratory, facilities, equipment, refrigerator plants, medical library, and professional supervision available to the students in the laboratories
6. The opportunities for student practitioners, availability of hospital patients, and amphitheater to observe surgery and clinical patients.

On the basis of these criteria, Flexner found a wide discrepancy in standards of medical education in the schools he visited. He concluded, based on his observations, that many medical schools were doing a disservice to the nation in preparing poorly educated physicians. He recommended that there be fewer medical schools.

Flexner's evaluations of the 155 medical schools led to dramatic changes in medical education that occurred in the next 15 years. He recommended that medical schools and hospitals enter into teaching relationships, that state boards reject applicants for medical degrees who graduate from medical schools that were inadequate, that examinations for state licensure be rigorous; and he hoped that "Perhaps the entire country may some day be covered by a health organization engaged in protecting the public health against the formidable combination made by ignorance, incompetency, commercialism, and disease" (p. 173). All of these recommendations were eventually implemented.

Evaluation research as used by Flexner was directed toward the improvement of an institution, specifically the medical profession. However, abuses of evaluation research exist as well.

Suchman (1967) identified several areas of potential abuse as listed below.

- **"Eyewash"** is an attempt to justify an ineffective program by deliberately selecting only those aspects that appear successful and overlooking the important parts of the program.
- **"Whitewash"** is an effort whereby the evaluators try to cover up program failure and inadequacies by avoiding these areas when evaluating the program. The evaluators may solicit "testimonials" in order to divert attention from the general failure of the program.
- **"Submarine"** or **"torpedo"** is a device to destroy a program regardless of its worth or usefulness in delivering health services. This often occurs in administrative power struggles when opponents are attacked along with their programs.
- **"Posture"** is used by evaluators when they want to appear scientific and objective when, in fact, they carry out a superficial and incomplete evaluation.
- **"Postponement"** is a tactic of using evaluation research, for example, to answer public reaction to scandalous conditions in an institution. The real purpose of this ploy is to defuse public outrage by substituting research for action.
- **"Substitution"** is an attempt to hide an essential part of a program that is an obvious failure and to shift emphasis to areas that are controversial.

From the foregoing examples, it is evident that evaluation research can serve not only to provide objective data, but also as a tactic to keep an inadequate program operative or to discredit an effective program.

When properly used, evaluation research can be useful (Weiss, 1972) in deciding whether to

- continue or discontinue a program
- improve an agency's practices and procedures
- add or drop specific program strategies and techniques
- use a program as a model for new agencies
- utilize more fully on a geographical basis, the services of a program
- accept or reject theoretical approaches underlining an agency's program.

These purposes are achieved only after the investigator has collected objective and valid data. The research steps include (a) the stated need for evaluation research; (b) a review of the literature, comprising a description of programs and criteria used; (c) an objective research design for collecting data through interviews, questionnaires, attitude scales, and clinical observation; (d) statistical analysis of records and examination of the physical plant; (e) comparisons of program with objective criteria; and (f) separate sections on results and discussion of findings.

Figure 3–13 identifies examples of potential areas for evaluation research in allied health, rehabilitation, and special education.

Strategies of Evaluation Research

The issue of researcher bias is of prime consideration in evaluation research. The underlying purpose of evaluation research is to apply objective assessment to a facility, agency, or treatment program. How does a researcher objectively evaluate an organization? How are criteria established for measuring the effectiveness of a program? Are criteria established by the evaluation research team based on ideal, theoretical considera-

TREATMENT FACILITIES	HEALTH MAINTENANCE ORGANIZATIONS (HMOs)
• General hospitals • Psychiatric facilities • Rehabilitation centers • Half-way houses • Residential treatment centers (RTC) • Independent living complexes • Special schools, sheltered workshops, clinics, therapy departments, and training centers	• Visiting nurse services • Outpatient clinics • Insurance plans • Group medical practices

EDUCATIONAL AND THERAPEUTIC PROGRAMS	EDUCATIONAL PROGRAMS FOR HEALTH CARE WORKERS
• Physical and mental disabilities • Developmental disabilities • Social disadvantages	• Certified assistants • Basic professional • Advanced professional

VOLUNTARY AND PRIMARY AGENCIES RELATED TO	GOVERNMENTAL AGENCIES
• AIDS • Alzheimer's • Arthritis • Cerebral palsy • Heart disease • Cancer • Crippled children • Muscular sclerosis • Muscular dystrophy • Traumatic brain injury • Mental retardation	• Division of Vocational Rehabilitation • Department of Health, Welfare, Correction • Social Security Administration • National Institute of Mental Health • United States Department of Education

Figure 3–13.   Potential areas for evaluation research in allied health, rehabilitation, and special education.

tions, or by the treatment agency being evaluated? What expertise in research is needed in evaluating the competence and abilities of health professionals? What controls should be established in the research methodology to reduce investigator bias?

A hypothetical example below explores the process of evaluation research as applied to a residential school for disturbed adolescents.

1. Stated purposes of evaluation are set forth, such as:
   a. Continued school certification or accreditation
   b. Evaluation of treatment effectiveness
   c. Direct and indirect costs per student treatment

    d. Widening of services to include more diverse client groups

    e. Change in delivery of services to reduce residential population and to include more day care or community-based treatment

    f. The overall decision to cease operation.

    Before evaluation research is undertaken, there must be a mutual understanding of the purpose between the evaluators and those being evaluated. If the purposes are unclear, or if there is a hidden agenda, then the research objectivity could become undermined, and the evaluation could serve more as a political maneuver than as a means to collect objective data. For example, if the evaluators seek to close a program by collecting negative or damaging information and by omitting any positive attributes, if they exist, then the evaluation is worthless as scientific research.

2. The formation of a research team of evaluators is dependent upon the stated purposes of the evaluation and the specific areas considered. Expertise and experience in program administration, budgeting, treatment techniques, special education, vocational rehabilitation, research methodology, interviewing techniques, and familiarity with educational requirements and job descriptions of professional and nonprofessional staff members are necessary to provide appropriate expertise and knowledge levels for the members of an evaluation research team. Evaluation research demands a sophisticated level of expertise that is essential in the research process. The responsibility of judging the effectiveness of the program is delegated to the research team. As the level of effectiveness is a relative judgment, it is important that each member of the evaluation team understand and accept the criteria being used as the "measuring yardsticks." Experience of the members of the team in working in other treatment agencies and familiarity with the evaluation process, either as a supervisor in a clinic or in an educational environment, are necessary requisites for doing evaluation research. The size of the research team, responsibility based on the areas of expertise and experience represented, and the availability of consultants are considered in forming an effective evaluation research team.

3. The descriptive date will include:

    a. history of the organization, including why it was established and names and backgrounds of founders

    b. flow chart of administration, including lines of responsibility, and departmental components

    c. description of the physical plant, including a detailed layout of the facilities

    d. staff resumes, including education and experience of administrators, treatment staff, and supporting personnel

    e. job descriptions of work responsibilities

    f. rehabilitation and treatment services offered, including but not limited to medical, psychological, educational, child care, and prevocational

    g. formal and informal meetings, conferences, and patient staffings

    h. intake policies, orientation, and discharge procedures

    i. follow-up care and evaluation of discharges

    j. relationships with community and outside agencies

    k. numerical data regarding maximum client capacity of facility, present number of clients, average length of residence, number of referrals, and discharges over time.

4. Criteria of effectiveness are established by the research team. The criteria are based on a priori standards or objectives furnished by the administrator of the program. Areas for criteria include:

   a. *treatment effect:* percentage of clients who have made successful and unsuccessful adjustments after discharge. (Definition of successful and unsuccessful outcome should be operationally defined.)

   b. *physical plant:* safety, health, and accessibility for those individuals with mobility impairment meeting Americans with Disability Act (ADA) requirements; and fire requirements

   c. *professional staff:* percentage of staff having professional educational backgrounds (resumes, number of years at facility, reasons for leaving)

   d. *staff ratio:* number of clients per treatment staff

   e. *staff salaries:* average salaries as compared to national average or salaries in comparable agencies

   f. *continuing education:* opportunities for staff to attend conferences, workshops, or inservices

   g. *discharges:* number over time and reasons for client discharge.

   Criteria can also be established by selecting characteristic patterns from programs considered to be successful models. However, flexibility in employing these models is necessary when applying criteria. The severity of the disability in clients serviced and the financial resources available to an agency are factors that must be considered when analyzing outside criteria.

5. Interviews with staff and residents of the facility provide the research team with qualitative data that are extremely important in assessing the overall morale of staff and the personal reactions of residents. Rating scales, in-depth interviews, questionnaires, self-report scales, and group sessions are some of the methods that can be used to assess these attitudes. It is extremely important that the interviewer and researcher involved with this aspect of data collection be objective in the process. The art of interviewing is to transform the highly subjective process of "getting insights into a systematic method for the collection of social data" (Festinger & Katz, 1953, p. 327). The limitations of the interview process should be recognized by the researcher. The very nature of communicating feelings and attitudes is limited by the natural suspiciousness of the interviewee and his/her reliance on memory to provide information. It is not the authors' intent to discuss in detail interviewing techniques, but it shall be sufficient to note that researchers utilizing interview information must be certain that the interviewers have had training. Leading questions, long and complicated questions, and rambling unrelated items, used many times by untrained interviewers, provide data that subsequently bias the results. (See Festinger & Katz, 1953, for further information.)

6. The next process in evaluation research is the synthesis of objective descriptive data and objective interview material. The Results section of the report should be separated from the Discussion and Conclusions. Results are raw data that are objective findings. Results should not be "flavored" by subjective analysis or "undone" by interpretations. The results should remain separate from critical analysis.

   Table 3–7 lists hypothetical data that would be included in a Results section.

Table 3–7 *Hypothetical Results Analyzing Flow of Individuals Through a Residential Treatment Program*

Variable	Number	Percentage
1. Capacity of Residence	55	100%
2. Average daily attendance of residents during last six months	50	90%
3. Average length of residence for each individual discharged in last six months	3 months	
4. Number of individuals in residence for over one year	15	30%
5. Number of direct care workers (treatment personnel)	10	
6. Number of full-time professional staff, excluding administrators	6	
7. Number of part-time consultants	3	
8. Number of full-time teachers	5	

7. The interpretative summary consists of a qualitative discussion of the results apart from the quantitative results. Qualitative or naturalistic information could include, for example, staffs' opportunities to innovate new programs, the informality of the communication process, the accessibility of administrators, the feelings of hope and optimism generated by the staff, the willingness of the agency to change the consumer with disabilities' involvement in treatment planning, the use of community resources, the integration of new technology with present methods, and the facilitation of professional growth through supervision.

8. The conclusions and recommendations of evaluation research are a vital part of the report. How does the research team decide that a treatment program is effective and should have continued support by the community? Or that a treatment program is ineffective, not responsive to the needs of a community, and should be terminated?

   During the last thirty years we have seen the decline and closing of large, isolated institutions that served individuals with physical and psychiatric disabilities who mainly came from poor families. These institutions were closed because they became custodial "warehouses" without providing for the needs of the individuals. However, when the institutions were supported by governmental agencies in the United States in the 1920s, and up until the 1960s, there were few alternatives for community-based treatment. Did evaluation research pay a role in the closing of institutions during the 1960s and 1970s?

   The criteria identified in evaluative research must be consistent with the needs of the target population. These needs relate to values in human society, such as economic independence, social relationships, educational development, self-esteem, and whatever else the research team or agency sets forth as the goals and objectives. It should be clear that if an agency is not meeting "stated needs" of those individuals who are being treated, educated, or serviced, and alternative agencies or facilities are available, then the community should not continue to support an institution's existence.

The following research models—heuristic, correlational, clinical observation, survey, and historical—are *ex post facto* in nature. Clinical observation is unique in that it can be either ex post facto (retrospective) or prospective. The data collection procedure in ex post facto research is retrospective because the presumed independent variable has already occurred. Kerlinger (1986) differentiates experimental research and ex post facto research on the basis of the lack of direct control by the researcher in ex post facto designs. For example, in experimental research the investigator hypothesizes "if X then Y" and manipulates the X. In ex post facto research the investigator observes Y (the dependent variable) and hypothesizes X (the independent variable). The researcher in ex post facto designs can only presume a cause-effect relationship in the past. In many ex post facto designs the investigator seeks historically to reconstruct cause-effect relationships.

3.4 Heuristic Research

Purposes of Heuristic Research

Kerlinger (1986) describes a heuristic view of science as that which "emphasizes theory and interconnected conceptual schemata that are fruitful for further research" (p. 8). The main purpose of heuristic research is to discover relationships between variables as a means of generating further investigations. In heuristic research, the researcher "fishes" for correlational relationships as a means to build a theory and design further research.

The researcher engaged in heuristic research seeks to discover significant relationships by correlating variables with a specific disease or factors affecting treatment. Research in cardiovascular diseases, learning disorders, mental illness, arthritis, cancer, and AIDS are appropriate areas for heuristic research, as well as investigations of space, time, and cost factors in the treatment environment.

Assumptions Underlying Heuristic Research

In engaging in heuristic research, the investigator assumes the following:

1. The heuristic researcher seeks to discover statistically significant relationships.
2. The researcher seeks data for theory building. The result of research provides the basis for theoretical formulations.
3. Deductive methods are used in analyzing a research problem.
4. The research problem is analyzed retrospectively; that is, the researcher starts with the presumed effect (dependent variable) and works back to the presumed causative factors (independent variables).
5. Results derived from heuristic research are not conclusive, implying that further research using prospective research is needed to substantiate cause-effect relationships.

Method of Heuristic Research

The use of factor analytic studies with computer technology enables an investigator to correlate many variables and to systematically analyze interactional patterns. This method is especially appropriate in analyzing psychophysiological illnesses where there are a combination of presumed causative factors rather than a single etiological factor. Warren Weaver (1947) describes research in the seventeenth, eighteenth, and nineteenth centuries as typifying the era of the two-variable problems in simplicity. In medicine in the early part of the twentieth century, a single etiological factor was correlated with the effects of disease (two-variable research). However, both modern medical research and social sciences research are engaged in investigating complex health problems that involve multiple causes. For example, drug addiction, mental retardation, arteriosclerosis, dementia, and dyslexia have multiple factor causations. An application of a two-variable model, where the investigator searches for the single cause of the disease, is inadequate in biopsychosocial research. On the other hand, heuristic research lends itself to the study of multiple factors that are interactive in nature. The Framingham studies of heart disease (Dawber, Meaders, & Moore, 1951) is an example of heuristic research. The strategy involved in these studies was to identify numerous risk factors that are significantly more frequent in patients with heart disease than in the normal population. The purposes of heuristic research are diagrammed in Figure 3–14.

Factors Correlating Significantly With a Disease

In heuristic research the investigator seeks to derive the major factors in a patient's lifestyle that correlate significantly with a disease and to assess their relative importance. Multiple regression and factor analysis are two statistical methods appropriate for analyzing the relative significance of identified variables in relation to the dependent variable.

A major problem in this research model is in the selection of a diagnostic group. It is critical that a screening criteria be used in selecting a research sample. The researcher

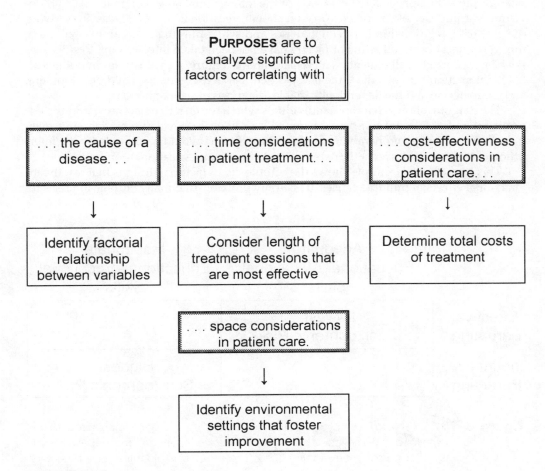

Figure 3–14.   Heuristic research.

cannot assume that a patient's diagnosis is accurate. There is much controversy in the diagnosis of chronic illnesses, such as asthma, schizophrenia, arthritis, and fetal alcohol syndrome (FAS) that requires the investigator to use rigorous methods for operationalizing diagnostic categories. After a screening criteria for subject selection has been developed and refined, the investigator's next problem is to select a population of subjects that will be the source for a representative sample.

Parallel to the process of subject selection is the compiling of investigative variables. These variables are derived from analyzing the following areas:

- **Demographic**: age, sex, occupation, educational level, marital status, income
- **Psychosocial**: personality, intelligence, attitude, life-style
- **Biochemical**: physiological, somatotype, nutritional, genetic.

Interactional Effects in Heuristic Research

Heuristic research requires the investigator to make an exhaustive search for variables that can potentially contribute to the onset of a disease. It is necessary for the investigator to take a holistic view of the problem of etiology, so as to avoid the trap of two-variable research that lacks an analysis of interactional effects. As an example, let us suppose, hypothetically, schizophrenia to be a result of the interactional effects of genetics, child development, and lack of competence in educational, vocational, or social areas. In studying the exclusive relationship between genetics and schizophrenia a researcher will have mixed results because other major factors have not been taken into account. Results cannot be generalized to all patients with schizophrenia. Figure 3–15 illustrates hypothetically the interaction between the three independent variables (genetics, child development, and competence) and the dependent variable (diagnosis of schizophrenia).

The diagram shows that those individuals who have effective parenting and the educational and vocational competence are the least likely to develop schizophrenia, even if they have a genetic vulnerability factor. Schizophrenia would result only by the interaction of three variables: genetic, parental, and educational-vocational competence.

This hypothetical example shows the complexity of factorial designs that test the interactional effects of multiple causes. It is highly probable that many chronic illnesses re-

	Adequate Educational–Vocational Skills	Inadequate Educational–Vocational Skills
Effective Parenting	Lowest Schizophrenic Risk	
Ineffective Parenting		Highest Schizophrenic Risk

Figure 3–15.   Risk of developing schizophrenia utilizing the genetic vulnerability factor. This figure shows a hypothetical interaction between independent and dependent variables in the risk of a person's developing schizophrenia. An explanation of the development of schizophrenia must take into account all major variables, not just a single variable.

sult from this type of interactional pattern. However, only by rigorous, painstaking research will it be possible to identify interactional effects. Heuristic research provides the framework to investigate multiple factors in the development of a disease process.

Analysis of Time Factor in Patient Treatment

What are the determining factors in planning treatment time for patients? (See Figure 3–16.) Why is 1 hour a week sufficient for one patient while 2 hours a week are prescribed for another patient? What proportion of treatment time is a function of pragmatic issues, such as the availability of a therapist? What consideration for time is given to the physical and emotional needs of the patient? How is treatment time planned for patient groups? All of these questions are suitable for research analysis. In general there have only been a few studies that have analyzed time factors in patient care. Yet time is one of the most basic factors in clinical treatment. An analysis of the factors considered in determining the length of time for treatments should consider both the ideal factors and the pragmatic issues. (See Table 3–8.)

Analysis of Cost Effectiveness Factors in Treatment

What are the real economic costs for treatment? What does it cost to treat a patient in a hospital as compared to an outpatient clinic? What are the costs for direct patient care by professionals as compared to nonprofessional healths technicians trained for specific health purposes? What is the cost of a massive public health prevention program as compared to existing costs for treating a specific disability group? What factors are considered in determining fees for health services? How are salaries for health workers determined? What is the economic worth of a health professional? These questions are typical of the pressing economic problems facing industrialized and developing countries where the demand for health care far outreaches the resources that countries can allocate for prevention and treatment. If a society is to determine rationally how its economic resources can be used most effectively for implementation, then it must examine objectively the underlying factors affecting the costs of health care.

Analysis of Space Factors in Patient Care

As with time and cost, space has received little attention by clinical researchers. Ethnologists and social anthropologists (e.g., Hall, 1966) analyzed the effect of space in animal

Table 3–8   *Analysis of Time Factors in Treatment*

Ideal	Pragmatic
1. Time needed for application of treatment method.	1. Amount of patients under care in proportion to the number of hours allocated for treatment (patient load).
2. Time needed to meet emotional needs of patients.	2. Traditional practices (therapy schedules).
3. Time needed to instruct patient.	3. Third-party reimbursement for service (insurance coverage).

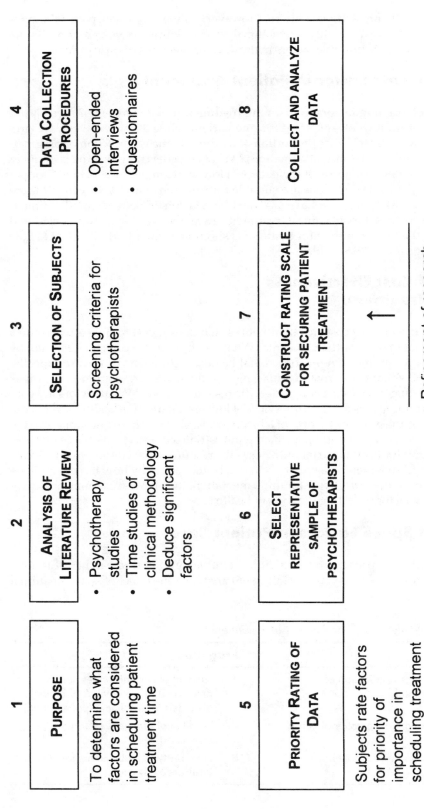

Figure 3-16. Analysis of time factors in psychotherapy.

behavior and health. There are a few studies that suggest a direct relationship between life space and psychological reactions.

In psychiatry it has been evident that space affects a patient's emotions and behavioral patterns. Goffman (1961) describes the syndrome of passivity and depersonalization as being the result of institutionalization. A contemporary definition of space is not limited to the traditional nineteenth century view that space represents *area*. Since Einstein's theory of relativity, space has taken on new meaning, implying in conceptual terms that space is the distance between two events. Space involves events or occurrences or movement. An individual's space represents the potential area for movement. In this concept of space, factors related to increasing or diminishing space are appropriate. Hospitalization, imprisonment, and institutionalization are situations where the patient, prisoner, or inmate are deprived of space and consequently have fewer movements and events. In treating a patient what considerations are given to space? Are wards or private rooms considered on any other basis than economic? Do groups occupying space limit the number of events or increase the movement of patients? Questions involving space are invariably linked to issues of group versus individual treatment. What is the relationship between the number of patients in a group, the area of movement and the events taking place in a group? Issues related to the size of patient groups in physical therapy clinics involve space factors.

A researcher employing a heuristic research model seeks to discover underlying factors affecting space. For example, how would a researcher analyze the problem of determining the space needs of geriatric patients in a nursing home? Figure 3–17 illustrates this example. The first step is to define operationally the space of geriatric patients.

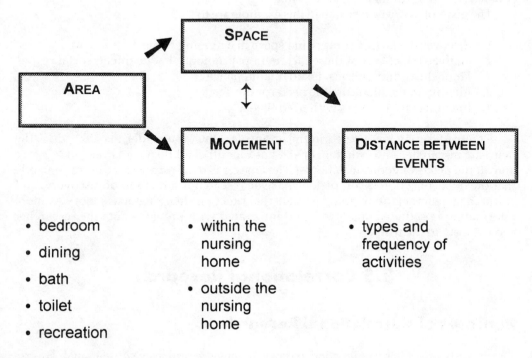

Figure 3–17. Analysis of space factors in a nursing home.

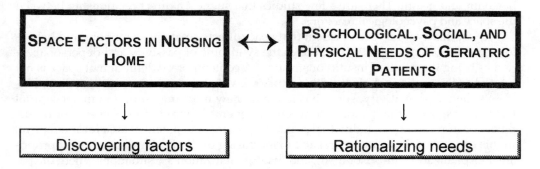

Figure 3–18. Integration of data with need theory. In this example, the data obtained from analyzing space factors in the nursing home with the needs of elderly patients (obtained through a literature review) is integrated.

The next step is to discover the physical, psychological, and social needs of geriatric patients. A review of the literature and a survey of existing programs would provide the data. Maslow's (1954) theory of a hierarchy of needs and Havighurst's (1952) activity theory could be applied to an analysis of psychological and emotional needs. Theories of aging and health could provide the framework for setting physical and health goals.

The third step in the research process is to integrate the data derived from analyzing space factors in a nursing home for patients who are older with the theoretical needs of patients. This is illustrated in Figure 3–18.

The goals of heuristic research in this example are to

1. discover the factors comprising space in a nursing home
2. analyze the effects of these factors in psychological adjustment, social relationships, and physical health maintenance
3. identify in the literature the needs of the aged
4. integrate space factors with need theory.

The reader may be puzzled in this example. How, the reader may ask, does the heuristic researcher know that he or she has identified all the factors related to space and all the needs of geriatric patients? The answer is that researchers cannot conclude that the data collection is complete. Heuristic research is a method of discovery, and research in general is an ongoing process that functions like a feedback loop. As more information is gathered, analyzed, and integrated with previous data the researcher comes closer to the truth.

3.5 Correlational Research

Purposes of Correlational Research

The majority of studies in education and psychology are primarily correlational. This research is analogous to experimental research in that the investigator tests a hypothesis.

However, unlike the experimental researcher the investigator does not manipulate independent variables, nor does he or she simulate a cause-effect relationship. In correlational research the investigator compares the relationships between variables and populations by measuring differences. It is applied very frequently to areas in the social sciences because the very nature of the problem limits the experimenter from inducing causal effects. If, for example, a researcher's purpose is to correlate characteristics in the individual who is alcoholic with causative factors, then he or she is limited to an ex post facto design where it is not possible to induce experimentally the onset of alcoholism. The researcher in this example is limited to a retrospective analysis of the assumed causes of alcoholism. Kerlinger (1986), in discussing the value of nonexperimental research, concludes ". . . social, scientific, and educational problems do not lend themselves to experimentation, although many of them do lend themselves to controlled inquiry of the nonexperimental kind" (p. 359).

A sequential analysis of correlational research is diagrammed in Figure 3–19. These steps are reviewed in the section below.

Identification of Research Variables

As clinicians in the health fields we are all concerned with the question of etiology. Why did this patient become schizophrenic? Why did this individual develop learning problems? What factors led to arthritis? What environmental factors interfered with school learning? These questions regarding etiology and relationships between variables are feasible for correlational research. The first step in correlational research is to identify the variables in a patient population to be studied. These variables are presumed causative factors that are genetic, neurophysiological, learned, or environmental. The variables are identified from observations by the clinician in contact with patients, by an examination of previous studies or theoretical papers, or simply by thinking the problem through. The presumed independent variables and presumed dependent variables are identified. Since the researcher does not actively induce the independent variables he or she can only assume an associational relationship.

Formulating Hypotheses in Correlational Research

The researcher formulates a hypothesis after reviewing the related literature. The hypothesis can be directional, for example, where a significant positive relationship between two variables is predicted. A hypothesis stated in a null form predicts no significant relationship. The decision whether to formulate a directional hypothesis or null hypothesis is based on direct or implied evidence from previous research.

Examples of directional hypotheses are as follows:

- Subjects who are blind have a significantly greater kinesthetic ability than subjects with normal vision.
- There is a positive significant relationship between self-concept and learning achievement in institutionalized children who are mentally retarded.
- Peptic ulcers are more frequent among male factory workers than comparable female factory workers.
- Children from dysfunctional low-income families have better perceptual abilities in the visual-motor areas than in the auditory areas.
- There is a higher percentage of cancer among asbestos workers than in the population at large.

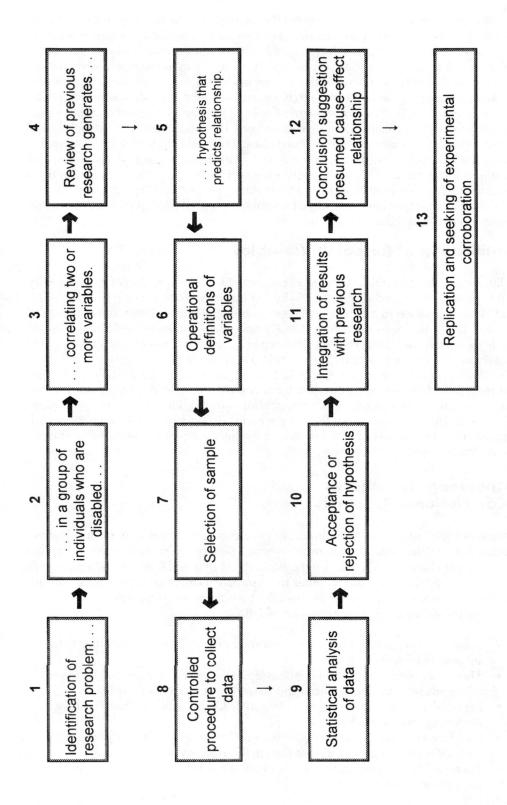

Figure 3–19. The sequential analysis of correlational research.

In all of the foregoing examples of directional hypotheses the variables are associated with a population. In analyzing the hypotheses one by one we find the following relationships. (See Table 3–9.)

In the foregoing hypotheses variables and populations are compared. Hypotheses can test the effects of multiple variables in one population or, conversely, the differences between multiple populations on one variable. A researcher cannot test multiple variables in multiple populations in one hypothesis. For example, it is fallacious to state a hypothesis such as the following: High cholesterol level and hypertension are more prevalent among cardiac patients than among a normal population. Each variable, high cholesterol level and hypertension, should be stated in a separate hypothesis.

In stating a null hypothesis the investigator states that there will be no statistically significant relationship between two variables. For example, a null hypothesis can be stated in the following way: There is no statistically significant relationship between smoking and heart disease. The decision whether to state a hypothesis in a directional form or as a null hypothesis should be an outcome of the literature review. If previous studies indicate directionality, then the researcher should state a directional hypothesis. On the other hand, if the researcher finds no evidence for a directional hypothesis in the a review of the literature, then a null hypothesis should be stated. In which form the hypothesis is stated has implications when analyzing the data statistically. For those readers without statistical background it will suffice to say that when a researcher is comparing statistically significant differences between two variables with a *t* test, a null hypothesis indicates a two-tail test of significance, and a directional hypothesis indicates usually a one-tail test of significance.

Operational Definitions of Variables

Before a hypothesis can be tested the investigator must operationally define the variables stated in the hypothesis. The operational definition includes the specific test or procedure used in measuring a variable. For example, if an investigator is measuring auditory perception, then a test such as the Wepman Test of Auditory Discrimination (Reynolds, 1987) would be indicated as the operational measure.

Table 3–9 *Associational Relationships Between Variables*

	Variables	Populations
1.	Kinesthetic ability	Blind Normal vision
2.	Self-concept	Institutionalized Children with mental retardation
3.	Peptic ulcer	Male factory workers Female factory workers
4.	Visual–motor perception Auditory perception	Children from low-income, dysfunctional families
5.	Cancer	Asbestos workers Typical

Selection of Sample

A screening criteria is necessary when selecting a sample. It is not sufficient simply to state that patients with diabetes or epilepsy will be compared. The investigator must be able to indicate how the patients have been diagnosed, the severity of the illness considered, and other variables identifying the population such as age, sex, occupation, socioeconomic status, education, and geographical area. The screening criteria devised by the investigator serve as a reference point in generalizing the results to a population. Universality and external validity depend upon the screening criteria devised for subject selection.

Data Collection Procedure

Can the test procedure be replicated? Has the investigator tried to reduce factors such as subject fatigue, anxiety, extraneous distractions, noncooperativeness, and any other factors that threaten the *internal validity* of the investigation? The test procedure should be described in detail by the investigator, including the time of day when the subjects are tested, the number in the group, the environmental conditions, the length of time for testing each subject, and the sequence in presenting the operational measures.

Interpretation of Results

In general, research has a cumulative effect. Usually, the results of one study are not sufficient to be conclusive. Many factors affect the results in correlational research that are not directly controlled by the investigator. These limitations affecting internal validity do not negate correlational research. The advantages of correlational research are that investigations can be easily replicated and subjects easily tested. Before an investigator proposes a conclusion based on the results of one study one must integrate the results with previous research. If the results are contradictory, then perhaps further research is indicated. If the results are consistent with previous literature, then it may be valid to suggest that conclusive evidence has been found. There is a need in research to be conservative, rather than premature.

Example of Correlational Research

1. **Bibliographical Notation**
    Matter, S., Weltman, A., & Stamford, B. A. (1980). Body fat content and serum lipid levels. *Journal of the American Dietetic Association, 77*, 149–152.

2. **Abstract**
    A sample of 112 men and 92 women who represented a sedentary, middle-aged population were evaluated for body weight, body composition, fasting serum triglycerides, fasting high-density lipoprotein (HDL), cholesterol, fasting low density lipoprotein (LDL) cholesterol, fasting very-low density lipoprotein (VLDL) cholesterol, and caloric intake. The results indicated that men and women designated as "over-fat" had a statistically significant higher serum cholesterol total and VLDL cholesterol than "normal-fat" individuals. In addition, nutrient distribution of caloric intake does not differ significantly between over-fat and normal-fat individuals.

3. **Justification and Need for Study**
    The investigators cited evidence to show the relationship between high concentrations of serum cholesterol in the blood and obesity and coronary heart disease.

They theorized that cholesterol transported by low-density lipoprotein may infiltrate the arterial intima and contribute to the atherosclerotic process, while cholesterol carried by high-density lipoprotein may on the other hand have a protective effect. The purpose of this study was to examine the relationship between dietary intake, body fat levels, and serum lipids in men and women of different body fat levels.

4. **Literature Review**

   Thirty-five references were cited in the study. Articles came from a wide variety of journals, such as *Lancet, Circulation, Journal of Chronic Diseases, Journal of Atherosclerosis, Clinical Endocrinology Metabolism, Journal of Applied Physiology, New England Journal of Medicine, American Dietetic Association,* and *American Journal of Clinical Nutrition.* The majority of articles cited were published during the 1960s and 1970s.

5. **Research Hypothesis or Guiding Questions**
   a. Is there a significant difference between normal-fat and over-fat groups on descriptive characteristics (age, height, weight, percentage of fat)?
   b. Is there a significant difference between normal-fat and over-fat groups in sources of caloric intake in protein, carbohydrate, fat and alcohol?
   c. Is there a significant difference between normal-fat and over-fat groups in serum lipid levels?

6. **Methodology**
   Subjects came from the greater Louisville, Kentucky area. Body fat and lean body mass were determined by hydrostatic weighing. Other methods used to measure variables were documented from the literature. For example, the cholesterol determination was based on the Liberman-Burchard reaction. The subject's usual daily caloric and nutrient intake were established by the dietary record method. Subjects were asked to record everything they ate and drank for any typical two days in a week. Subjects were divided into two groups: over-fat and normal-fat. Body fat contents of 25% for men and 35% for women were used to label the over-fat groups. The 204 subjects selected for the study consisted of 112 sedentary, middle-aged men (mean = 45 years) and 92 sedentary, middle-aged women (mean = 40 years). The t test for independent samples was used to determine significant mean differences between the variables examined. The level of statistical significance was chosen at $p < .05$.

7. **Results**

   Women had significantly higher values for body weight and body composition. Caloric intake for the over-fat and normal-fat groups were not significantly different. Normal-fat individuals had significantly lower total serum cholesterol and triglyceride intake than over-fat individuals.

8. **Conclusions**

   The following conclusions were presented by the authors:

   "Our findings suggest that (a) Men and women designated as 'over-fat' by hydrostatic weighing techniques have statistically significant higher serum triglycerides, serum cholesterol (total), and VLDL cholesterol and exhibit a trend for higher LDL cholesterol level than 'normal'-fat individuals; (b) nutrient distribution of caloric intake does not differ significantly between overfat and normal-fat persons; and (c) caloric intake is slightly elevated in overfat individuals" (p. 151).

9 . **Limitations of the Study**
   a. The authors did not describe how the subjects were recruited for the study. Does the sample represent a middle-aged sedentary population?
   b. Only one method was used to determine excess body fat. To test reliability and validity of method it is suggested that another method be used to corroborate findings.

10. **Sample of References Cited in the Study**

Nestel, P., & Goldrick, B. (1976). Obesity: Changes in lipid metabolism and the role of insulin. *Clinics in Endocrinology and Metabolism, 5*, 313.

Katch, F., Michael, E. D., & Horvath, S. (1967). Estimation of body volume by underwater weighing: Description of a simple inexpensive method. *Journal of Applied Physiology: Respiratory, Environmental, and Exercise Physiology, 28*, 811.

Reed, R. R., & Burke, B. S. (1954). Collection and analysis of dietary intake data. *American Journal of Public Health, 11*, 1015.

Rifkind, B. M., & Berg, T. (1966). Relationship between relative body weight and serum lipid levels. *British Medical Journal, 1966*, 208.

3.6 Clinical Observation and Qualitative Research Methods

It is not by chance that many of the important contributions in the social sciences have emerged from clinical observation methods (Dukes, 1965). Sigmund Freud in his search for an understanding of the psychodynamics of mental illness, Arnold Gesell's (1928) rigorous observation of child development, Jean Piaget's (1926) conceptualization of cognitive development through detailed analysis of clinical responses, and Jules Henry's (1971) naturalistic observation of families of children with emotional disturbance have all made a significant impact in the social sciences. Clinical observation as a research method has the potential to contribute greatly to the fields of allied health, rehabilitation, and special education.

Table 3–10 lists some of the major studies in the social sciences based on clinical observation research methods.

Clinical observation research employs four methods: individual case study, developmental observation, field observation (ethnography), and operations research. The definition, purposes, procedure, and application to allied health, rehabilitation, and special education are listed in Table 3–11.

Case Study—(Qualitative Research)

There is much criticism of the case study approach as a model for research. The main criticism is directed toward the subjectivity of the researcher and the inability to generalize to a population on the basis of one subject. The most important purpose of the case study is in the intensive investigation of one individual. Through a thorough study the researcher can examine factors that ordinarily would be difficult either in an experimental study involving a group of subjects or in a correlational study. To illustrate, let us suppose an investigator is interested in finding why patients who are older and living in a nursing home develop feelings of hopelessness and disengage from the life stream and society. The researcher poses the question: What factors in an older person's life contribute to feelings of hopelessness and disengagement? In this study the investigator is limited to an ex post facto research model. It would be possible to answer this question by comparing a group of patients who are older who display feelings of hopelessness with another group of patients who are older and who are actively independent. In this hypothetical study the researcher could test whether individuals who have personality characteristics of dependency will feel more hopeless than a similar geriatric sample who characteristically are more independent. The reader will recognize this research model as correlational. However, in a correlational model the researcher is restricted by the test instruments used in measuring the variable of hopelessness and by the limita-

Table 3-10 *Major Contributions from Clinical Observation Methodologies in the Social Sciences*

Social Scientist	Major Works	Methods	Publication Dates	Fields of Investigation
Sigmund Freud and Josef Breuer	*Studies in Hysteria*	Case study	1895	Psychiatry
Margaret Mead	*Coming of Age in Samoa*	Field observation	1928	Cultural Anthropology
Arnold Gesell	*Infancy and Human Growth*	Developmental observation	1929	Child Development
Jean Piaget	*The Psychology of Intelligence*	Developmental observation	1947	Cognitive Development
Stanton and Schwartz	*The Mental Hospital*	Operations Research	1950	Psychiatry
Robert White	*Lives in Progress*	Case study	1952	Personality
Jules Henry	*Pathways to Madness*	Field observation	1965	Family Casework
Rene A. Spitz	*The First Year of Life: A Psychoanalytic Study of Normal and Deviant Development of Object Relations*	Developmental observation	1965	Child Psychiatry
Joseph Church	*Three Babies: Biographies of Cognitive Development*	Case study	1966	Cognition
Oscar Lewis	*La Vida*	Field observation	1966	Cultural Anthropology
Bruno Bettelheim	*The Empty Fortress*	Case study	1967	Child Psychiatry
Robert Coles	*Children of Crisis*	Field observation	1967	Social Psychiatry
Eric Berman	*Scapegoat*	Field observation	1973	Family Casework
Mary Ainsworth et al.	*Patterns of Attachment*	Clinical observation	1978	Social Psychology
Jack Fadely and Virginia Hosier	*Case Studies in Left and Right Hemispheric Functioning*	Case study	1983	Perception
Stephen Marks	*Three Corners: Exploring Marriage and the Self*	Case Study	1986	Family Relationships

tions in controlling for the individual differences among subjects. The case study approach allows the investigator the freedom to search for individual factors that could easily be overlooked in a correlational study, but on closer investigation prove to be a critical variable in the onset of an illness. The flexibility of a case study and the creativity afforded to the researcher compensate for the apparent lack of external validity, or the ability to generalize to a representative population.

Table 3-11   *Applying Clinical Observation Methods to Allied Health, Rehabilitation, and Special Education*

Methods	Purposes	Procedures for Collecting Data	Application to Fields
Individual case study	Understanding of underlying dynamics of illness	• interviewing • testing • examination of personal documents • case research	Investigation of • health problems • chronic diseases • individual factors
Developmental observation	Description of the sequential, hierarchical processes in human development	• objective observation in a controlled setting • mechanical audiovisual recordings	• Examination of normal and abnormal patterns in development
Field observations (ethnography)	Examination of the interaction between members of a social group, educational group, or family	• naturalistic observation • process recordings of interactions • unobtrusive measurement	Description of group interaction in: • dysfunctional families • half–way houses • residential treatment program (RTC's) • educational classrooms • socioeconomic units
Operations research	Analysis of administrative administrative problems in organization systems	• flow charts of organizational structure • job descriptions • communication patterns • decision–making process	Examination of interrelationships between systems • political • economic • health care • educational

The general outline of case study research is similar to all aspects of research in that the researcher justifies the need for investigation, reviews previous literature, states guiding questions for data collection, and objectively obtains data. In contrast to experimental and correlational research, in the case study the researcher does not state a statistical hypothesis or collect group data from a representative sample of a population. The general format of a case study follows.

Need for the Study

In this section the investigator explores the multiple effects of a health problem, its incidence within a population, and its relationship to the health professions. The investigator should discuss also the appropriateness of using a case study model in contrast to an experimental or correlational design. If a case study is used as a pilot study or preliminary study, such as to collect data about a problem before undertaking a larger study, then it should be so stated. However, a case study should not be used in place of an experimental or correlational study. For example, a case study is more appropriate than experimental or correlational methods in an in-depth study of a complex chronic disability. The investigator should also consider the indirect effects of a health problem, such as economic loss to society due to the inability of the patient with disabilities to work and the emotional and family turmoil that accompany chronic disability. The number and percentage of a population affected by a health problem should be documented. What statistics are available regarding mortality rates, hospitalization admissions, and physician visits? What evaluation tests and treatment methods are provided by allied health professionals at present and what is the potential of generating therapeutic techniques? These questions are pertinent in demonstrating the need for a study. The investigator should also discuss in this section what the possible implications of the results from a case study could provide. Investigations into the dynamic factors affecting the onset of arthritis, schizophrenia, delinquency, stuttering, dementia, and attention deficit-hyperactivity disorder are particularly appropriate for case study research.

Review of Literature

The investigator should do an extensive review of the literature on the disability examined in the case study. Research related to etiology and treatment is particularly important in a case study. The literature review should provide the investigator with a general overview of the current state of knowledge. Research journals, textbooks, and conference proceedings should be reviewed. (For a more detailed discussion on reviewing literature see Chapter 5.) The investigator should be guided by an outline in deciding what aspects of the disability to include and the extensiveness of the review.

The literature review should include also an examination of case study methods for collecting data, such as interviewing, reliability of case records, medical history recording and psychological testing. These areas are especially important to the investigator who is unfamiliar with the case study methods.

Research Methodology

In this section variables are operationally defined, a screening criteria for subject selection is delineated, a procedure for interviewing and testing subjects is stated, test instruments are identified, and reliability and validity data are reported. A screening criteria should be based on a rationale considering representative statistical data for a target population. For example, if an investigator is interested in doing a case study of a youth who is delinquent, he or she would consider sex, age when most delinquency occurs, socioeconomic group factors, school status, cognitive level, family, and delinquent acts committed. The variables identified should be obtained from a review of the literature, statistical abstracts, and clinical observations. From these sources the researcher operationalizes the screening criteria as outlined in Table 3–12.

The investigator should also consider exclusional criteria, that is, factors that should not be present in the subject. These could include the absence of brain damage, mental illness, or language difficulty or language difference. After the researcher has decided upon inclusional and exclusional criteria the next task is to plan a procedure for selecting subjects. This entails contacting a juvenile facility, court, or agency working with delinquent youth. The cooperation of the agency is crucial to the research. The participant and the parent or guardian must be told of the purposes of the study through informed consent. The plan for collecting data is another important part of the research methodology. This includes the following questions:

- At what setting will the study take place?

Table 3-12 *Example of Screening Criteria (Youth who Are Delinquent)*

Age:	16-year-old
Gender:	Male
Socioeconomic factor:	Working-class family
Intelligence:	Average nonverbal I.Q.
Family:	Dysfunctional, nonintact, due to divorce, separation, or parent desertion
School Status:	Special education setting
Geographic Area:	Urban
Behavior:	Delinquent, with vandalism, truancy, and deviant behavior that results in adjudication, probation, or referral to residential treatment setting

- What psychological tests, evaluation instruments, questionnaires, and interview schedules will be employed?
- During what period of time will the study take place (e.g., hours of day, school time or evening, time of year)?

Results

The data gathered for a case study include the subject's history, results of testing and collateral information from case records, interviews with family members, and clinical reports obtained from health personnel. Difficulties can arise in a case study that threaten the researcher's objectivity. Robert White (1952) in his classical study *Lives in Progress* felt "It is impossible to study another person without making evaluations, and it is hard to keep the evaluations from being seriously distorted by one's personal reactions to the subject" (p. 99). This limitation of a case study must be controlled by the investigator. One way to control for investigator bias is to have more than one independent history taken of the same subject. In this way investigator bias can be isolated. Another method is to make the investigators aware of their own rigidities, assumptions, and prejudices ". . . through increased familiarity with their own personalities" (p. 100).

Most investigators, in reporting a case study, use a chronological outline starting from the subject's early childhood to current state. A topical biography is another way to organize data. For example, in a case study of a subject with arthritis, the investigator may want to report data under subject headings, such as possible etiological factors (joint injuries, allergies, emotional disturbances, endocrine disorders) or treatment intervention (occupational therapy, physical therapy, chemotherapy, and psychologic counseling). An interpretive summary and recommendation for further research follow the reporting of results.

In short, case study research is a viable method for obtaining objective data pertaining to the life of an individual with disabilities. It is an idiographic approach to research that considers the individual differences in etiology of disease and specific adaptations in coping with a disability.

Example of Case Study (Qualitative Research)

1. **Bibliographical Notation**

   Stein, F., & Nikolic, S. (1989). Teaching stress management techniques to a schizo-phrenic patient. *The American Journal of Occupational Therapy, 43*, 162–169.

2. **Abstract**

   The authors wrote the following abstract:

   This paper describes a stress management training program used with a 26 [sic]-year old schizophrenic man attending an outpatient day care program. In a seven-session program, the patient was taught to use various techniques in muscle relaxation and biofeedback to decrease anxiety and to cope with stress. The patient's improvement on 7 of the 20 items of the State-Trait Anxiety Inventory demonstrated the effectiveness of even a short-term stress management program. (p. 162)

3. **Justification and Need for Study**

   The authors cited evidence for a biological basis for schizophrenia related to elevated dopamine levels. As dopamine increases, the occurrence of schizophrenic episodes increase. Initial research has suggested that some schizophrenics can be taught ways to cope with psychosocial stressors. If this is possible, then the number of schizophrenic episodes might be reduced. The purpose of this study was to "teach stress management techniques to a schizophrenic man to help him reduce his anxiety level." (p. 163)

4. **Literature Review**

   Twenty-five references were cited in the study. Articles came from a wide variety of journals, such as *Journal of Consulting and Clinical Psychology, British Journal of Psychiatry, Perceptual and Motor Skills, Journal of Nervous and Mental Disease, Occupational Therapy in Mental Health, and Mental Health Special Interest Section Newsletter.* The majority of articles cited were published during the 1970s and 1980s.

5. **Research Hypothesis or Guiding Questions**

   The guiding question explicitly stated was "Can anxiety in schizophrenic patients be reduced through stress management training?" (p. 162)

6. **Methodology**

   The client was a 27-year-old single man who had been diagnosed with undifferentiated schizophrenia. His first hospitalization had been at age 19, and repeated hospitalization had occurred from that time. He was on neuroleptics and received occupational therapy for "poor grooming, inappropriate socializations, conflict with sexual identity, and impaired thought processes" (p. 163). "The patient agreed to stress management training because he had experienced intense levels of stress in the past and wanted to learn to deal with stress more effectively" (p. 163).

   Anxiety was measured through the S-scale on the State-Trait Anxiety Inventory (STAI; Spielberger, 1983). Qualitative measurements of coping behavior were measured through the Stress Management Questionnaire (SMQ; Stein, 1987). The program was carried out in six 1-hour weekly sessions using "practical stress management techniques that could be generalized to everyday living" (p. 165). The STAI was used as a pre- and posttest during all sessions except the first one. The patient was asked to complete the SMQ and use techniques learned during the sessions during the week. "A follow-up session to administer the SMQ and attain therapeutic closure was held 2 weeks after the sixth session" (p. 166).

   A one-sample *t* test was used to compare pre- and posttest scores on the STAI. The nonparametric sign test was used to examine changes in scores on the STAI over five sessions. The level of statistical significance for both statistical analyses was chosen at $p < .05$. Qualitative analysis of the SMQ was obtained regarding symptoms experienced, stressors, and activities to reduce stress.

7. **Results**

    Significant changes in anxiety were noted over the sessions. The patient's mean posttest score on the STAI was statistically significantly lower than his pretest score. In addition, he "significantly reduced his anxiety on 9 of the 20 items [on the STAI] during the course of the study" (p. 166). Finally, changes in symptoms, stressors, and ways to reduce stressors changed over time.

    > In summary, on the pretest [for the SMQ] during Session 1, the patient's primary symptom of stress was talking excessively, his primary stressor was being watched by others, and his primary activity to relieve stress was walking. In the follow-up Session 7, the patient's primary stress symptom was chest pains, his primary stressor was doing new things for the first time, and his stress-relieving activity was listening to music. (p. 167)

    Two years after this study, the first author informally followed up on the patient's whereabouts and functioning. At that time, the patient had had no relapse and was maintaining successfully in the community.

8. **Conclusions**

    Stein and Nicolic concluded the following:

    1. A short-term stress management program using a combination of biofeedback and relaxation techniques can be used successfully with some individuals with schizophrenia.
    2. The role of occupational therapists in a psychiatric setting can be enhanced by having them teach tress management techniques to individuals with schizophrenia.

9. **Limitations of the Study**

    Since this was a case study, further research must be done if the findings are to be generalized to a larger population of individuals with schizophrenia.

10. **Major References Cited in the Study**

    Benson, H. (1975). *The relaxation response*. New York: William Morrow.

    Acost, F., Yamamoto, J., & Wilcox, S. (1978). Application of electromyographic biofeedback to the relaxation training of schizophrenic, neurotic, and tension headache patients. *Journal of Consulting and Clinical Psychology, 46*, 383–384.

    Hawkins, R., Doell, S. & Lindseth, P. (1980). Anxiety reduction in hospitalized schizophrenics through thermal biofeedback and relaxation training. *Perceptual and Motor Skills, 51*, 475–582.

    Stein, F. (1987). *Stress management questionnaire*. Unpublished manuscript, University of Wisconsin-Milwaukee.

Operations Research

Ackoff and Rivett (1963) describe the three essential characteristics of operations research: "(1) systems orientation, (2) the use of interdisciplinary teams, and (3) the adaptation of scientific method" (p. 10). Operations research was developed in Great Britain during the Second World War mainly for the purpose of using radar effectively in combatting German air attacks (Crowther & Whiddington, 1948). Subsequently during the 1950s large corporations employed operations research teams to analyze production methods as a way of increasing efficiency. Norbert Weiner's (1948) contribution in cybernetics and the application of the feedback principle expanded systems theory to biological, sociological, and psychological dimensions. Using the technology of cybernetics, the methodology of operations research, and systems theory, researchers have examined the physiology of respiration (Pribran, 1958), equipment design, and human engineering (United States Department of Defence, Joint Services Steering Committee, 1963), political life (Easton, 1961), and the city as a system (Blumberg, 1972).

Efficiency in industrial production has been one of the areas where operations research has been widely applied. The goal of the efficiency expert in a factory is to minimize expenditures and maximize production. By analyzing the industrial system of production the operations researcher can determine where costs can be reduced and production increased. Factors such as competitive costs of raw materials and plant machinery, redeployment of labor, employee morale, and distribution of goods are all considered in operations research. Essentially, operations research analyzes a system by identifying all those factors that affect input or raw materials, and output or finished product. The feedback in this system represents the critical analysis of input and output and the resultant changes in the total system of production.

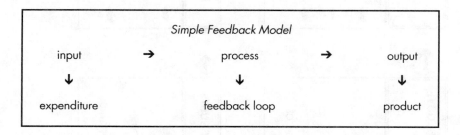

The concept of operations research and systems theory can also be applied to research problems in health care. For example, hospital management provides an excellent area for operations research. For hospital administrators, the problems of expanding costs and depersonalized care for inpatients have become increasingly more aggravated during the last two decades. While society seeks improved expanded health care for larger portions of the population, hospitals have to find more efficient methods to service more clients and to provide them with sophisticated diagnostic methods for detecting and treating illnesses with the most advanced technology. Specifically, these problems include (a) architectural design, (b) medical equipment, (c) hospital staffing, including availability of consultants, (d) cost sharing for using expensive machinery such as for kidney dialysis, and (e) any other problems "concerned with the design, improvement and installation of integrated system of men, materials and equipment" (Rushmer, 1972, p. 101). Operations research as applied to the fields of allied health and rehabilitation uses observational data and systems analysis to solve identification problems. Health problems appropriate for operations research include the following:

- The lack of health care workers in rural areas
- Depersonalization of patients in custodial institutions
- Inadequate funding for chronic disabilities
- Underutilization of general hospitals in rural areas
- Recurrence of chronic illness
- Inefficient emergency care in urban hospitals.

In all the foregoing problems, the underlying assumption is that a system, a unified interconnected whole, exists. The systems researcher analyzes the specific components of the system and their interrelationships. In these examples the systems are identified as rural health, custodial institution, legislation process, general hospitals, chronic illness, and emergency care. The process of operations research is outlined in Figure 3–20.

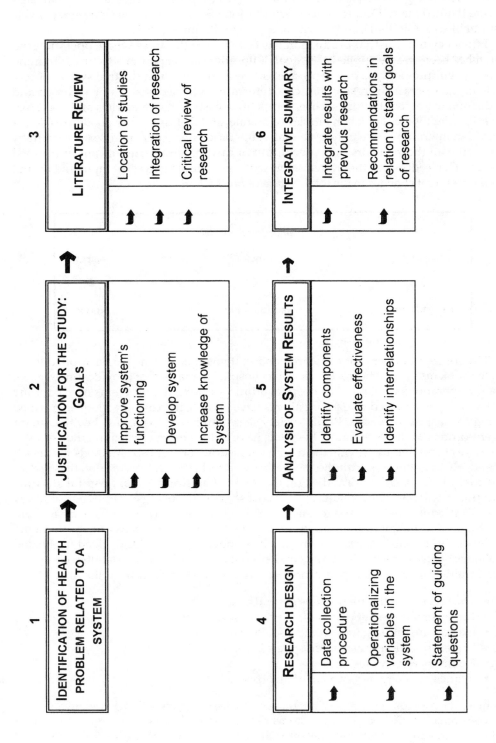

Figure 3-20. The process of operations research.

Developmental Observations

"Experimental observation, with conditions so clearly defined that they can be duplicated and so delimited that only a single variable remains for study is, scientifically, a goal to work toward" (Gesell, 1928, p. 23). This description stated over three-quarters of a century ago remains the hallmark of research on child development. Developmental observation research is concerned with the rigorous, controlled investigations into the process, stages, and hierarchial steps in human development. How does speech develop? What are the sequential stages in the areas of language, ambulation, social relationships, cognition, and reading? These and other questions are examples of research problems that lend themselves best to developmental observation methods. The investigator seeks to identify the processes involved in development, the approximate ages when landmarks are reached, and the forces in the child, such as genetic and environmental that shape development.

A key assumption in developmental research is that human behavior unfolds at critical stages. For example, in Table 3–13 some examples of approximate ages are given for achieving a developmental landmark in language. The typical child is expected to pass a test item related to chronological age. The child's rate of development is relative to the norm response for specific chronological age groups. The basic assumption in the DDST-R test is that human development progresses in a linear direction originating from genetic forces. In this model the child is ready at specific ages to learn to walk, play games cooperatively with other children, write, speak, or perform any number of other developmental tasks. Environmental experiences provide the opportunities for development to occur.

Stating the Guiding Question

The first task of the researcher is to state a research question that generates data. Piaget (1926) in the first sentence of his book *The Language and Thought of the Child* states: "The question which we shall attempt to answer in this book may be stated as follows: What are the needs which a child tends to satisfy when he talks?" (p. 1). Gesell and Thompson (1923) in their research on infant behavior also began with a guiding question: "When does this orthogenetic patterning of the human individual begin?" (p. 9).

Table 3–13 *Denver Developmental Screening Test—Revised*[a]

Developmental Skills	Hierarchial Sequential Activities from Birth to 6 Years
Gross–Motor:	Lifts head at 2 months to walks backward (heel to toe) at 6 years.
Fine–Motor:	Visually tracks objects to midline at 2 months to draws a man with six distinct parts at 6 years.
Language:	Responds to bell at 2 months to defines six words at 6 years.
Personal–Social:	Regards face at 2 months to dresses without supervision at 5 years.

[a]*Note*. From normative data, age levels were established as to when children develop individual skills. Normal limits (upper and lower) were validated for each hierarchical activity.

Note: Adapted from *The Denver Developmental Screening Test–II* (DDST–II) by W. R. Frankenburg, J. B. Dodds, P. Archur, H. Shapiro, & B. Bresnick (1990), Denver: Denver Developmental Materials.

The potential areas for research using developmental observation are considerable. An outline of the broad areas of development and specific research questions, listed in Table 3–14, demonstrates the wide perspective in doing developmental research.

These questions listed in Table 3–14 represent only a fraction of the potential research appropriate for developmental observation. The area of development selected by a researcher and the research questions generated provide the engine for the study. The research process is to justify the need for the study.

Need for Study in Developmental Observation

For the allied health practitioner and special educator, developmental research provides the data for evaluating patients. Is this patient functioning within normal limits? In order to answer this question, data regarding normal development are needed. Developmental studies therefore provide "yardsticks" for interpreting a patient's level of development. As well as providing valuable data for the therapist evaluating a patient, developmental data can be used in constructing sequential treatment programs. In children with developmental disabilities, such as cerebral palsy, mental retardation, childhood autism, and severe social deprivation, data from developmental observations are used by therapists to program treatment. The rationale behind this approach is that development progresses sequentially in the typical child, but is delayed, incomplete, or impaired in the child with a developmental disability. The developmental therapist reconstructs the sequential stages in an area of development and treats the child by facilitating progress through each stage. Steps along a linear developmental progression are programmed for the individual child starting at his or her base level of performance.

The results of developmental observation research have a direct effect on evaluating and treating children with developmental disabilities. After delineating the need for the study the researcher designs an observational method for collecting data.

Observational Methods for Collecting Data

The technique of observation of infant behavior is not a subject that lends itself to free and easy generalization. Nor does the question, what is the best technique, permit a simple answer. Observation methods must vary considerably with the age of the infant and, of course, with the objectives in view. (Gesell, 1928, p. 23)

Table 3–14 *Suggested Areas for Research Questions*

Areas of Development	Examples of Research Questions
Social	What are the sequential stages that lead to cooperative play in children?
Emotional	What are the origins of anxiety?
Cognitive	What types of logic are used by 3-year-old children?
Language	What is the most favorable age for learning a second language?
Academic	What cognitive processes are related to reading?
Moral	What factors facilitate moral learning in 8-year-old children?
Motor	What are the sequential stages of development in eye–hand coordination?
Feeding	What is the relationship between obesity in infancy and obesity in adolescence?

The observational method selected by the developmental researcher should provide objective descriptive data that are representative of the child's repertoire of behavior. This is accomplished by providing the child with a stimulus that will elicit the desired behavior. Schematically this is represented in Figure 3–21.

The stimulus is selected after the researcher operationally defines the area of development in terms of the behavioral response. Tests for assessing a child's level of development such as the McCarthy Scales of Children's Abilities (McCarthy, 1972) and the Miller Assessment for Preschoolers (MAP; Miller, 1988) are examples of this method. In the McCarthy Scales, motor ability is operationally defined by the following tests:

Developmental Factor	Operational Definition
Leg Coordination	Child performs motor tasks that involve the lower extremities, such as walking backwards or standing on one foot.
Imitative Action	Child copies simple movements, such as folding one's hands or looking through a tube

Questions arise in this context. How does the researcher know that:

* All aspects of a developmental factor are being measured?
* The operational definition of a developmental factor is valid?

These questions are pertinent in developmental research, and they demand a rationale from the investigator.

In reporting developmental data, the researcher should describe factors in the child that affect the results. These factors include sex, age, intelligence, education, and experiences. The selection and control of these factors by inclusion in the research eliminates ambiguity in interpreting the results.

As well as operationally defining the developmental factors and controlling for variables within the child, the researcher must construct an objective environment for col-

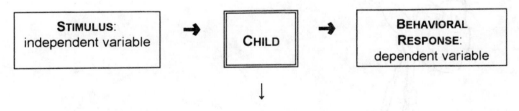

Figure 3–21. Schematic representation of observational research. Notice that the subject is provided with a stimuli in order to elicit a particular response. The data collected is the behavior elicited by the stimulus.

lecting valid data. The basic experimental environment in developmental research is shown in Figures 3–22 and 3–23.

This arrangement for observation is a standard procedure. Adaptations in this method include the use of a photographic dome as developed by Gesell (1928) or the use of experimental rooms with one-way mirrors, where the observer is not seen by the subject.

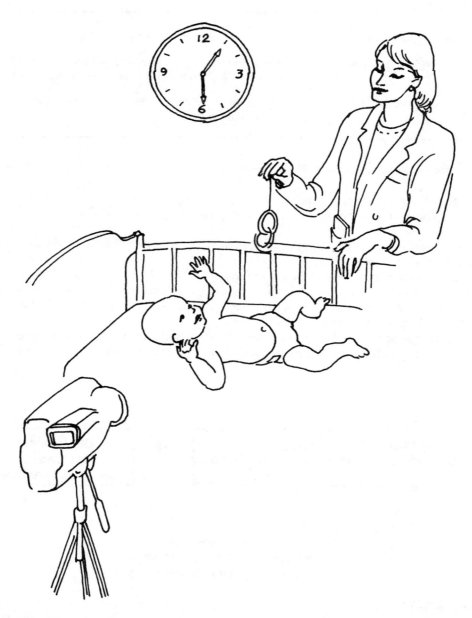

Figure 3–22.   Position of the camera and baby when taking observational data.

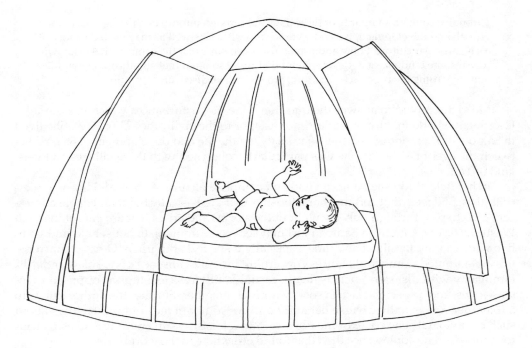

Figure 3–23. Illustration of a photographic dome, used in observational research.

Longitudinal Research (Prospective Designs)

Are there developmental factors over a period of time that cause changes in a person's anatomical and physiological processe, predisposing him or her to illness? Does prolonged exposure to smog cause lung cancer? Do obese adults develop heart disease when they are middle-aged at a higher rate than nonobese adults? Do children who have high IQs become leaders in the society when they are adults? What is the prognosis for high-risk children who come from socially disadvantaged environments? What is the relationship between occupational hazards and the later onset of disease? These problems are all affected by time factors. Longitudinal research is a method used in observing the effects of independent variables on dependent variables over a determined period of time. The investigator uses longitudinal research to predict an outcome based on the presence of causative factors. For example, a team of researchers may study groups of individuals over a period of 20 years from young adult to middle age and observe whether certain groups are more vulnerable to heart attacks than other groups.

Field Observation (Ethnography)— Qualitative Research

About the same time that Gesell was experimenting with his photographic dome, cultural anthropology developed scientific methods for collecting data describing the everyday lives of primitive people. Franz Boas, the noted anthropologist, wrote in the foreword to Margaret Mead's classical study *Coming of Age in Samoa* (1928) the following, which summarizes field research:

Through a comparative study of these data and through information that tells us of their growth and development, we endeavor to reconstruct, as well as may be, the history of each particular culture. Some anthropologists even hope that the comparative study will reveal some tendencies of development that recur so often that significant generalizations regarding the processes of cultural growth will be discovered. (p. xiii)

Mead attempted to answer the question "Are the disturbances which vex our adolescents due to the nature of adolescence itself or to the civilization?" (p. 6–7). She lived in Samoa for six months, and there she analyzed the life and development of 68 girls between the ages of 8 and 20. She was particularly concerned with three villages on the island of Tau.

In her field study she paints a vivid and complete picture of the island life of adolescent girls. She feels that certain characteristics that are basically Samoan enable adolescent girls to pass through puberty without the storms and crises that are part of living in Western society. Chiefly, a Samoan girl may leave her immediate household and go to live with another family at any time, especially if she feels put upon. Other characteristics are a limited number of choices concerning life roles, absence of double standards, familiarity with disasters such as death, casual family relationships as opposed to intense ones, and a specific place in society for each member. Further, the author points to a tolerance for sexually diverse behavior and concomitant lack of guilt feelings about such behavior, absence of extreme poverty, and a less stressful environment as reasons for a more serene adolescence than that found elsewhere in the world.

Mead's pioneering research lead to the field of ethnography: to reconstruct accurately a particular culture and to search for patterns that can be generalized to a specific population. The observations occur in a natural setting, such as in a primitive village, urban neighborhood, family home, playground, street corner, Israeli kibbutz, or mental hospital. Examples of field studies are Stanton and Schwartz's (1954) analysis of the interactional communication patterns among staff members in a mental hospital, Bruno Bettleheim's (1969) investigation of the child-rearing patterns among families living in an Israeli kibbutz, and Oscar Lewis' (1965) study of a Puerto Rican family coping with slum life in New York City. (See also Hall, 1966.)

Jules Henry's (1971) in-depth study of five families where a child with psychosis is present is a bleak and brilliant example of field observation. He proposes that the main difference between "them and us" is "that they [families with a child with psychosis] seem to go to extremes and do too many things that are upsetting" (p. xx). Henry details communication patterns, physical interaction, and positions of power in each of the five families. He faithfully records the emotional content of the parents' attempts at communication and their effects on the children in these families. In order to record accurately, he lived with four of the five families for a short time and relied on a trained observer to supply similar observations about the fifth family.

The five studies involved field visits to each family once a week. Rapport was established when the investigator informed each family that this kind of observation would perhaps aid other children with psychosis. He maintained confidentiality in the study by altering some of the details of family life and all of the names of the families.

The Application of Field Observation (Ethnography) to Allied Health and Rehabilitation

What research problems are appropriate to field observations? Research involving the culture of the individuals with disabilities living in specialized environments such as half-way houses, psychiatric hospitals, communities for individuals with physical disabilities, and residential institutions for the individuals with profound mental retardation are potential areas of investigation. In the field study the investigator structures observations to examine the social interactions among patients and between patients and staff. The investigator must be as unobtrusive as possible in the environment so that one's presence does not affect the behavior of those being observed. The major advantage of the field observation is that data obtained from this method are not affected by artificial laboratory conditions. Another advantage is that the investigator observes behavior directly rather than eliciting verbal responses, such as through group personality tests. A third advantage is that the observer, who is not a part of the culture and who is objective, is able to recognize patterns and behaviors that are not easily recognized by those within the culture.

A study entitled *Clinical Observation of Ghetto Four-Year-Olds: Organizational, Involvement, Interpersonal Responsiveness and Psychosexual Content of Play* by Borowitz, Costello, and Hirsch, (1971) is a good example of field observation methodology. In this study, children were observed while playing in semistructured settings. The play sessions were filmed on 16 mm silent movie film while being tape-recorded simultaneously. The data were analyzed later by independent raters using play behavior scales developed by the authors.

Purposes of Field Observation

The main purpose of field observation or ethnography is to describe accurately the social structure of a group. The investigator observes the interactions between members of a group, records their responses, describes their formal codes for communications, and analyzes the structure that shapes their behavior (Frederick, 1928; Mead, 1928).

Which research method would be appropriate for examining the interactions in a residential school for individuals with profound retardation? It is not possible to construct experimental conditions or control for all of the possible variables that could affect the dependent variable, which is, in this example, the rate of development in the child who is profoundly retarded. The only valid method is to observe, like an ethnographer in a natural setting, the transactions between people in an institution.

Method of Field Observation

The investigator using field observation research is guided by research questions that focus on the important issues in a social structure such as education, vocational preparation, child-rearing practices, sexual expression, ethical standards, peer relationships, leisure patterns, and recreation. Broad areas selected for field observation are decided before the investigator collects data. The preparation for field observation is detailed in the Research Design section. Here the investigator decides:

- The total time period for field observation
- The methods used in establishing rapport with the group
- The broad areas in a social structure to be investigated
- The observational recording devices to be used
- Methods for preserving the confidentiality of group and obtaining informed consent
- Test instructions for collecting data (e.g., rating scales, questionnaires, and attitude surveys).

3.7 Survey Research

Definition of Survey Research

Survey research, as defined in this text, is the descriptive study of populations. The main purpose of survey research is to obtain accurate objective descriptions about a specific universe of people or entities, such as a group of individuals with disabilities, or the curriculum requirements in audiology. The major task of the survey researcher is to obtain reliable and valid data from a representative sample of a population. In some cases the researcher will be able to survey the total population or universe without relying on a representative sample.

Purposes of Survey Research

Health, social, and educational planners use descriptive survey research as the basis for developing health strategies, programs, and physical plants. The changing needs of populations as derived from needs assessments can contribute to the planning of health centers, special residential schools for individuals with disabilities, allied health training programs, welfare centers, mental health clinics, and day care centers for senior citizens. Survey research should play an essential part in assessing the needs of a population where the planning of services is involved. Where poor planning exists, such as in hospitals that have a high percentage of empty beds or health clinics that are under- or overutilized, one could expect that survey research was not used in assessing the needs of the potential population to be serviced.

Along with community planning, survey research is an important tool for learning about the general attitudes of people. Many studies are sponsored by governmental agencies and legislators to solicit general opinion on topics such as national health insurance, malpractice in health, legalization of abortion, ethics in research, and other controversial issues where majority opinion is used to formulate national policy and to guide the enactments of laws.

Survey research need not be limited to questioning individuals. Methodologies in survey research assessing the physical characteristics of groups are also applicable. Recently, governmental grants in health research have funded studies that screen a population for the presence of a disability. Children are surveyed for auditory and visual impairments. Diabetes tests, chest X-Rays to detect tuberculosis and lung cancer, cardiovascular screening utilizing blood cholesterol counts, blood pressure measurements, and testing for HIV are some of the examples of survey research utilizing physical measurements to screen for health defects in large populations. Public health agencies use survey research as a means of identifying trends in the incidence of diseases and health problems. The information comprising the survey data is obtained from physicians, hospitals, clinics, and other health agencies that compile disease statistics. Table 3–15 from the Morbidity and Mortality Weekly Report is an example of epidemiological statistics, that is, data showing cases of specified notifiable diseases in the United States.

Statement of Problem in Survey Research

The first step in survey research is to state the problem in question form. The problem should be researchable, requiring measurable data that can be collected and analyzed. In stating a problem in survey research the investigator must operationally define the population to be surveyed in terms of geographical area and demographic characteristics,

Table 3–15 *Summary Cases of Specified Notifiable Dise...*

Disease	
Acquired Immunodeficiency Syndrome	
Anthrax	
Botulism	
foodborne	
infant	5...
other	5
Brucellosis	86
Cholera	17
Congenital Rubella Syndrome	7
Diphtheria	N.A.
Encephalitis, postinfectious	150
Gonorrhea	379,397
Haemophilus influenzae (invasive disease)[b]	1,201
Hansen Disease	169
Leptospirosis	41
Lyme disease	7,540
Measles	
imported	56
indigenous	220
Plague	10
Poliomyelitis, paralytic[c]	N.A.
Psittacosis	50
Rabies, human	2
Syphilis, primary and secondary	25,117
Syphilis, congenital, age < 1 year[d]	1,493
Tetanus	40
Toxic shock syndrome	212
Trichinosis	15
Tuberculosis	21,199
Tularemia	120
Typhoid fever	332
Typhus fever, tickborne	445

[a]*Note.* Data taken from the *Morbidity and Mortality Weekly Report* (MMRW, 12/24/93, p. 974). Data are cumulative through the week ending December 18, 1993, (50th week).

[b]*Note.* Of 1147 cases of known age, 372 (32%) were reported among children less than 5 years of age.

[c]*Note.* Two cases of suspected poliomyelitis have been reported in 1993; 4 of the 5 suspected cases with onset in 1992 were confirmed; the confirmed cases were vaccine-associated.

[d]*Note.* Reports through second quarter of 1993.

such as age, sex, socioeconomic level, education, and marital status. The identified population must be rigorously defined; otherwise there can be confusion in the *external validity* or in generalizing the results from the representative sample to the larger population. This, of course, is not a problem when the total population is surveyed. The following are hypothetical questions related to survey research:

atus of clients who have been discharged
hey had been for a least 1 year?
ints of professional programs in rehabili-

dividuals with spinal cord injuries per-

teristics of individuals using community

dentary office workers?
ividuals with disabilities held by various

 JY

After identifying a researchable problem, the target population, and the variables to be measured in the sample, the investigator formulates the procedure for collecting data and the measuring instruments. Sampling procedures (discussed in more detail in Chapter 6, Research Design and Methodology) should be objective and unbiased and provide a true description of the population. Random sampling, where the investigator selects a sample out of the total population, is the best method to achieve an unbiased, representative sample. The *external validity* of the results are, of course, increased as the percentage of the population sampled increases. For example, a random sample of 50% of the population will be more accurate than a random sample of 30% of the population. Sampling *stratified samples* also increases the external validity. However, the determination of how large a sample to include in a survey is many times based on practical considerations such as the cost of the survey and the time allocated to the research project.

The principle methods for collecting data in survey research are the personal interview, mail survey, and telephone. Table 3–16 lists the relative merits of these three procedures.

Selection of Questionnaire

In selecting a measuring instrument for data collection, the survey researcher often finds him- or herself in the position of devising a self-made questionnaire. Whether the questionnaire is custom-designed for a study or has already been published, the researcher must account for the reliability and validity of the instrument. Before the investigator devises the instrument, a thorough search of published questionnaires should be undertaken. Buros' latest edition of *Tests in Print* and other compendiums of tests and questionnaires, as well as abstracting journals, are excellent sources for locating specific measuring instruments for study.

Surveys involving the measurement of physical variables in human research are also dependent on the reliability and validity of the instruments used. Procedures are employed for increasing the validity of a subject's response, such as taking three blood pressure readings or two different grip strength readings. Usually, the instruments used in collecting data are reliable and valid, such as the X-Ray, electrocardiogram, and blood typing; but sometimes, because of subject anxiety or variability due to external circumstances, one test result can cause inaccurate data. Figure 3–24 describes the sequential steps in undertaking survey research.

Table 3-16   *Relative Merits of Principal Survey Methods of Data Collection*

Personal Interview	Mail	Telephone
Advantages		
Most flexible means of obtaining data	Wider and more representative distribution of sample possible	Representative and wider distribution of sample possible
Identity of respondent known	No field staff	No field staff
Nonresponse generally very low	Cost per questionnaire relatively low	Cost per response relatively low
Distribution of sample controllable in all respects	People may be more frank on certain issues (e.g., sex)	Control over interviewer bias easier; supervisor present essentially at interview
	No interviewer bias; answsers in respondent's own words	Quick way of obtaining information
	Respondent can answer at leisure; has time to "think things over"	Nonresponse generally very low
	Certain segments of population more easily approachable	Call-backs simple and economical
Disadvantages		
Likely to be most expensive of all	Bias due to nonresponse often indeterminate	Interview period not likely to exceed 5 minutes
Problems of interviewer supervision and control	Control over questionnaire may be lost	Questions must be short and to the point; problems difficult to handle
Dangers of interviewer bias and cheating	Interpretation of omissions difficult	Certain types of questions cannot be used (e.g., thematic apperception)
	Cost per return may be high if nonresponse very large	Nontelephone owners as well as those without listed numbers cannot be reached
	Certain questions, such as extensive problems, cannot be asked	
	Only those interested in subject may reply	
	Not always clear who replies	
	Certain segments of population nonapproachable (e.g., those who can't read)	
	Likely to be slowest of all	

Note. Taken from *Research Methods in Economics and Business* by R. Ferber and P. J. Verdoorn, 1962, p. 210, The Macmillan Company. Copyright, 1962, The Macmillian Company. Reprinted with permission.

Constructing a Questionnaire in Survey Research

The questionnaire is the most commonly used and most frequently self-devised measuring instrument. Simply defined, a *questionnaire* is a standardized list of factual questions or elicited opinions. The purpose of a questionnaire is to obtain information directly from subjects so as to make generalizations to a larger population. The three components of a questionnaire are:

1. Content (e.g., demographic variables, personality characteristics, behavioral patterns, health history)
2. Form of question (e.g., forced-choice or open-ended)
3. Level of data collected (e.g., factual or attitudinal).

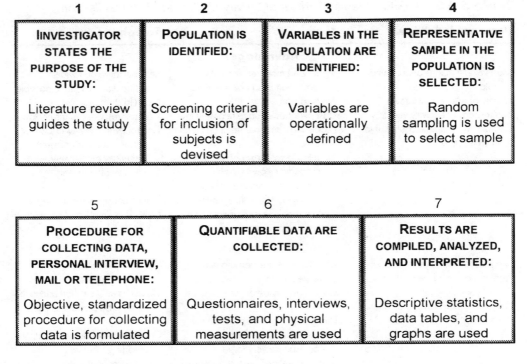

Figure 3–24.   Sequential steps in survey research.

The steps in creating a questionnaire are listed in Table 3–17.

Item Construction

In constructing items the researcher should be aware of the following:

- The choices available to the subjects should be exhaustive. On some items a place for "other, please specify" should be provided.
- The choices should be mutually exclusive.
- The items presented should be unambiguous and precise. A pilot study testing the reliability of items is essential.
- Items should ask only one question. Avoid double-barreled questions.
- The respondent should have enough information to answer the item.
- The researcher should have a rationale for each item asked. The questionnaire should not be padded with irrelevant items.
- Negative questions should be avoided.
- Leading questions that force a response should be omitted. The respondents should not be in a position to give expected answers or opinions. Examples of questionnaire items using various formats are described below:

1. *Likert-type scales* rate subjects by their agreement or disagreement with a statement on a scale usually of 1–5 or 1–7. For example, if an investigator is interested in surveying the attitudes of the general

Table 3-17   *An Example of the Steps in Creating a Questionnaire*

State research question
- What are the role functions of public school occupational therapists?

Carry out literature review
- Locate studies on public school occupational therapists (OT)

Identify key areas
- Description of school
- Student characteristics
- Major diagnoses treated by OT
- Treatment techniques employed by OT
- OT treatment goals
- Treatment modalities used in OT
- Outcome measures and quality assurance
- Description of OT personnel
- OT facilities and space

Devise survey format
- Forced-choice check off
- Ranking priorities
- Avoid open-ended questions
- Allow opportunity for comment

Expert evaluation
- Send questionnaire to three public school OTs asking them to evaluate each item and make suggestions for improvement
- Send questionnaire to research design expert

Revise questionnaire
- Base revisions on expert recommendations
- Questionnaire should not take longer than 10 to 15 minutes

Final draft
- Before mailing questionnaire, have local public school OT complete questionnaire
- Work out final "bugs" and consider aesthetics of format

public in respect to research on children, an item such as the following could be considered for inclusion in the study:

All experimental research with children is unethical.						
1	2	3	4	5	6	7
Disagree Very Strongly	Disagree Strongly	Disagree	No Opinion	Agree	Agree Strongly	Agree Very Strongly

2. *Multiple-choice questions* can be used to elicit opinions or attitudes. Suppose a researcher is interested in surveying a group of patients with post myocardial infarction on their attitudes toward their disability. The following multiple-choice question is one example:

If I had a severe pain in my chest I would first do the following:

1.   Call my private physician.
2.   Call an ambulance.
3.   Call the emergency rescue unit of the police.
4.   Lie down and rest.
5.   Other, please specify.

---

3.   *Rank order items* are used by researchers as a way of finding out priorities of choices. For example, a survey soliciting perceptions of treatment from former patients with psychiatric problems could include the following item:

From the list below of mental health workers rank in order the most important persons who helped you improve in the hospital. Start numbering with 1 as the person who helped you most; 2, the second most helpful person and so on:

Mental Health Worker	Rank
Attendant	_____
Nurse	_____
Occupational Therapist	_____
Psychiatrist	_____
Psychologist	_____
Social Worker	_____

Other: Please specify occupation:

4.   *Incomplete sentences* are used in questionnaires to measure informational level, personality traits, and attitudes. For example:

Children with mental retardation are different from normal children in . . .

---

5.   *Multiple adjective checklists* can be used to elicit effective perception such as in the following example:

Circle the appropriate adjectives:

In general older patients in nursing homes are:

independent	dependent	active
passive	happy	sad
sick	healthy	well nourished
poorly fed	supervised	neglected

---

6. *Open-ended questions* are used in the interviews when the researcher wants the subject to discuss a particular issue in detail. Examples of such questions are:

- What is your opinion of national health insurance?
- Do you think that adults with mental retardation should be allowed to marry?
- Should prisons be eliminated?

Depending on the ingenuity and creativeness of the researcher other types of questionnaire items can be constructed, such as true-false questions, analogies, and rating scales. As with constructing any test instrument, it is critical that the investigator check the reliability and validity of the questionnaire before collecting data.

Application of Survey Research to Allied Health

In the last 75 years the allied health professions have expanded their role from those of health providers and health maintainers to those of health planners and researchers. The future role of the allied health professions in the planning of regional health services and health programs in schools and the community, and in determining the costs of health care relates to the areas of research indicated in Figure 3–25.

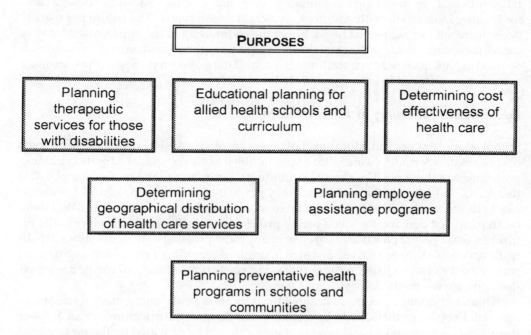

Figure 3–25.   Application of survey research to allied health.

Distribution of Health Care

One of the essential purposes of survey research is to guide the direction and planning of health services in a community. Health planners are continually faced with the need for hard data before they can recommend the construction of a health facility or hospital or the allocation of additional financial resources to a community health agency. Community health planning is therefore vitally linked to survey research. Legislators and developers who are persuaded by community pressures for new facilities need data to justify their positions. Survey research has taken on new importance in the current debate on whether the federal government should be responsible for the total health needs of the population. The data provided by survey research such as the distribution of health personnel, the proportion of hospital beds for a designated population, and the number of various services provided in defined health catchment areas can enable legislators to decide whether the present system of delivering health services is adequate for the country, or whether a national system for health care would meet the needs of the population more equitably. Survey research is not intended to provide data regarding the effectiveness of a health delivery system. Rather, this is the intent of evaluation research.

Planning Therapeutic Services

Community organization of health services is a good example of the applicability of survey research to the needs of a population. Questions such as What are the health needs of a community? and What are the health resources available? are areas that can be directly examined through survey research. Survey research in health is comparable to market research in advertising. In market research the individuals in a corporation collect data regarding the need for a product in the community and the community's attitude toward the introduction of new merchandise. Health planners have sometimes failed miserably in surveying a community before introducing a half-way house, a clinic for treating individuals with additions, or a child health center. The failure has usually been the result of unexpected resistance of the community to the apparent visibility of individuals with social or physical disabilities in a neighborhood. Survey research can be used to anticipate negative attitudes of a community or even to expose the unrealistic fears that are attached to individuals with disabilities.

Educational Planning in Allied Health

School administrators and educational planners are often asked by deans and presidents of colleges to determine the need for a specific allied health or special education training program. Are there positions in the community for occupational therapists, physical therapists, and special educators when they graduate from a new program? Do vacancies in these professions exist in hospitals and community clinics at present? Will there be an increased demand for allied health professionals and special educators in the future? In what geographical areas are the needs most pressing? These questions are directly accessible through survey research. Questions regarding level of training (i.e., associate, bachelors, graduate, postgraduate, and continuing education) can be answered through a survey methodology.

Other important concerns of health educators are course content, clinical reasoning, and skill knowledge that should be considered in designing curriculums. What areas of theoretical content, ability, and level of training should be provided by the professional educational program? In designing curriculums, health educators must be aware of the expectations of administrators. Have graduates of an allied health or special education program been adequately prepared to provide services needed by individuals with disabilities? On what basis does the educator determine the content of a training program? The need for continual feedback and interaction between educators and health administrators is necessary if there is going to be meaningful development of the professions. The educator must decide whether the education provided is directly related to the needs of the individual with disabilities or whether the education is general. If the education of the health professional is directed toward clinical practice and specialization, then educators must be responsive to the community's demands. Survey research can provide the technology to gather data from the community to answer many questions in educational planning.

Occupational Health Planning

There is an increasing need to investigate the prevention of occupational injuries; the relationship between mental health and job satisfaction; and the study of environmental conditions, such as noise, ventilation, chemical contamination, and radiation. The distribution of accidents and the statistical relationship between occupation and disease are related to the application of survey research to occupational health. Knowledge of activity patterns, nutritional needs, and protective equipment of workers can be provided by allied health professionals in consultation with industrial researchers. Occupational health planning should not be done in a vacuum. There are obvious needs for descriptive data regarding frequency of diseases or accidents and the attitudes of workers toward using ergonomic methods before preventive programs can be implemented.

Research in occupational health and education must also consider psychosocial factors, such as the relationships between personality and accident-proneness; the effects of boredom, low morale, and poor motivation on job satisfaction and mental health, and the effects of job modification factors on productivity and health.

Preventive Programs in Schools and Communities

For the child from a low income or socially disadvantaged family, school represents the greatest potential escape from a life of deprivation and misery. The school is one of the few institutions that can help the child overcome parental neglect or other disadvantages. It was not by happenstance that during the 1960s social reformers saw the need for Head Start programs, work-study curriculums, nutritional programs, and vocational education to be incorporated into schools geographically located in inner city slums and poor rural regions. Survey research has been used in the past as a means to justify the existence of new programs in the schools. However, there has been a backlash to the abuse of survey research in areas where data have been gathered and the needs of a community substantiated, without any program implementation. Community leaders are now suspicious of researchers who come into a neighborhood for the purpose of determining the need for services and promise to start new programs, only to leave without any follow-up.

Allied health professionals and special educators have much to contribute in the areas of nutrition, health education, career planning, recreation, and developmental screening in schools and community centers. Survey research can provide the data for planning these services. However, community support and follow-up are necessary if survey research is to have any impact on planning preventive programs.

Example of Survey Research

1. **Bibliographic Notation**

   Cartwright, L. R., & Ruscello, D. M. (1979). A survey on parent involvement practices in the speech clinic. *ASHA: A Journal of the American Speech and Hearing Association, 21*, 275–279.

2. **Abstract**

   This report summarized the results of a national survey on parent involvement that was sent to 198 clinics and training institutions throughout the United States and Canada. A questionnaire sought information relative to the existence of programs for parent involvement; components employed in existing programs; and the participation of graduate clinicians in training institutions with parent programs. Approximately 68% of the sample returned their questionnaires for analysis. A majority of the respondents felt parent involvement was an important supplemental service; however, only slightly more than half of the replies indicated that they had a formalized parent involvement program. Many of the remaining facilities did incorporate certain parent involvement components, even though a formalized program was not employed. In most cases where formal programs exist, the individual clinical supervisors exercise a large measure of control in the enactment of parent involvement activities. There are a number of training institutions that provide student clinicians with supervised practicum experiences and other related training in parent involvement.

3. **Justification and Need for Study**

   The investigators cited evidence for the increasing interest in parents assisting in the management of their children's speech and language problems. "This increased concern for parent involvement prompted us to study the scope of parent-related programs in clinics and graduate training institutions throughout the United States and Canada" (p. 275).

4. **Literature Review**

   Recent articles and papers from 1974 to 1978 primarily from the speech and hearing literature are cited by the investigators. The investigators conclude that "The preceding data suggest that the speech-language pathologist has recognized the importance of parent participation and actively sought this participation in a number of different ways" (p. 275).

5. **Research Hypotheses for Guiding Questions**

   Three specific questions were investigated:

   1. Are parent involvement programs employed in clinics and other training institutions?
   2. What are the primary components of existing parent involvement programs?
   3. What is the role of graduate students in training institutions with such programs?

6. **Methodology**

   The following questionnaire was sent to 1,998 clinics and student training institutions whose programs had been certified by the American Board of Examiners in Speech Pathology and Audiology (pp. 278–279).

   Parent Involvement Questionnaire

   1. a. Is an organized parent involvement program available in your facility?

      Yes   No

      b. Is the parent involvement program administered in a similar fashion among supervisors or clinicians?

Yes   No

   c.   Does each individual supervisor or clinician implement his/her own parent involvement program?

Yes   No

2. a.   Are parent conferences scheduled during the course of the semester?

Departmental Policy: Yes   No

Discretion of Individual Supervisor or Clinician: Yes   No

   b.   If yes, how often are conferences scheduled?

Daily_____   Weekly_____   Twice a Semester_____

Depends upon the individual supervisor or clinician._____.

3. a.   Do parents observe their children during therapy?

Departmental Policy: Yes   No

Discretion of Individual Supervisor or Clinician: Yes   No

   b.   If yes, how often during a semester do they observe?

Once_____   Twice_____   Four Times_____ More Often_____

Depends upon individual supervisor or clinician_____.

4. a.   Do parents receive verbal feedback regarding the child's progress on a regular basis?

Departmental Policy: Yes   No

Discretion of Individual Supervisor or Clinician: Yes   No

   b.   If yes, how frequently does the feedback occur?

Daily_____   Weekly_____   Twice a Semester_____

Depends upon individual supervisor or clinician_____.

5. a.   Do parents receive written feedback regarding the child's progress on a regular basis?

Departmental Policy: Yes   No

Discretion of Individual Supervisor or Clinician: Yes   No

   b.   If yes, how frequently does the feedback occur?

Daily_____   Weekly_____   Twice a Semester_____

Depends upon the individual supervisor or clinician_____.

6. a.   Do parents view videotapes of their children participating in therapy?

Departmental Policy: Yes   No

Discretion of Individual Supervisor or Clinician: Yes   No

   b.   If yes, how often are videotapes viewed?

Once a Semester_____   Twice a Semester_____   More Often_____

Depends upon the individual supervisor or clinician_____.

7. a.   Are pamphlets, books or other written materials available for use by the parents?

Departmental Policy: Yes   No

Discretion of Individual Supervisor or Clinician: Yes   No

   b.   If yes, which materials have been particularly beneficial for use with parents?

   c.   Are materials provided free of charge?   Yes   No

Discretion of Individual Supervisor or Clinician: Yes   No

8. a.   Are tapes and films available for use by parents?

Departmental Policy: Yes   No

Discretion of Individual Supervisor or Clinician: Yes   No

   b.   If yes, which materials have been particularly beneficial for use by parents?

9. a.   Are parent discussion groups a part of your clinical program?

Departmental Policy: Yes   No

Discretion of Individual Supervisor or Clinician: Yes   No

   b.   If yes, do you feel that most parents interact differently in group discussions?

Yes   No

10.   Are home practice activities assigned on a regular basis?

   a.   Departmental Policy: Yes   No

   b.   Discretion of Individual Supervisor or Clinician: Yes   No

11. a.   Is specific training offered to parents prior to administration of home programs?

Departmental Policy: Yes   No

Discretion of Individual Supervisor or Clinician: Yes   No

   b.   Are the parents required to demonstrate a proficiency with the task before the home program is administered?

Departmental Policy: Yes   No

Discretion of Individual Supervisor or Clinician: Yes   No

12. a.   Do student clinicians actively participate in the parent involvement program?

Departmental Policy: Yes   No

Discretion of Individual Supervisor or Clinician: Yes   No

   b.   If yes, does the student clinician have the major responsibility of parent contact (i.e., conferences, home programs, etc.)?   Yes   No

   c.   If yes, does the student clinician carry out these duties without direct supervision?

Departmental Policy: Yes   No

Discretion of Individual Supervisor or Clinician: Yes   No

   d.   Is the student required to register for a specific course that deals with parent interaction?

Departmental Policy: Yes   No

Discretion of Individual Supervisor or Clinician: Yes   No

e. If no, is the student required to participate in any informal training procedures regarding parent interaction?

Departmental Policy: Yes   No

Discretion of Individual Supervisor or Clinician: Yes   No

13. If you have any comments regarding parent involvement that would be beneficial in establishing our program, we would appreciate any input.

7. Analysis of Results

The following results excerpted from the study were based on a total of 115 replies (58%) of the population surveyed (198 clinics).

a. Nine percent ($N = 102$) indicated that their facilities considered parent involvement to be an essential part of clinical services.

b. Of the above 102 clinics, 51% had organized parent involvement programs.

c. Fifty-seven percent of the clinics specified that parent conferences were an integral part of the services provided.

d. In nearly 79% of the clinics parental observation of therapy is a clinical policy requirement.

e. Ninety-three percent of the respondents reported that verbal feedback in informing parents of their child's performance in training was part of a general policy.

f. Twenty-seven percent of the respondents reported that written feedback was a clinical policy.

g. Parent discussion groups were reported to be used in 54% of the total sample.

h. In 36% of the clinics the assignment of home practice with the parent is a policy of the facility.

i. Student participation in parent involvement programs is an established policy in 66% of the training institutions (total $N = 77$).

8. Conclusion of Study

"The results of the questionnaire certainly bespeak of the fact that parent involvement is an important consideration in the treatment of children with communication disorders" (p. 277).

9. Stated Limitations of the Study

a. It is not clear whether the sample of respondents represent the total population of clinics providing speech pathology and audiology services.

b. The geographical distribution of respondents was not included. The results could have been biased to certain areas in the United States or Canada.

c. The methodology in designing the questionnaire was omitted. Can we assume that the questionnaire is a reliable and valid instrument?

10. Major References in the Study

Baker, B. L. (1976). Parent involvement in programming for developmentally disabled children. In L. L. Lloyd (Ed.). *Communication assessment and intervention strategies* (pp. 691–733). Baltimore: University Park Press.

Bennen, L. M., & Henson, O. F. (1977). *Keeping in touch with parents: The teacher's best friend*. Austin: Learning Concepts.

Goodwin, W. M., Simmons, J. O., & Hall, M. K. (1977). *A sequential approach to parental involvement in children's treatment programs*. Paper presented at the Annual Convention of the American Speech and Hearing Association, November, 1977, Chicago, Illinois.

McDonald, J. D., Blott, J.P., Gordon, K., Spiegel, B., & Hartman, M. (1974). An experimental parent-assisted treatment program for preschool language-delayed children. *Journal of Speech and Hearing Disorders, 39*, 345–412.

Ruscello, D. M., & Cartwright, R. (1978). Active parent involvement in a university speech and hearing clinic. *Communique, 3*, 13–15.

Ruscello, D. M.,Cartwright, L. R., Sholtis, D., & Fitzpatrick, B. (1978). *Parent involvement in the speech clinic.* Paper presented at the Annual Convention of the American Speech and Hearing Association, November 1978, San Francisco, California.

Schumake, J., & Sherman, J. (1978). Parent's intervention agent. In R. L. Schiefelbusch (Ed). *Language intervention strategies* (pp. 239–315). Baltimore: University Park Press.

3.8 Historical Research

Definition and Comparison to Other Research Methods

Historical research is a method for reconstructing events that happened in the past. As applied to health care, historical research pertains to (a) the chronology of events in medicine, rehabilitation, health, and special education, (b) the interrelationship between these events, and (c) the critical factors influencing them. In studying historical data in health research, the investigator examines the individuals who were significant in shaping events and creating change, and the institutions or organizations that were part of the historical process. The scientific approach to collecting historical data is similar to all methods of research in that the investigator proposes a research problem, states guiding questions, collects data, interprets the results, and arrives at conclusions and implications. The main differences between historical research and other types of research models are in the format of guiding questions and in the use of related literature. In historical research the guiding questions serve as the generating rationale for collecting data and the literature review provides the data, whereas in experimental and correlational research the literature review generates hypotheses.

Format of Historical Research

The outline of historical research is as follows:

Part I   The statement of problem and the need for the study
Part II   Assumptions, guiding questions, procedures, and methods for collecting data
Part III   The results, the collection of data from primary and secondary sources
Part IV   A discussion of the results based on previous data from other studies
Part V   Conclusions, implications of results, and recommendations for further study.

Part 1: The Statement of the Problem

What are potential areas for historical research in allied health and special education? How does one determine its significance? These are issues of concern for the historical researcher or historiographer planning a study. Jacques Barzun (1974), in a discussion of psychohistory, states that the primary purpose of the new history is explanation, and the ulterior motive is action. He states, "The type of explanation sought is the scientific; that is, showing a connection ('durable link') between the facts and a definable cause. Classification, then analysis, then prediction is the sequence that leads naturally to action" (p.

60). Barzun suggests that the historiographer's main motive is to obtain evidence in support of a cause. In effect the historical researcher is a tool for change. This approach to medicine and health care can lead to research supporting causes that advocate change in the delivery of health care, public health education, the training and preparation of health professionals, and the training of special educators. The vulnerability of this approach is that the researcher could subjectively determine what evidence to cite. The historiographer should start with a relevant problem and objectively collect data.

Using the psychohistorical method in allied health research can generate the relationships outlined in Table 3–18 between the motive of the researcher and the problem investigated.

Part II: Assumptions, Guiding Questions, and Methodology

After narrowing the area of investigation to a researchable question, the researcher states any assumptions underlying the study. These assumptions are the researcher's preliminary opinions, attitudes, and knowledge in the area. For example, if a researcher is interested in what factors led to the development of the rehabilitation movement in the twentieth century, tentative assumptions could be proposed. These are:

- The rehabilitation movement developed in response to the health needs of the individual who is chronically disabled.
- The rehabilitation movement was facilitated by governmental legislation related to social security.
- The industrialized countries were first to educate specialized rehabilitation workers.
- The First and Second World Wars generated the need for developing a technology for restoring function in soldiers who were severely wounded.
- The first leaders in the rehabilitation movement were social reformers.

Continuing with the above examples, the researcher generates the following questions.

- What was the historical chronology of the rehabilitation movement?

Table 3–18 *Relationships Between Researcher's Motive and Investigated Problem*

Motive of Researcher	Statement of Problem
• Establishing the allied health professional as an independent practitioner	• How did the independent health practitioner emerge historically?
• The individual with mental retardation should be educated in community schools	• What factors led to the institutionalization of the individual with mental retardation from 1900 to 1950?
• Public health education should include medical knowledge	• What is the history of health education in public schools?
• Primary health care should be a right of every individual	• Historically, what is the relationship between the practice of health care and individual rights?

- How did social welfare programs influence rehabilitation legislation?
- How did advances in medical treatment influence rehabilitation of individuals who were chronically disabled?
- When did the allied health professions emerge and affect the rehabilitation movement?
- What scientific technology facilitated advances in rehabilitation medicine?
- Who are the leaders and supporters of the rehabilitation movement?

These guiding questions provide the content areas for the literature search and collection of data. The plan for collecting the data should be carefully formulated. The research plan is the outline of primary and secondary sources to be used in the data collection procedure. These sources include the following:

- Published books, periodicals, newspapers, and pamphlets
- Unpublished conference proceedings and minutes of meetings
- Official records and vital statistics
- Governmental documents, archives, and publications
- Personal letters, diaries, and memoirs
- Collateral interviews of eyewitnesses
- Tape recordings and films.

Part III: Data Collection

The essential task of the historiographer is to collect reliable and valid data. By obtaining various sources of information one is able to cross-check the data, thereby substantiating one's conclusions. Primary sources that represent "first hand" data, such as eyewitnesses and contemporary documents, are the best evidence for the historical researcher. In comparison, secondary sources are the interpretations and critiques of historical evidence. Primary sources are the raw data for historical research, whereas secondary sources serve as supportive evidence. In researching a problem the investigator should seek evidence that is direct, objective, and verifiable. It should be clear that one unit of datum is not conclusive. The "personal equation," which is the observer's effect on what is being observed and measured, must be controlled by the investigator's substantiating evidence from more than one primary source as eyewitness account.

Secondary sources such as encyclopedias, textbooks, and critical essays are useful in initially obtaining an overview of an historical problem. These sources represent the generally accepted versions of historical events that have been "retold" in a reductive manner. The critical historiographer need not accept any evidence until primary data can substantiate the facts.

Part IV: Discussion of Results and Part V: Conclusions and Recommendations

The raw data of an historical study must be critically analyzed by the investigator for its validity before any conclusions or generalizations can be made. The historiographer must examine every document and piece of evidence with a skeptical eye, seeking substantiating proof for the authorship and the accuracy of its contents. *External criticism* of a document is a testimony of its authenticity. The Hippocratic writings are an example of unknown authorship and unknown copyright date. It is important for the historical researcher to substantiate the author of every document, the date it was written, and the place it originated or where it was presented as evidence for external validity. Indirect means for collecting evidence are frequently used by historians. These methods include archeology and paleography (e.g., study of ancient manuscripts and examination of art objects). Ancient medical instruments used in surgery were discovered through archeological evidence.

The next step of the historical researcher is to establish the validity or truth contained in a document. This process is called *internal criticism*. The purpose of this process is to establish as near as possible the actuality of an event. How accurate was the observer? Are the interpretations and perceptions correct?

Historical surveys of medical progress are frequently filled with interpretative statements that go beyond the evidence and selective omissions that fail to give a true perspective of events or individuals who had an impact on treatment. It is left to the historical researcher in medicine to carefully evaluate the biases of the authors when interpreting evidence. Generalizations and synthesizing statements should be carefully documented. In examining the causes of medical events the historiographer takes a multidimensional point of view looking at the influences of contemporary practices of treatment, discoveries, patterns of disease, governmental intervention, war, and natural disasters. One variable rarely changes the course of history.

A good example of historical research is a scholarly manuscript by Saul Benison (1972), "The History of Polio Research in the United States: Appraisal and Lessons." In this article Benison documents the chronological events that led to a safe and effective vaccine for preventing polio. He analyzes the problem from three perspectives: (a) time of events, (b) settings where research took place, and (c) individuals and scientists who had an impact on the problem and facilitated progress in the development of a vaccine. These three factors are detailed in Table 3–19.

In documenting the chronology of events and the individuals who made important contributions to the development of a successful polio vaccine, Benison used the following primary sources:

- contemporary accounts of the early polio epidemics from 1894 to 1910
- autobiographical notes
- history of the Rockefeller Institute
- foreign journals
- scholarly articles by Flexner and associates
- conference proceedings
- research articles
- Bulletin of the History of Medicine
- National Foundation Archives
- history of Warm Springs
- private communication
- minutes of committees
- files from the National Foundation
- biographical essays
- final reports of research grants
- congressional hearings.

In total, Benison used 117 citations in documenting his article. It is interesting to note that he concludes that the development of a successful polio vaccine was a cooperative effort by researchers in major universities funded by two private organizations—The

Table 3-19   *History of Polio Research in the United States*

Time	Event	Setting	Contributors
1984	Polio epidemics identified in U.S.		
1907	Initial research in polio	Rockefeller Institute	Flexner
1910–1913	Poliovirus implicated	Rockefeller Institute	Flexner and associates
1920–1930	Transmission of polio	Rockefeller Institute	Olitsky, et al.
1938	Warm Springs Foundation	Georgia	Roosevelt, et al.
1938	Electron microscope	Germany	Borries
1946	Immunization of monkeys	Johns Hopkins	Morgan
1948–1951	Identification of poliovirus	U.C. Calif. Johns Hopkins U. of Pittsburgh	Kessel Bodian Salk
1949	Cultivation of poliovirus	Harvard	Enders, et al.
1952	Salk vaccine	U. Pittsburgh	Salk
1954	Mass vaccinations	U. Michigan	Francis
1958	Sabin vaccine	U. Cincinnati	Sabin

Note. Adapted from "The History of Polio Research in the United States: Appraisal and Lessons" by S. Benison, 1972, pp. 308–343.

Rockefeller Foundation and the National Foundation—with external support from the United States Public Health Service. Benison's "lesson" in the article is that modern medical progress is a cooperative effort where researchers from diverse settings are supported by the federal government, private foundations, and voluntary heath agencies.

The historical research article by Benison is an example of rigorous documentation providing strong external validity. Benison's article should serve as a model for research in allied health.

Potential areas for historical research in allied health are listed below:

- biography
- development of a technological innovation in allied health
- development of social attitude toward health (e.g., medical research, abortion)
- chronological analysis of the treatment of a disease
- history of a health profession
- history of a hospital, health facility, organization, or institution
- economic history of health care delivery
- history of movements in health (e.g., rehabilitation and normalization)
- interpretive analysis of history into stages, phases, cycles, and periods.

CHAPTER
4

The Research Problem

The great working hypotheses in the past have often originated in the minds of the pioneers as a result of mental processes which can best be described by such words as "inspired guess", "intuitive hunch", or "brilliant flash of imagination."—J. B. Conan, *Science and Common Sense* (p. 48)

••

Operational Learning Objectives

By the end of this chapter, the reader should be able to

1.   identify a feasible research topic in an area of clinical practice, administration, or education
2.   write a paragraph justifying the need for a research study
3.   identify a feasible research problem
4.   formulate relevant questions pertaining to a research problem
5.   identify possible psychological blocks in the investigator and flaws in research design that could potentially deter the research
6.   outline a general plan for data collection

••

4.1 The Need for Problem-Oriented Research in Allied Health and Special Education

During the last 50 years, health research in the United States has multiplied beyond the volume that could have been predicted a century earlier. One hundred years ago a medical scientist could easily have read most of the published research in a wide range of health specialties. A scholar in the sciences in the nineteenth century would also be familiar with the literary and artistic worlds. Today it is impossible. C. P. Snow (1964) in his discussion of the two worlds of science and humanities was one of the first to recognize the isolating effect of specialization in the twentieth century. Scientists and humanists now

133

live in two cultures, deprived of the sharing and communication that existed in the eighteenth and nineteenth centuries. Specialization and the narrowing of interest in scientific topics have led to a multiplicity of professional associations and published journals.

Recently there has been much criticism of the quality and relevance of research that fills the thousands of scientific journals that are published monthly, semimonthly, and quarterly. Out of the numerous articles published yearly, how many contribute directly or indirectly to social progress or to an understanding of humankind and our environment? Research in the social sciences is most vulnerable to criticism as the need for progress in these areas is most pressing. The gap between research in the social sciences and its impact on social problems has led to criticism of applied research. Yet one need only examine the history of medical progress to realize the tremendous gains science has made through applied research. There is also a strong need for basic research in areas that may not seem relevant at the moment, as with cellular research and microbiology, where theory and basic research carried out 50 years ago have led to practical results in understanding the immune system. There is a need for basic research into life processes, such as in DNA, muscle metabolism, and in neurological and cognitive areas of human development. The need also exists for problem-oriented research that can be applied in the areas from health, medicine, special education, and rehabilitation to mental illness, delinquency, poverty, drug addiction, and unemployment. A study begins with establishing the need, significance, and implications of the results to existing psychosocial and biological problems.

4.2 Selecting a Significant Problem

How does a researcher select a significant area for investigation? What factors in an individual's personal life, education, or professional experience generate a research interest? William Harvey in the introduction of his book *On the Motion of the Heart and Blood in Animals,* written in 1628, describes his purpose in investigating the problem of circulation of blood in the following quotation.

> Since, therefore, from the foregoing considerations and many others to the same effect, it is plain that what has . . . been said concerning the motion and function of the heart and arteries must appear obscure, inconsistent, or even impossible to him who carefully considers the entire subject, it would be proper to look more narrowly into the matter to contemplate the motion of the heart and arteries, not only in man, but in all animals that have hearts; and also by frequent appeals to vivisection, and much ocular inspection, to investigate and discuss the truth. (p. 73)

Harvey selected the problem of investigating the circulatory system after he evaluated the previous studies as contradictory and inconclusive. His motivation to study the problem was based on his desire to bring clarity to an area of medicine that is vital to human survival. This desire to clarify is an important motivating force in the researcher. There are numerous examples in the history of scientific research of individuals seeking to understand the basic anatomical and physiological processes of man. Other motivating forces can also generate research.

- Individuals can pursue a research area because they seek insight into a disease or disability that has touched their own life or a family member or close friend. Ignaz Semmelweis, a relentless investigator, in 1847 pursued the causes of puerperal fever (i.e., blood poisoning associated with childbirth) after the death of a friend. Louis Braille, blinded at the age of four, became a teacher of the blind and in 1824 devised a reading method for the blind.

- A clinician becomes a researcher after becoming aware of the need for more effective treatment methods or diagnostic instruments. There are many instances in the history of medicine where practitioners became part-time researchers and through their efforts made notable contributions. For instance, Freud's interest in psychotherapy grew out of his frustration with neurology and anatomical brain research. He used clinical research to verify his hypotheses and to explore the inner psychological environment of man.

- A dramatic increase in the incidence of a disease produces national priorities for research. In the United States in the last 25 years there has been a significant amount of research effort in the areas of cancer, cardiovascular disease, and AIDS. These areas have received added attention and interest by researchers partially because of the dramatic increases in the incidence of these illnesses, and partially because of the availability of federal grant support. It is no secret that a research investigator's career can become determined by national politics and priorities.

  The abuse of federal grant support in the opportunism of research can also become an overriding problem in neglecting research areas that are significant yet receive little interest from the granting foundations and governmental agencies.

- An interest in a content area is generated by an inspiring teacher. There is no doubt that universities are an ideal place for research as they can play an active yet neutral role in facilitating research efforts. Universities need not be caught in political decisions.

- A student develops an interest in a research area through intellectual curiosity spurred by intense reading and study. As the student gains more understanding in a specific area, more questions are raised, which motivate research.

From these motivating forces and others, the researcher selects an area of investigation. From this point how does one maintain momentum and nurture research interests sometimes in the face of insignificant results and tedious, laborious work? The story of Fleming's discovery of penicillin in 1929 is an example of persistence. The impetus for Fleming's investigation was the catastrophic rate of death that occurred during the First World War from infected wounds. Fleming sought a chemical substance that would destroy the pathogenic germs entering the body from an open flesh wound. After 10 years of painstaking laboratory work that involved growing bacterial colonies and observing the reactions of chemicals, he was successful in discovering a powerful therapeutic agent that would eventually change the course of medical practice. There were two landmark events in his work. The first occurred in 1922 when he noticed that a foreign chemical substance prevented a bacterial colony from growing. At this point in his work he was unable to isolate or identify the chemical substance. In 1928, Fleming noticed that a bacterial culture of staphylococci had accidentally become contaminated by mold. He found that the mold produced a substance that retarded the growth of the bacteria. The chemical substance was later identified by an American mycologist, Thom, as *Penicillium notatum*. After the substance was identified, Fleming was able to produce penicillin in the laboratory and experiment with its effect on bacteria and normal human tissues. However it was not until 1943, about 20 years after Fleming's original investigations that penicillin became mass produced in Great Britain and the United States. In analyzing Fleming's discovery, it is important to note that a combination of persistence and responsiveness to accidental discovery was the key factor. Fleming first asked a researchable question: Is there a chemical substance that can stop the growth of harmful bacteria in the bloodstream without destroying normal human tissue? He persisted in his efforts on the problem over a period of 25 years until his successful discovery of penicillin.

Compared to medicine, research originating from allied health and special education fields is in the beginning stages of development. Potential directions for research abound in the areas of evaluation and treatment and in the areas of professional education and administration. These areas can be described as two triangles as depicted in Figure 4–1.

In Diagram I of the figure, research originates out of the relationship between the evaluation and treatment of a specific disability. By analyzing a disability, the clinical researcher tries to determine where the major gaps in knowledge exist. For instance, in evaluating and treating the patient with arthritis, are there effective evaluative instruments? What treatment methods have been demonstrated to be effective? What factors in the patient's life affect the course of the illness? From this analysis the researcher can identify a research problem. This same process of generating research is evident also in analyzing the educational and administrative aspects in a health profession as depicted in Diagram II of the figure. The need for research is justified when a researcher can establish the significance of the results. A researcher should clearly state the implications of the study, relating it to the evaluation or treatment of a specified disability or the educational or administrative practices that could be affected by the results. Before data are collected the researcher should be able to think through the impact of the results. An *if* (results positive or negative) . . . *then* (recommendations and options taken) . . . contingency is the initial strategy proposed by the researcher.

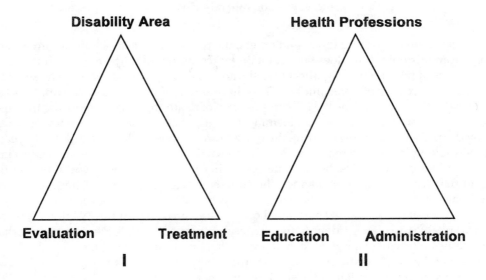

Figure 4–1.   Potential directions for research in allied health and special education. Note that the relationship between evaluation and treatment leads to research in disabilities, while the relationship between education and administration leads to research in health professions.

4.3 Identifying Problems Resulting From a Disability

In selecting a disability area for research, the investigator can be guided by one's own clinical experience in an area of specialization. For example, the significance of a problem can be gauged by the leading causes of death and the leading causes of hospitalization. The 14 leading causes of death in 1990 and 1993 in the United States in order of rank are shown in Table 4–1.

For the researcher these disabilities and diseases represent significant problems. Evaluation and diagnosis are ongoing concerns for the therapist. Methodological research such as in diagnostic hardware, clinical observational methods, screening procedures, and objective tests can become the focal point of an investigation. The development of specific treatment techniques that can be generalized to a population with disabilities represents another fertile direction for researchers. Treatment techniques such as language programs, exercise, diet, special education, and biofeedback are a few examples of research areas generated from examining the needs of populations with disabilities.

Table 4–1   *Fourteen Leading Causes of Death for 1990 and 1993*

Cause	1990		1993	
	Number	**Rank**	**Number**	**Rank**
All causes	2,148,463	—	2,252,000	—
Heart disease	720,058	1	936,000	1
Malignant neoplasms	505,322	2	529,060	2
Cerebrovascular disease	144,088	3	149,090	3
Injuries, including motor vehicles	91,983	4	85,410	4
Chronic obstructive pulmonary disease	86,679	5	99,520	5
Pneumonia and influenza	79,513	6	77,800	6
Diabetes mellitis	47,664	7	54,280	7
Suicide	30,906	8	29,680	9
Chronic liver disease and cirrhosis	25,815	9	24,660	11
HIV infection	5,188	10	36,460	8
Homicide and legal intervention	24,932	11	24,540	12
Nephritis, nephrotic syndrome, and nephrosis	20,764	12	24,980	10
Septicemia	19,169	13	20,250	13
Atherosclerosis	18,047	14	17,020	14

Note. The table shows the number and rank for the top causes of death in the United States in 1993. The data include all races and are based on the National Vital Statistics Report. Taken from the *Monthly Vital Statistics Report,* Vol. 42, No. 12, May 13, 1994, U.S. National Center for Health Statistics.

4.4 Identifying Significant Issues in Professional Education

Who should become the speech–language pathologists, physical therapists, occupational therapists, school psychologists, special educators, rehabilitation counselors, nurses, and physicians? Are there specific abilities, personalities, intellectual potentials, or academic achievements that are necessary before entering a professional preparatory program? What is the rationale for each prerequisite? How are admission requirements for schools decided upon? Who are the decision makers and shapers of policy in medical schools, nursing schools, and schools for allied health professionals? These questions examine the assumptions underlying the education of health professionals. The recruitment, screening, and selection of students pose realistic problems to the health educator that should provide significant areas for investigation.

Along with the selection process, the content and methods of educating health professionals require reexamination by researchers. The educational technology includes the classroom teaching methods, curricula content, audiovisual aids, clinical education, and student evaluation. Examples of these potential areas of research in educating health professional students are listed in Table 4–2.

Administration of clinical programs, personnel policies, budgetary planning, physical plant layouts, and job satisfaction are often neglected areas of research because of the indirect relationship to patient treatment. However, the effect of administrative policies has sometimes more impact on the course of a patient's disease than the direct effects of treatment. Public health policies to mass vaccinate a population, the geographical placement of a health facility, and the lowering of staff morale are all critical areas of concern that have important implications in the total health needs of a patient.

4.5 Justifying the Research Problem

Once a research area is identified by the investigator, statistical data should be cited (see Table 4–3 as an example of statistical data) that indicate the extent and proportion of the

Table 4–2   *Factors in Educating Health Professionals*

Classroom Teaching Methods	Curricula Content	Audiovisual Aids	Clinical Education	Student Evaluation
• Lecture • Seminar • Workshop • Cooperative learning experiences	• Anatomy and phyisology • Interpersonal processes • Evaluation and treatment techniques • Clinical reasoning • Problem-based learning	• Closed circuit television • Computer-assisted instruction • Films • Distance education • Interactive television	• Internships (one year) • Affiliations (Specialty area) • Clerkships (undergraduate experiences) • Competency-based education • On-the-job training (learning by working)	• Individual counseling • Grades–Pass/Fail • Causes for termination

Table 4–3   *Number of Selected Reported Chronic Conditions per 1,000 Persons*

Impairment	All Ages
Visual impairments	35.7
Color blindness	12.6
Cataracts	26.7
Glaucoma	9.9
Hearing impairment	94.6
Tinnitus	30.9
Speech impairment	12.3
Absence of extremities (excludes tips of fingers or toes only)	6.3
Paralysis of extremities, complete or partial	5.8
Deformity of orthopedic impairment	125.7
Back	74.3
Upper extremities	17.8
Lower extremities	51.0

Note. Data obtained from "Current Estimates from the National Health Interest Survey, 1992," *Vital and Health Statistics*, January, 1994, p.83.

problem. A problem involving one of the ten leading causes of death or hospitalization is obviously significant. However, how does one justify investigating a rare disease that affects very few people? On the other hand should the freedom of an investigator be restricted by governmental agencies deciding which areas to fund research? The question of research significance does touch on societal values. Priorities are established by nations in areas of health that realistically affect research efforts. It is assumed that the individual scientist should have the freedom to pursue any area of investigation as long as it does not endanger the lives of any subjects. Yet, research should not be isolated from the pressing needs of a society. If, for example, breast cancer becomes a problem of epidemic proportions in the United States in the late 1990s, then the society should justly allocate a large percentage of its health resources to those researchers seeking means to reduce the incidence of breast cancer. Establishing research priorities in a democratic society involves the participation of a broad spectrum of groups who represent the policy makers, clinicians, consumers, and researchers. Governmental agencies, universities, pharmaceutical companies, and private foundations are the primary sources for the financial support of research, and thus, the policy makers for research. The recipients of research grants are those clinical practitioners, educators, and administrators who have convinced policy makers of the significance and validity of their research proposals.

In summary, the researcher justifies an investigation by establishing the need for a study based on an analysis of a health problem and the implications of the results. The need for an investigation is documented by the following statistical data:

- The *incidence* (initial occurrences) and *prevalence* (existing cases in the population) of a disability, derived from statistical data.
- The leading causes of death as reported by National Centers for Health Statistics.

- The number of first admissions and readmissions to a hospital caused by a disability. Information obtained from state public health agencies.
- The number of physician and outpatient visits reported as the result of a disability.
- The days lost at work because of specific health problems, compiled from Department of Labor Statistics.
- The incidence of social disabilities (i.e., alcoholism, drug addiction, adult crime, juvenile delinquency, and child abuse). This information should be available through the state public health agency and the state attorney general's office.
- The number of health workers employed in the United States as provided by professional organizations, the *Occupational Outlook Handbook* (published by the United States Department of Labor), and state employment agencies.
- Statistics on the number of hospitals, outpatient clinics, state institutions for individuals with mental retardation and mental illness, rehabilitation centers, and other patient care facilities, usually available from public health agencies or through directories published by municipal and state organizations and private social service agencies.

4.6 Narrowing the Investigation

Problem-oriented research is a process of asking questions and gathering data. The investigator generates a question and intellectually ponders the possible outcomes. This ability to formulate research questions and to predict outcomes is an essential part of the research process. The Socratic method of teaching is based on this principle of questions and answers that invariably lead to other questions and answers until a topic is exhausted. Brainstorming a problem is another method for generating questions by creative free association. The researcher must be able to freely generate questions that on initial examination may seem unrelated or unfeasible. Many great discoveries, when they were first reported publicly, seemed like "hair-brained" ideas that would never work. Roentgen, a physicist, accidentally discovered X-Rays when examining the results of passing electricity through a vacuum tube. He then proceeded to ask himself questions regarding its applicability to medical diagnosis. People in the streets on hearing of Roentgen's discovery in 1895 were incredulous. Many felt that X–Rays would be used like a camera to spy on people or to expose them. On the other hand, medical scientists later raised questions regarding the potential of X-Ray in diagnosis and in the treatment of cancerous growths.

This process of asking questions and observing the outcome is the essential part of research. At first the question may be general, ill-conceived, unclear, and incongruous. As the researcher mentally explores what is actually being asked, the research question becomes sharper until, as Graham Wallas (1926) stated:

> Our mind is not likely to give us a clear answer to any particular problem unless we set it a clear question, and we are more likely to notice the significance of any new piece of evidence, or new association of ideas, if we have formed a definite conception of a case to be proved or disproved. (p. 84)

The persistent effort on the part of the researcher to brainstorm a problem, to think it through, to ponder silently, or to discuss it with a colleague brings the researcher closer to a solution. For some investigators the problem incubates, while for others the problem stirs. Whatever the style is, the researcher must be able to stay with a problem while trying to overcome the apparent pitfalls and cul de sacs created. Many a researcher is stymied by the assumption of others that the problem is too complex or impossible to solve or by the knowledge that others have failed. The investigator must be able to ward off the prophets of failure and to risk effort in working through the problem. For example, low back pain is a significant health problem that affects a large number of sedentary and manual workers in the western nations. It directly affects industrial production, psychological well-being, and participation in sports and general activities. Although it is widespread in the population, and it has significant implications, practitioners have been only partially successful in treating this disability. Experienced clinicians observe that low back pain is an elusive syndrome that is difficult to diagnose and sometimes difficult to separate from malingering or psychosomatic effects. Other clinicians are hesitant to investigate the problem because of the subjective nature of measuring pain. Others state that the neurophysiology is too complex to investigate. These reactions to low back pain should not deter research. The investigator entering into an area of research can become overwhelmed by the immensity of a problem. However, the investigator need not try to solve all aspects of a problem, including objective diagnosis and successful treatment. The researcher should attempt to "slice off" that part of a research problem that is feasible within the limitations of time and resources available. The process of formulating a research problem by a clinician is summarized in Figure 4–2.

Let us examine hypothetical examples of research questions derived from significant health problems. (See Table 4–4.) These research questions are derived directly from an

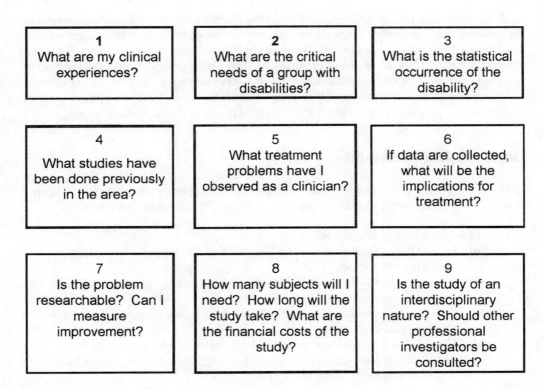

1 What are my clinical experiences?	2 What are the critical needs of a group with disabilities?	3 What is the statistical occurrence of the disability?
4 What studies have been done previously in the area?	5 What treatment problems have I observed as a clinician?	6 If data are collected, what will be the implications for treatment?
7 Is the problem researchable? Can I measure improvement?	8 How many subjects will I need? How long will the study take? What are the financial costs of the study?	9 Is the study of an interdisciplinary nature? Should other professional investigators be consulted?

Figure 4–2.   Clinical formulation of a research problem.

Table 4–4 *Hypothetical Research Questions Related to Disability*

Disability	Research Question
Cerebral palsy:	Is development sequential and hierarchical in children with motor lesions in the cerebral cortex?
Mental retardation:	How does the environmental facilitate or restrict learning?
Social deprivation:	How is language acquisition affected by parental auditory stimulation and feedback?
Stroke rehabilitation:	What psychological factors significantly affect recovery of function?
Diabetes:	What is the interrelationships between diet, exercise, weight, body type, and insulin production in the body?
Hypertension:	Can blood pressure rates be self-regulated through biofeedback techniques?
Depression:	What is the role of exercise in increasing serotonin?
Learning disability:	What are significant factors in facilitating reading?
Multiple sclerosis:	What are the effects of stress on "triggering" episodes?
AIDS:	What factors are helpful in reducing symptons?
Traumatic brain injury:	What issues need to be addressed if school re-entry is to be successful?

analysis of a health problem. The specificity of the question depends on the uniqueness of the investigator's interests. After the researcher identifies an area of investigation and documents the significance of the study, he or she is faced with the task of narrowing the area of investigation into a feasible chunk within a designated time span. Some researchers devote their entire professional life to a specific area of research. Others drastically change their research areas as they broaden their interests. For some the selection of an initial topic for research can be the starting point of many years of investigation.

Determining Feasibility

In the process of narrowing the investigation to a feasible project, the investigator should, as a preliminary procedure, carefully examine the following questions:

1. How long will data collection take?
   a. Laboratory experiments—the length of time required for collecting data for each subject.
   b. Interview time—time for each subject multiplied by total number of subjects equal total interview time.
   c. Mail survey—researcher must account for response time and possibly a second mailing.
   d. Correlational study—individual or group testing time periods.
   e. Methodological—consideration of time for constructing instrument and obtaining reliability and validity data.

2. What measuring instruments are available for testing constructs and variables?
3. Are subjects readily available? Where can subjects be obtained?
4. What expertise is required by the researcher for administering tests and carrying out the research procedures?
5. Are all variables operationally defined (i.e., measurable by a test or a procedure)?
6. What are the financial costs of the research?
7. How long will it take for approval by the institutional review board (IRB) of ethical standards?

4.7 Psychological Blocks in Selection of a Research Problem

Many times graduate students confronted with the task of completing a thesis, dissertation, or study that involves collecting primary data are stymied in selecting a researchable topic. Students often belabor the process and frequently change their research area. In the process of selecting a feasible research problem, the student can become frustrated and immobilized. In overcoming these psychological blocks, the student should be able to mentally deduce the consequences of a research study and forecast its potential significance. The following examples are typical of the psychological blocks that interfere with selecting a research problem.

- A research topic is dropped prematurely because the investigator fails to locate enough published studies related to the topic.
- The investigator is overwhelmed by the multiplicity of studies published in an area and concludes that further research is not necessary because the area has already been researched. The investigator drops the topic without rigorously evaluating the validity and conclusiveness of results.
- The research topic selected is too broad, considering the time constraints of an investigator. Instead of narrowing the research topic to a feasible study the investigation is terminated.
- A preliminary investigation of a research area reveals difficulty in measuring an outcome variable of improvement. The investigator drops the investigation without seeking to construct an instrument that could reliably and validly measure the variable.
- An investigator is motivated to explore a research area with the goal of making an important and original contribution to the body of knowledge. The investigator refuses to delimit a study after realizing the amount of time necessary to complete the study and subsequently terminates the investigation.

Selecting a researchable problem should be an ongoing process where the prospective investigator explores the relevance, feasibility, applicability, and significance of a study. The following worksheet guide lists the areas that a researcher should be aware of in the process of selecting and narrowing a researchable problem.

4.8 Worksheet Guide for Selecting a Research Problem

Guiding Question

1. What is the target population?
   a. group with disabilities
   b. allied health profession
      • student
      • clinician

2. What are the perceived needs of the population?
   a. investigating causes of disability
   b. evaluation and diagnostic methods
   c. student performance
   d. evaluation of therapists' effectiveness
   e. investigation of treatment techniques
   f. evaluation of personnel factors

3. What are the important published studies relevant to responses 1 and 2?
   a. journal articles
   b. annual reviews
   c. textbooks
   d. statistical compendiums

4. Are independent and dependent variables identifiable?
   independent variables (presumed causes):
   dependent variables (presumed effects):

5. What are the possible consequences of research (between too broad and too narrow)
   a. for treatment
   b. for education
   c. for administration

6. Can research variables be operationally defined?

7. What explanation or theory accounts for the presumed relationship between variables?

8. What research models are relevant to the study? State research question relative to research model.
   a. experimental (pretest, posttest)
   b. methodological (construction of instrument)
   c. evaluation (evaluation of health care system)
   d. correlation (relationship between variables)
   e. survey (description of population)
   f. historical (reconstruction of events)
   g. clinical or naturalistic observation (dynamic analysis of subject)
   h. heuristic (discovery of relationships)

9. a. State the research problem.
   b. State the hypothesis in null or directional form.
   c. State the guiding question.

10. To which groups are the research findings directed?
    - clinicians
    - individuals with disabilities
    - students
    - academicians
    - program administrators

11. Feasibility check
    a. Where can subjects be obtained?
    b. How many subjects are necessary?
    c. What tests, instruments or apparatus will be necessary to measure outcome?
    d. What are financial costs?
       - travel
       - mailings and address labels
       - tests
       - protocols
       - clinical time
       - apparatus
       - computer analysis
       - books and duplicating
       - clerical and typing
       - laboratory analysis of findings

12. Analysis of time (List the projected time sequence for completion of research phases)

Date for initiation of study	Date for review of literature	Date for preparing for data collection	Date for approval from IRB	Date for collecting results	Date for writing discussion	Date for completion of study

4.9 Why Research Proposals Are Disapproved

The following list of major reasons for the disapproval of research proposals are based on the authors' experiences as raters on governmental and university committees. The list is summarized in Table 4–5.

- *The research problem is insignificant and the results will have little impact on clinical practice currently or in the future.* An example of an insignificant problem is an investigation of the relationship of low birth weight with the incidence of cerebral palsy. A literature search in this area already confirms that low birth weight is one among many risk factors for cerebral palsy. However, not all infants with cerebral palsy are born prematurely nor are all infants

Table 4–5   *Reasons Why Research Proposals Are Denied*

- The research problem is insignificant and the results will have little impact on clinical practice currently or in the future.
- The hypothesis presented is not supported by scientific evidence and seems speculative.
- The research problem is more complex than the investigator presents and it needs to be narrowed down.
- The anticipated results from the study will be of only local significance and lacks external validity or generalizability.
- The research proposed has too many elements that are uncontrolled.
- The research methodology seems overcomplex and difficult to replicate.
- The proposed outcome measures are either inappropriate, unstandardized, unreliable, or invalid.
- Extraneous variables are left uncontrolled and may have an influence on the results.
- Overall design of the study seems incomplete and not well thought through.
- The statistical tests suggested for analyzing the data are not appropriate.
- Selection of subjects for the study is not representative of a target population.
- The treatment procedure under investigation has not been adequately defined in enough detail to replicate.
- The literature review seems outdated and lacks landmark studies in the area of investigation.
- The equipment identified in the study is outmoded or unsuitable.
- The investigator has not proposed adequate time for completion of the study.
- Resources are inadequate to complete the study.
- The setting and environment for the study is unsuitable.
- The investigator has not considered the ethical nature of the study, such as stating the potential physical and psychological risks to participants in an informed consent form.

with low birth weight destined to have cerebral palsy. This study will have little impact on our understanding of the causes of cerebral palsy and will not provide insight into the prevention and treatment. The projected results from this type of study would have a splintering effect where one variable is linked to a disability that has already been found to have multiple causes. A better study in a related area would be to examine the effects of low birth weight on one area of development such as motor function. In this way the investigator can narrow the research and control for extraneous variables that could have a potential effect on the results.

- *The hypothesis presented is not supported by scientific evidence and seems speculative.* As a hypothetical example, a researcher proposes that a computer software program in cognitive rehabilitation is effective in treating patients with closed head injuries. The investigator equates improvement with the patient's ability to learn a computer game. The investigator does not demonstrate through a literature review that there is a carryover of this computer skill to the learning of functional skills in independent living. A better study is to investigate the types of skills that are facilitated while learning with a computer.

- *The research problem is more complex than the investigator presents and it needs to be narrowed down.* For example, a researcher proposes to examine the effects of sensory integration therapy on children with attentional deficits. Both variables are complex and must be operationally defined. Sensory integration therapy includes a number of components in treatment whereas attention deficit-hyperactivity disorder is a complex disorder with multiple causes. A better study is to identify one aspect of sensory integration therapy, such as controlled rotary vestibular stimulation, and evaluate its effectiveness with a measurable variable such as motor proficiency as assessed by the Miller Assessment for Preschoolers (MAP; Miller, 1988).

- *The anticipated results from the study will be of only local significance and lacks external validity or generalizability.* An example of a flawed proposal is when a researcher designs a survey of job satisfaction for teachers in a local elementary school without considering the generalizability to a larger sample or population. The data collected from this study would have only local interest and could not be generalized to teachers in other schools. In a better study of job satisfaction among teachers, the researcher would determine first the demographics of an average teacher, considering age, gender, and educational level. These variables could be used to determine if the local school teachers are representative of a larger population. The survey would be designed with the intentions of applying it to a more general sample. Questions would be generated that examine the broad issues of job satisfaction among teachers in general, rather than looking at local issues that affect job satisfaction in that particular school.

- *The research proposed has too many elements that are uncontrolled.* For example, a researcher wants to study the effects of in utero exposure of alcohol on children born with Fetal Alcohol Syndrome (FAS). The amount of alcohol exposure is unknown and is dependent on the mother's self-report which is often unreliable. In addition, the home environment and genetic makeup are variables that may play a part in the child's behavior. These variables are difficult to measure and are often neglected by the researcher. A better approach is a retrospective case study analysis and presentation of FAS from a woman at risk for alcoholism, exploring the dynamics of the case.

- *The research methodology seems overcomplex and difficult to replicate.* For example, a researcher wants to examine the relationship between cocaine use in fathers and metacognitive abilities. Several instruments are used; however, only a few of these instruments have been linked to metacognition. In addition, variables such as family makeup, educational achievement, and personal use of cocaine are ignored in the analysis. It is probable that these variables would influence one's ability to use metacognitive skills. A better study would be to group subjects by variable (e.g., personal cocaine use and educational achievement). In addition, using only one or two instruments known to be related to metacognition will result in more accurate data collection.

- *The proposed outcome measures are either inappropriate, unstandardized, unreliable, or invalid.* A researcher investigating the effects of exercise on depression creates a scale for depression without testing for its reliability or validity. A better approach to measurement is to use more than one instrument to measure outcome (*triangulation*). For example, the investigator can use a physiological measure, a standardized test, and a patient self-report. These three measures will increase the internal validity of the study in assessing outcome.

- *Extraneous variables are left uncontrolled and may have an influence on the results.* For example, a researcher wants to examine the effect of a specific treatment method on improving motor skills. While the researcher is careful to administer pre- and posttests, extraneous variables, such as practice at home, additional interventions, or sessions per week, are not included in the analysis. These variables will most certainly affect the results. A better study would be to take frequent measures of performance, perhaps at the beginning and end of each therapy session, in order to determine changes in skill level. Another possibility is to have the researcher qualitatively describe changes in the subjects.

- *Overall design of the study seems incomplete and not well thought through.* In this example, elements of the research proposal are missing, such as controlling for extraneous variables that could possibly influence the results, or a large section of the literature review is omitted. It is important for the researcher to work with an outline that lists the essential components of a research proposal.

- *The statistical tests suggested for analyzing the data are not appropriate.* An investigator has collected ordinal data such as ranking of students on an achievement test. Rather than using a nonparametric tests, such as the Spearman Rank Order Correlation used for ordinal type data, the researcher inappropriately applies a parametric test, such as the Pearson Correlational Coefficient statistical test used for interval scale data. The statistical test applied should be based on the measurement scale of data. The assumptions of parametric statistics such as normality of data distribution should be followed. The appropriate statistics are based on the assumptions underlying the statistical tests.

- *Selection of subjects for the study is not representative of a target population.* If it is known that the incidence of closed head injuries is higher for males than females by more than 2 to 1, and that over 50% of clients with closed head injuries are between the ages of 15 and 24, then the investigator should try to select subjects that reflect these statistics. This is especially true for studies where the investigator intends to generalize results to a representative sample. However, there are studies where the investigator is interested in examining a nonrepresentative sample that is a portion of the target population, such as females or children with closed head injuries. Then the investigator must delineate clearly the target population in the title of the study.

- *The treatment procedure under investigation has not been adequately defined in enough detail to replicate.* An investigator identifies the independent variable as counseling; however, not enough detail is given regarding how counseling will be used. Therefore, this study cannot be replicated.

- *The literature review seems outdated and lacks landmark studies in the area of investigation.* In reviewing the literature it is wise to first examine secondary texts or to survey articles in the area to identify the major landmark studies that are often cited. An up-to-date literature review can be found also by scanning the current journals in a subject area and by looking at the journal's yearly index.

- *The equipment identified in the study is outmoded or unsuitable.* For example, a test that has been standardized on adults is used for children. This is inappropriate and unsuitable for the study.

- *The investigator has not proposed adequate time for completion of the study.* In out-lining the proposal for a study the researcher should set up a time line graph that breaks down the components of the study into time periods. For exam-ple, doing a literature search, designing a questionnaire, obtaining approval from an Institutional Review Board, collecting and analyzing data, and writ-ing the conclusions, are some of the time dimensions in the study.
- *Resources are inadequate to complete the study.* For example, a research plan in-cludes the need to obtain information from parents of children in a study. Funds are requested for one evaluator to complete the diagnostic tests and one interviewer to obtain information from parents. Although there are an adequate number of personnel selected, the funds requested for support are insufficient to complete the study.
- *The setting and environment for the study, is unsuitable.* In this instance, the in-vestigator attempts to complete a complex study without securing an appro-priate environment for the study, such as a fully equipped laboratory or testing area that is free from distracting noise.
- *The investigator has not considered the ethical nature of the study, such as stating the potential physical and psychological risks to subjects in an informed consent form or has not received approval from an Institutional Review Board (IRB) regard-ing human subjects.* For example, a researcher begins to collect data for a study on educational characteristics of students with Fetal Alcohol Syn-drome before the IRB has approved the research design. This is unethical, and data collected cannot be used in the final analysis.

CHAPTER
5

Review of the Literature

That "the library"—as yet unspecified—is the repository of by far the largest part of our recorded knowledge needs no demonstration. The author of an active article on West Africa who reports that the annual rainfall in Fernando, Pa. is 100 inches found this information in the library—in a book. It is most unlikely that he measured the rain himself.—Jacques Barzun and Henry Graff, *The Modern Researcher*, (p. 63)

Operational Learning Objectives

By the end of this chapter, the reader should be able to

1. identify the main purpose of a literature review
2. initiate a computer-based library search, such as MEDLARS, PsychLIT, or ERIC
3. compare and contrast referral and primary sources
4. initiate a search of the literature, identifying relevant research articles
5. critically evaluate the validity of research studies
6. outline a comprehensive search of the related literature

5.1 Need for a Literature Review

Good research is part of a cumulative process where information expands in many directions. Breakthroughs in knowledge do not occur suddenly. The scientist exploring solutions to problems first masters the previous literature to determine (a) what has been accomplished, (b) where the cul de sacs are, and (c) what research is in the forefront of knowledge. A search of the literature involving the location of relevant studies is a critical part of the research process. It is impossible to conceive of a scientist devising a research plan without first examining previous findings. The literature search is not only a method of uncovering, it is also a way for the researcher to attain an historical perspective and overview of a problem.

Scientific research is a force that advances knowledge. For many scientists discovery of new information or technology is a process of juxtaposing research from diverse fields in relation to an identifiable problem. Norbert Weiner (1948) in his work on cybernetics, which eventually led to the invention of the computers, attained success by brainstorming with engineers, psychiatrists, educators, and physicists. They were able to intermingle their ideas and stimulate one another to examine a problem from many perspectives. Weiner, for this experience, developed a theory of thinking based on the integration of physical science theory with behavioral observations. The investigator exploring the literature should not only examine studies directly related to a problem, but also should try to find studies from other fields that have an indirect or implied relationship to the research question.

If, for example, a researcher is interested in examining the relationship between staff morale and treatment effectiveness, he or she would need to search the literature in management psychology if a preliminary search reveals a lack of studies in allied health. The diversity of findings adds strength to a study, especially if corroboration of data appears from many directions. The Hawthorne effect, which was first noted in factory workers, is now widely accepted as a factor in clinical treatment. Spinoffs from research in the space programs, such as the advances in nutrition, computer programming, temperature control, and monitoring of vital bodily functions, are examples of applying data generated from a seemingly unrelated field.

The main goals of the investigator in searching the literature are to

- make an exhaustive search for related studies
- identify the landmark studies that have an important impact in the area investigated
- evaluate the validity of the research findings
- integrate and synthesize the results into subject areas
- summarize the findings from previous studies, highlighting areas where results are either inconclusive or controversial.

These goals are part of the overall preliminary process of research that precedes data collection. A conceptual view of the literature search is shown in Figure 5–1.

5.2 Locating Sources of Related Literature

Nearly 4,000 periodicals are currently published every year in medical and health related areas. The task of searching the literature would be enormous if the investigator only relied on reviewing individually each and every periodical. How can the investigator quickly obtain a list of studies that are relevant so as to narrow the search and reduce the number of hours examining the card catalogs and library stacks? For the compulsive investigator seeking to identify every study conceivable, the task could be endless. Realistically the investigator accepts the limitation that some published and unpublished studies will not be located. For example, studies published in foreign journals that have not been translated, recent unpublished papers presented at conferences and institutes, ongoing research where the investigator has not published the findings, and research studies by students presented in unpublished theses, dissertations, or special studies may

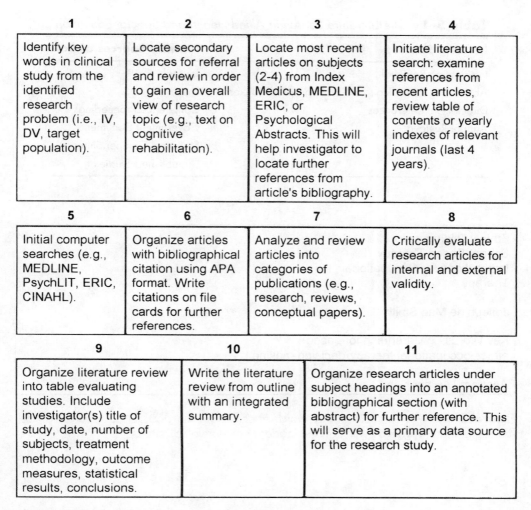

1	2	3	4
Identify key words in clinical study from the identified research problem (i.e., IV, DV, target population).	Locate secondary sources for referral and review in order to gain an overall view of research topic (e.g., text on cognitive rehabilitation).	Locate most recent articles on subjects (2-4) from Index Medicus, MEDLINE, ERIC, or Psychological Abstracts. This will help investigator to locate further references from article's bibliography.	Initiate literature search: examine references from recent articles, review table of contents or yearly indexes of relevant journals (last 4 years).

5	6	7	8
Initial computer searches (e.g., MEDLINE, PsychLIT, ERIC, CINAHL).	Organize articles with bibliographical citation using APA format. Write citations on file cards for further references.	Analyze and review articles into categories of publications (e.g., research, reviews, conceptual papers).	Critically evaluate research articles for internal and external validity.

9	10	11
Organize literature review into table evaluating studies. Include investigator(s) title of study, date, number of subjects, treatment methodology, outcome measures, statistical results, conclusions.	Write the literature review from outline with an integrated summary.	Organize research articles under subject headings into an annotated bibliographical section (with abstract) for further reference. This will serve as a primary data source for the research study.

Figure 5–1.   Conceptual review of the literature search.

not be found. These are realistic limitations on every study. However, with the availability of computer systems for information retrieval the present day investigator is able to locate a vast portion of the literature.

The literature search is divided into two areas: referral sources and primary sources of data. These two areas are outlined in Table 5–1.

The first step in searching the literature is to locate where the relevant studies are reported, that is, in which journal, source book, or dissertation. The referral source supplies bibliographical information locating a specific study. The use of key words allows the student or researcher to identify more easily those studies that cover a particular topic. Frequently, the key words for a specific article are listed immediately before or after the abstract. This is illustrated in Figure 5–2, where the key words (children, decision making, ethics, occupational therapy, school-based) have been listed before the abstract. A student or researcher looking for related articles would use one or more of these key words in the computer search.

Table 5–1   *The Literature Search in Allied Health and Special Education*

Referral Sources	Primary Sources of Data
Information Retrieval Systems	Journals
Abstracting Periodicals and Bibliographic Indexes	Theses
Directory of References	Conference Proceedings
Annual Reviews	Government Documents
	Statistical Compendiums
	Unpublished Studies

Ethical Dilemmas in
School-Based Therapy:
Implications for Occupational
Therapy

Josephine Mae Smith

Key Words: children•school-based•
ethics•occupational therapy•decision-making

Abstract: An analysis . . .

Figure 5–2.   An example of key words listed before the abstract and journal article. The use of these keywords will lead the reader to other related articles.

Each data base has its own thesaurus or subject authority list that contains key words or concepts by using a controlled vocabulary. The controlled vocabulary provides a structure for classifying articles into given topics. An outline of the MEDLARS structure of categories is listed in Table 5–2. These categories are divided into subcategories and Medical Subject Headings (MeSH), allowing for a very specific search of terms.

Subjects or key words used by each base can be found in a thesaurus (e.g., ERIC Thesaurus; Psychological Thesaurus). The thesaurus is available in hard copy as well as on the CD-ROM as part of the search process. The researcher or student will want to refer to the appropriate thesaurus to obtain the correct term for the database being used. For more specialized words, such as names of tests, specific intervention theories (e.g., direct teaching, Fernald method), the exact term will suffice to locate the articles.

Most database search systems use *Boolean logic* as the strategy to build search statements. Boolean logic uses the logical operators *and, or,* and *and not* to represent relationships between topics in a symbolic manner. (See Figure 5–3). Some systems use also the search operators of *with* and *in*. The use of the term *with* identifies those articles in which the connected terms are used in the same field (e.g., dyslexia with children), whereas the use of the term *in* specifies the particular field. By combing search terms with these logical operators, the researcher can limit or enlarge the search. For example, if a researcher

Table 5–2   *MEDLARS Category Headings*

A.   Anatomy
B.   Organisms
C.   Diseases
D.   Chemicals and Drugs
E.   Analytical, Diagnostic, and Therapeutic Techniques and Equipment
F.   Psychiatry and Psychology
G.   Biological Science
H.   Physical Sciences
I.   Anthropology, Education, Sociology, and Social Anthropology
J.   Technology, Commerce, and Industry
K.   Humanities
L.   Information Sciences
M.   Named Groups
N.   Health Care
Z.   Geographical

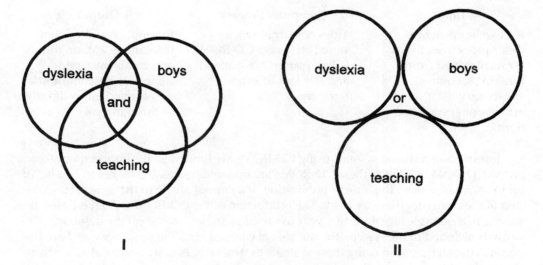

Figure 5–3.   An example of Boolean thinking. In this example, the researcher is interested in information about dyslexia *and* boys *and* teaching. The articles retrieved from the search will be found in the intersection that contains all three terms. In the second example, articles about dyslexia, boys, or teaching will be found. The first example is a more specific search that yields a smaller number of articles.

is looking for articles regarding the etiology and treatment of dyslexia, the search term would be written as

dyslexia and etiology and treatment.

Use of these terms as well as the delimiter *and* would limit the search to only those articles in which both the etiology and treatment of dyslexia have been discussed. Articles that contain only etiology or only treatment will not be obtained. If, on the other hand, the researcher is interested in articles that describe either the etiology or the treatment of dyslexia, the search statement is written as

dyslexia and etiology or dyslexia and treatment.

Articles that examine the etiology or the treatment of dyslexia, or both the etiology and treatment of dyslexia will be obtained. Thus, this search statement produces a larger list of citations, including the citations from the first search statement. Because each system uses a slightly different search technique, it will be necessary to obtain specific information about search strategies for the system being used.

5.21 Information Retrieval Systems

Automated systems for storing and retrieving information have revolutionized libraries. Through computer technology, research librarians are now able to provide a printout of studies and their sources. The studies, sources, and key words are stored on disks, allowing for direct random access and interactive searching. In using a computer-based retrieval system the research proceeds in the following manner:

Input	Computer Process	Output
Researcher provides descriptors from list of terms obtained from thesaurus, controlled vocabulary list, previous articles, or specialized terms.	Titles of journal articles stored on disk or CD-ROM (silver platter) are scanned and relevant titles are retrieved.	Printout of studies (containing author, title, source, abstract, and sometimes the entire article) are obtained, either directly or through mail.

Information retrieval systems using CD-ROMs are limited by the information stored on the CD-ROM. Although these CD-ROMs are updated frequently, there can be a lag of up to six months from the time of publication of a journal article to the time of its inclusion in the computer memory bank. The production of the CD-ROM is delayed, also, resulting in a possible lag of up to a year in the information stored on the database. The journals included in the system, the number of citations, and the years reviewed are important considerations in using these systems for research. A more up-to-date list of articles can be obtained through on-line databases; however, these are costly and most students do not have access to them.

In spite of these limitations, computer-based retrieval systems should be one of the first referral sources used to locating relevant literature. There are two major advantages in using them: (a) the amount of time saved from laboriously reviewing individual journals or printed lists of journal articles (e.g., Psychological Abstracts, Medicus Indicus), and (b) the ability to limit the articles by combining a number of key terms (e.g., Fetal Alcohol Syndrome, children, and Native Americans). On the other hand, computer-based retrieval systems are not inclusive as indicated in the foregoing, and they should not be the sole method of locating bibliographical references. The major information retrieval systems relevant to research in medicine, rehabilitation, health care, and education are described below.

MEDLARS

The Medical Literature Analysis and Retrieval System (MEDLARS) is a database system using computer systems (ELHILL and TOXNET) and which contains over 18 million citations in more than 40 databases derived from over 3700 journals indexed for *Cumulative Index Medicus*, as well as about 700 selected journals indexed in the *Index to Dental Literature* or the *International Nursing Index*. Citations are available as far back as 1964. Articles are indexed using a list of over 15,000 medical subject headings (MeSH). Use of one or more of these MeSH headings allows an individual to search for articles and obtain citations of articles on a particular topic. Table 5–3 has an example of a printout for a complete MEDLINE Unit Record. Although any or all of these data elements can be printed within the computer printout of the search, usually the researcher requests only the author, title, source (location of the article), MeSH headings, and abstract.

The MEDLARS system consists of a number of different online databases. MEDLINE (acronym for MEDlars onLINE) is the most widely used medical database. MEDLINE and its companion databases (MED86, MED83, MED80, MED77, MED72, and MED66) contain citations in all languages for all areas of biomedicine. SDILINE is a monthly update and contains citations of newly indexed articles to be published in the monthly *Index Medicus*. Because of its cost and complexity, the online MEDLINE service is available only to individuals with user numbers and to medical libraries. A CD-ROM (called the Silver Platter), available in some medical libraries, allows students and researchers to independently search for citations without using the more expensive and more complex online services. The CD-ROM is updated regularly.

There are 32 specialized online databases included in MEDLARS. These databases include such subjects as acquired immunodeficiency syndrome (AIDS) and related subjects (AIDSLINE), drugs being used in clinical trials for AIDS (AIDSDRUGS), biotechnological journals not covered in MEDLINE (BIOSEEK), major cancer topics (CANCERLIT), nursing and allied health literature (CINAHL), and bibliographic citations regarding toxicological, pharmacological, biochemical, and physiological effects of drugs and other chemicals (TOXLINE, TOXLIT, and the TOXNET system).

The computer base for this system is located in the National Library of Medicine in Bethesda, Maryland. Over 400 medical schools and hospital libraries in the United States have access to the MEDLARS system. A back-up system of eight regional medical libraries in the United States provides MEDLARS searches for health scientists in hospitals that do not have computer terminals. These federally designated regional medical libraries also provide consultative services and interlibrary loan privileges to other medical libraries within their region. The regional medical libraries are listed below:

- Toll-free phone number for all regional medical libraries: 1–800–338–7657

- **Middle Atlantic Region**
  The New York Academy of Medicine
  1216 Fifth Avenue
  New York, NY 10029
  Phone: 212–876–1232 or 8763
  FAX: 212–534–7042
  Serves the states of DE, NJ, NY, PA

- **Southeastern/Atlantic Region**
  University of Maryland
  Health Services Library
  111 South Greene Street
  Baltimore, MD 21201–1583
  Phone: 401–706–7545 or 2855

  FAX: 410–706–0099
  Serves AL, FL, GA, MD, MS, NC, SC, TN, VA, WV, the District of Columbia, Puerto Rico, and the U.S. Virgin Islands

- **Greater Midwest Region**
  University of Illinois at Chicago
  Library of the Health Sciences
  1750 W. Polk St.
  Chicago, IL 60612–7223
  Phone: 312–966–8974 or 2464
  FAX: 312–996–2226
  Serves IA, IL, IN, KY, MI, MN, ND, OH, SD, WI

Table 5–3 *Sample MEDLINE Unit Record*[a]

Unique Identifier
94328060
Authors
Hoehn TP. Baumeister AA.
Institution
Department of Psychology and Human Development, Peabody College, Vanderbilt University, Nashville, TN 37203
Title
A critique of the application of sensory integration therapy to children with learning disabilities. [Review]
Source
Journal of Learning Disabilities. 27(6):338–50, 1994 Jun–Jul
Abbreviated Source
J Learn Disabil. 27(6):338–50, 1994, Jun–Jul
County of Publication
United States
MeSH Subject Headings
Child, Child, Preschool, Cognition, Comorbidity, Evaluation Studies, Female, Human, Language, Learning Disorders/ep [Epidemiology], Learning Disorders/rh [Rehabilitation], *Learning Disorders/th [Therapy], Male, Motor Activity/ph [Physiology], Occupational Therapy/mt [Methods], *Occupational Therapy/st [Standards], *Psychomotor Performance/ph [Physiology], Self Concept, Sensation/ph [Physiology], Sensation Disorders/ep [Epidemiology], Sensation Disorders/rh [Rehabilitation], Sensation Disorders/th [Therapy], Support, U.S. Gov't, P.H.S.
Abstract

Sensory integration (SI) therapy is a controversial—though popular—treatment for the remediation of motor and academic problems. It has been applied primarily to children with learning disabilities, under the assumption that such children (or at least a subgroup of them) have problems in sensory integration to which some or all of their learning difficulties can be ascribed. The present article critically examines the related issues of whether children with learning disabilities differentially exhibit concomitant problems in sensory integration, and whether such children are helped in any way by means specific to SI therapy. An overview of theoretical contentions and empirical findings pertaining to the first issue is presented, followed by a detailed review of recent studies in the SI therapy research literature, in an effort to resolve the second issue. Results of this critique raise serious doubts as to the validity or utility of SI therapy as an appropriate, indicated treatment for the clinical population in question—and, by extension, for any other groups diagnosed as having "sensory integrative dysfunction." It is concluded that the current fund of research findings may well be sufficient to declare SI therapy not merely an unproven, but a demonstrably ineffective, primary or adjunctive remedial treatment for learning disabilities and other disorders. [References: 106]
ISSN
0022–2194
Publication Type
Journal Article. Review. Review, Tutorial.
Language
English
Grant Numbers
HD27336 (NICHD)
Entry Month
9411

---

[a]*Note.* From MEDLINE data base, Unique Identifier # 94328060
Note. Bolded terms along the top are called field names. A researcher can ask for any or all of these field names when searching for citations. Only the field names pertinent to the citation are included in the record.

- **Midcontinental Region**
  McGoogan Library of Medicine
  University of Nebraska Medical Center
  600 South 42nd Street
  Omaha, NE 68198–6706
  Phone: 402–559–7078 or 4326
  FAX: 902–559–5482
  Serves CO, KS, MO, NE, UT, WY
- **South Central Region**
  Houston Academy of Medicine
  Texas Medical Center Library
  1133 M.D. Andrian Boulevard
  Houston, TX 77030
  Phone: 713–790–7027 or 750–7020
  FAX: 713–790–7030
  Serves AR, LA, NM, OK, TX
- **New England Region**
  University of Connecticut Health Center
  Lyman Maynard Stowe Library
  263 Farmington Ave.
  Farmington, CT 06034-4033

Phone: 203–679–2547 or 4500
FAX: 203–679–1305
Serves CT, MA, ME, NH, RI, VT
- **Pacific Northwest Region**
  Regional Medical Library, ESLIC
  University of Washington
  Box 357155
  Seattle, WA 98195–7155
  Phone: 206–543–5531 or 8262
  FAX: 206–543–2469
  Serves AK, ID, MT, OR, WA
- **Pacific Southwest Region**
  University of California, Los Angeles
  (UCLA)
  Louise Darling Biomedical Library
  10833 Le Conte Avenue
  Los Angeles, CA 90024–1798
  Phone: 310–825–5781 or 1200
  FAX: 310–825–5389
  Serves AZ, CA, HI, NV, and U.S. Territories
  in the Pacific Basin

The location of medical libraries providing MEDLARS services are available from the National Library of Medicine. Since the use of automated information retrieval systems has been expanding at an extremely rapid rate, it is important for the researcher to keep abreast of the innovations and changes occurring in this field. The costs and services connected to the MEDLARS system vary throughout the country.

In addition to the MEDLARS system, the National Library of Medicine houses a National Information Center on Health Services Research and Health Care Technology (NICHSR). One of the goals of NICHSR is to make results of health services research more assessable to practitioners and health providers through additional databases and full text retrieval systems. In addition, they provide a complete list of health services research organizations through the DIRLINE database. More information regarding NICHSR can be obtained by calling 1–800–272–4787 or contacting them through the internet at nichsr@nlm.nih.gov (NICHSR Fact Sheet, 1994).

ERIC

ERIC is an acronym for Educational Resources Information Center. The database is available on CD-ROM (Silver Platter) in most university libraries and contains citations for more than 70,000 publications in educational journals and technical reports, documents of program descriptions, curricular materials, and papers presented at national conferences. An online edition, updated monthly, is available for those with access to an online major information retrieval services (e.g., Dialog or Bibliographic Retrieval Services [BRS]). Unpublished articles cited in ERIC are available as ERIC documents on microfiche in many university libraries. As with MEDLINE, the records for each citation include a number of fields (e.g., author, title, citation, language, year of publication, search descriptors, and target audience). A thesaurus of descriptors is available in hardback and as part of the CD-ROM for those unsure of the proper search term.

PsychLIT

PsychLIT and PsychINFO are online databases also available on CD-ROM. Together they provide information regarding literature in psychology and related fields. These fields include psychiatry, sociology, anthropology, education, pharmacology, physiology, linguistics, and psychopharmacology. Journal articles, technical reports, dissertations, and books and articles in books are included in the database. As with ERIC, a thesaurus of descriptors is available in hardback and as part of the online database or CD-ROM. The CD-ROM, available in most libraries, is updated regularly.

CINAHL

This database covers English-language journals and literature in nursing and allied health, including emergency services, health education, and social services in health care. A listing of new books available in nursing have been included since 1984. The database also lists publications from U.S. nursing associations. Although not a part of MEDLARS, the format of citations and search strategies are based on the MEDLARS MeSH subject headings. The database is available on CD-ROM and is updated regularly.

REHABDATA and ABLEDATA

These databases, sponsored by the National Rehabilitation Information Center, list citations of research reports, monographs, and other material that focuses on rehabilitation of individuals with physical or mental disabilities. ABLEDATA provides information regarding produces and technical aids in areas of personal care, therapeutic, sensory, educational, vocational, and transportation. ABLEDATA can be reached by a toll-free number, 1–800–344–5405.

CHID

This database, which stands for Combined Health Information Database, contains citations of items in the areas of arthritis, diabetes, digestive disease, high blood pressure, and health education/health promotion methods. Journals, books, pamphlets, audiovisuals, unpublished reports, and program descriptions are available. Full-text resource guides are also available.

Other Databases

Other databases which may be useful for researchers who are health providers and special educators include SocLit, a database for sociology and related fields; OT Source, which provides information about occupational therapy activities; and AGELine, a database specializing in social gerontology. Access to these databases may be limited by online services (e.g., Dialog and BRS). Because additional databases are being developed, the reader may want to explore library sources and online services for additional information.

5.22 Bibliographic Indexes and Abstracting Periodicals

There is a growing trend in the medical, educational, and allied health fields to group together published articles under specific headings or separate publications. Consequently indexes to the literature on arthritis, cardiovascular disease, stroke, gastroenteritis, cancer, and dyslexia, special teaching methods, and others are being published with the aid of computer technology. Because of the change in technology and the use of CD-ROMs and online services, these sources are quickly being discontinued. However, until they disappear, these sources can provide an additional means of obtaining information.

When using a bibliographic index the researcher should be aware of the specified journals cited and the frequency of publication. Although more tedious to use, these indexes supplement the CD-ROMs because of their more frequent updates. Articles referenced after the production of the CD-ROM will be listed in the monthly updates.

Bibliographic indexes and abstracting periodicals are hard copy sources for lists of recent studies from a multitude of journals grouped under a specific subject heading. Usually they include concise summaries (abstracts) of articles or investigations. The purpose of the abstract is to provide the reader with a quick overview of the problem under investigation, the methods used in data collection, the results reported, and the conclusions. The abstract is an intermediary step between the bibliographical citation and the complete journal article. Since the abstract is a self-contained summary, it can provide the researcher with all the information desired in a specific research area. More frequently, researchers use abstracting periodicals to select pertinent articles for further examination. Bibliographic indexes and abstracting journals most frequently used by allied health and special education providers are listed below.

- *Index Medicus* is published monthly as a bibliographic listing of references to current articles from over 3,000 worldwide biomedical science and clinical medicine journals. There is a separate bibliography of medical reviews. This index is the major index for journals in basic biomedical sciences and clinical medicine. Since 1976, the index has also published selected conference publications and multiauthored monographs. The index is the hard copy of MEDLARS. Citations use both author and subject headings. Journal articles are cited under the same major MeSH terms as found in MEDLARS (see Table 5–2), with an additional list of about 9,000 technical terms arranged in subheadings. These subheads are arranged alphabetically, with cross references in categorized lists. A search for articles in a specific topic is more arduous with this index than with MEDLARS since the researcher must examine all the articles under a given subject rather than narrowing the search through the use of delimiting terms such as *and, and not,* or *or.* However, use of this index allows the searcher to find the most recent articles not yet included on the CD-ROM.
- *Cumulated Index Medicus*, published since 1960 by the National Library of Medicine in conjunction with the U.S. Department of Health, Education, and Welfare (DHEW), Public Health Service, and National Institutes of Health, includes the culmination of the 12 monthly issues of *Index Medicus.*
- *Abridged Index Medicus* is a monthly bibliography, based on articles from English-language journals. This bibliography is designed for the individual practitioner and libraries of small hospitals and clinics. The *Cumulated Abridged Index Medicus* contains the cumulation of the monthly issues.
- *Cumulative Index to Nursing and Allied Health Literature (CINAHL)* is available through CINAHL, P. O. Box 871, Glendale, CA 91209. This is the hard copy edition of the CINAHL database. The index includes references to all the major nursing periodicals published in the English language. Journals, book reviews, pamphlets, illustrated material, films, filmstrips, and

recordings are cited. Over 250 periodicals are indexed and nonnursing data-bases (e.g., PsychLIT, ERIC) are scanned for articles of specific interest to nurses and allied health professionals.

- *International Nursing Index*, available through the American Journal of Nursing Company in cooperation with the National Library of Medicine, contains over 200 international nursing journals. In addition, nursing articles from over 2000 nonnursing journals currently listed in the *Index Medicus* are scanned.

- *Excerpta Medica Abstract Journals* is by far the most complete medical abstracting service in the world. Numerous abstract journals are published monthly under separate covers. The world medical literature consisting of almost 3,000 current journals are reviewed. Of particular interest to allied health students and dietitians are Arthritis and Rheumatism, Cancer, Cardiovascular Disease, Chest Diseases, Drug Dependency, Epilepsy, Gerontology and Geriatrics, Neurology, Occupational Health, Psychiatry, Public Health, and Rehabilitation and Physical Medicine.

- *Nutrition Abstracts and Reviews* is prepared by the Commonwealth Bureau of Nutrition, Aberdeen, Scotland. It provides over 100,000 abstracts and citiations by title each year. Major headings include technique, chemical composition of foodstuffs, human diet in relation to health and disease, and book reviews.

- *Health Education Research* contains abstracts of theses and dissertations from colleges offering graduate programs in health education. Studies are listed by areas that include community and public health, curriculum development, education, health careers, health institutions, environmental health, and nutrition and weight control, among others.

- *Hospital Literature Index*, first published in 1945, cites studies on administration, planning, and financing of hospitals and related health care institutions, and the administrative aspects of the medical, paramedical, and repayment fields. It is published quarterly.

- *Vocational Rehabilitation Review* is a cumulative index of articles from the major vocational rehabilitation journals.

- *Resources in Education (RIE)* and *Current Index to Journals in Education (CIJE)* are the hardback counterparts to the ERIC database. Each is published monthly and then synthesized into semiannual and annual indexes. RIE cites documents not printed in journals (e.g., conference papers and proceedings, informational handouts), most of which are available on microfiche or from the ERIC Document Reproduction Service (1–800–227–ERIC). CIJE, on the other hand, abstracts journal articles in education and related fields.

- *Education Index*, first published in 1932, contains articles from educational periodicals, conference proceedings, and yearbooks related to the following subject areas: (a) preschool, elementary and secondary schools, college, and adult education; (b) teacher education; (c) counseling and guidance; and (d) curriculum development and application of educational materials. Within these subject areas are included studies from the arts, applied science and technology, audiovisual education, business education, comparative and international education, exceptional children, special education, health and physical education, language and linguistics, mathematics, psychology, mental health, religious education, social studies, and education research.

- *Psychological Abstracts*, the hardcopy format of the *PsychLIT* database, provides international coverage of journals, books, government research reports, and disserations in all disciplines of psychology. The information is arranged by subject with author and subject indexes provided. *Psychological Abstracts* contains nonevaluative summaries of the world's literature from more than 850 journals, technical reports, monographs, and other scientific documents. Each monthly issue contains abstracts listed under numerous major classifications including the following: General Psychology, Psychometrics and Statistics, Perception and Motor Performance, Cognitive Processes and Motivation, Neurology and Physiology, Developmental Psychology, Cultural Influences and Social Issues, Social Behavior and Interpersonal Processes, Communication, Language, Personality, Professional, Personnel, Physical and Psychological Disorders, Treatment and Prevention, Educational Psychology, and Applied Psychology.

- *Sociological Abstracts* is the hardcover edition of the online service. Over 150 journals from sociology are represented in *Sociological Abstracts*, published five times a year. Articles of particular interest to allied health are included under subheadings such as sociology of health and medicine, demography and human biology, and social problems and social welfare.

- *Social Work Research and Abstracts*, previously entitled *Abstracts for Social Workers,* contains abstracts from journals related to the field of social work. These abstracts are grouped under major headings (e.g., fields of service, social policy and action, service methods, the social work profession, history of social work, and related fields in the social sciences. Subheadings of particular interest to allied health professionals and special educators include aging, health and medical care, mental retardation, mental health, interprofessional relations, and psychiatry and medicine.

- *DSH Abstract* (Deafness, Speech and Hearing Publications, Inc., Gallaudet University, Washington, D.C.) contains abstracts of articles related to hearing, hearing disorders, speech and speech disorders, published quarterly. Foreign journals are reviewed.

- *Dissertation Abstracts*, (University Microfilms, Xerox Co., Ann Arbor, Michigan) contains abstracts from the doctoral dissertations in most of the reputable colleges and universities in the United States and Canada. Disserations are available through three sources (microfilm, photocopy, and computer output). The computer service DATRIX (Direct Access to Reference Information: Xerox service) provides lists of dissertations relevant to a particular subject heading. Dissertations are classified into two broad areas: Sciences/Engineering and Humanities/Social Sciences.

- *Biological Abstracts* and *Biology Digest* report the world's bioscience research. These periodicals are published semimonthly with the cooperation of individual biologists, biological industries, and biological journals. Approximately 8,000 journals from 102 different countires are indexed in areas related to life science, genetics, anatomy, physiology, environmental pollutants, nutrition, psychiatry, and public health. The articles are arranged by topic, with author, biosystem, and subject indexes.

- *Science Information Exchange (SIE)* originates from the Smithsonian Institution, Washington, D.C. Current scientific research in agriculture, biology, medicine, physical sciences, psychology, and sociology are indexed. Two-hundred-word abstracts of ongoing research projects sponsored by government agencies, private foundations, universities, and state and municipalities are available to the researcher on request. The purpose of the computer-based information system is to assist researchers in obtaining current information on who is working on specific projects and areas of content specialties.

- *Science Citation Index (SCI)* is an international, interdisciplinary index to the literature of science, medicine, agriculture, technology, and the behavioral sciences. This index does not provide abstracts of articles. Rather, the references to articles within a given topic are referenced. "Thus, if you know a key article, it is easier to retrieve other relevant articles published subsequently. This is useful for updating your article collection" (Davis & Findley, 1990, p. 267). An online version of *SCI* is available.

- *Current Contents*, published weekly by the Institute of Scientific Information, Inc., publishes access to the table of contents of the world's most important journals. It provides complete bibliographic information, title, word, and author index, and author and publisher addresses. Separate editions cover life sciences; social and behavioral sciences; clinical medicine; engineering technology and applied sciences; and the arts and humanities. A computer disk is available as well as a hard copy.

- *Research Grants Index* is published annually by the U.S. Department of Health, Education, and Welfare (DHEW), Public Health Service, National Institutes of Health, Division of Research Grants. The index contains information about health research currently supported by various agencies of DHEW, thereby allowing scientists and administrators of science programs to identify current research activities in areas relating to their own endeavors.

- *Annual Reviews Inc.* is published yearly and contains integrated summaries of topical issues by recognized authorities. They publish the following Annual Reviews of interest to the researcher in allied health and special education:

> Annual Review of Neuroscience
>
> Annual Review of Genetics
>
> Annual Review of Medicine
>
> Annual Review of Gerontology and Geriatrics
>
> Annual Review of Psychology
>
> Annual Review of Rehabilitation
>
> Annual Review of Nutrition

5.23 Sources for Health Statistics

Statistical information is an essential part of the literature search. The incidence of diseases, hospitalization rates, occupational accidents, infant mortality rates, and the leading causes of death are examples of data compiled by government agencies and published in periodicals available to researchers. A common source of primary statistical information is the National Center for Health Statistics, Public Health Service, HRA, Rockville, MD 10852. They periodically issue the following series of statistical reports:

OUTLINE OF REPORT SERIES (FOR VITAL AND HEALTH STATISTICS)

Originally Public Health Service Publication No. 1000

Series 1: Programs and collection procedures: Reports that describe the general programs of the National Center for Health Statistics and its offices and divisions, data collection methods used, definitions, and other material necessary for understanding the data.

Series 2: Data evaluation and methods of research: Studies of new statistical methodology including experimental tests of new survey methods, studies of vital statistics collection methods, new analytical techniques, objective evaluations of reliability of collected data, and contributions to statistical theory.

Series 3: Analytical studies: Reports presenting analytical or interpretive studies based on vital and health statistics, carrying the analysis further than the expository types of reports in the other series.

Series 4: Documents and committee reports: Final reports of major committees concerned with vital and health statistics and documents, such as recommended model vital registration laws and revised birth and death certificates.

Series 10: Data from the health interview survey: Statistics on illness, accidental injury, disability, use of hospital, medical, dental, and other services, and other health-related topics, based on data collected in a continuing national household interview survey.

Series 11: Data from the health examination survey: Data from direct examination, testing, and rneasurement of national samples of the population provide the basis for two types of reports: (a) estimates of the medically defined prevalence of specific diseases in the United States and the distributions of the population with respect to physical, physiological, and psychological characteristics; and (b) analysis of relationships among the various measurements without reference to an explicit finite universe of persons.

Series 12: Data from the institutional population surveys: Statistics relating to the health characteristics of persons in institutions and on medical, nursing, and personal care received, based on national samples of establishments providing these services and samples of the residents or patients.

Series 13: Data from the hospital discharge survey: Statistics relating to discharged patients in short-stay hospitals, based on a sample of patient records in a national sample of hospitals.

Series 14: Data on health resources: manpower and facilities: Statistics on the numbers, geographic distribution, and characteristics of health sources including physicians, dentists, nurses, other health manpower occupations, hospitals, nursing homes, outpatient and other inpatient facilities.

Series 20: Data on mortality: Various statistics on mortality other than those included in annual or monthly reports—special analyses by cause of death, age, and other demographic variables, also geographic and time series analyses.

Series 21: Data on natality, marriage and divorce: Various statistics on natality, marriage, and divorce other than those included in annual or monthly reports with special analyses by demongraphic variables, also geographic and time series analyses and studies of fertility.

Series 22: Data from the national natality and mortality surveys: Statistics on characteristics of births and deaths not available from the vital records, based on sample surveys stemming from these records, including such topics as mortality by socioeconomic class, medical experience in the last year of life, and characteristics of pregnancy.

For a list of titles and reports published in these series, write to: Office of Information, National Center for Health Studies, Public Health Service, HRA, Rockville, MD 20852

The World Health Organization of the United Nations has compiled the following statistical compendiums:

- *World Health Statistics Report* is published quarterly by the World Health Organization, Geneva, Switzerland. It reports articles both in English and French and contains two parts: statistics on diseases and specific topics of current interest, such as certain causes of death and morbidity.
- *World Health Statistics Annual* is a result of a joint effort by national health and statistical administrations of various countries, and the statistical office of the United Nations and the World Health Organization. It consists of

three parts: (a) Volume I, vital statistics and causes of death; (b) Volume II, infectious diseases, causes, death, and vaccination; and (c) Volume III, health personnel and hospital establishments. It is printed simultaneously in English and French.

Other statistical compendiums include the following:

- *Demographic Yearbook*, published by the statistical office of the United Nations, Department of Economic and Social Affairs, New York. Statistics compiled from 250 countries of the world are included. Topics include population rates, mortality rates by disease, life expectancy tables, and marriage, divorce, and migration statistics.
- *American Statistics Index: A Comprehensive Guide and Index to the Statistical Publications of the United States Government*, published by Congressional Information Service, Inc. As this index contains all data collected by the federal government in various subjects, a researcher might find this a useful tool.
- U.S. Bureau of the Census
- U.S. Bureau of Labor Statistics
- U.S. Department of Agriculture

5.24 Directories of References

Directories of references are books that provide a comprehensive source for locating studies in specified fields. They provide lists and short reviews of available textbooks, journals, bibliographies, dictionaries, atlases, databases and government documents. The following directories are a sample of the many reference resources available to the clinical researcher. The main limitation of directories is the rapidity with which new sources of information are created, which makes it almost impossible for a directory to be up to date. It is important in using a directory that the researcher be very aware of the copyright date.

- Armstrong, C. J. (Ed.). (1993). *World Databases in Medicine*. London: Bowker-Saur. As its preface states:

    World Databases in Medicine is the first in a series of directories whose overall aim is to map the databases in twenty-three clearly defined subject disciplines—twenty-three disciplines which encompass all of mankind's knowledge. As its name implies, this directory like the others to follow, is attempting worldwide coverage and includes databases from Australasia, CIS, Europe, Scandinavia and the Far East as well as from UK and North America. (p. v)

    The book provides comprehensive information about each database, including commentaries and reviews about the database and links to similar databases. Journals and periodicals connected to databases are also identified, making it easy for the reader to find hard copy material.
- Blake, J. B., and Roos, C. (Eds.). (1967). *Medical Reference Works 1679–1966: A Selected Bibliography*. Chicago: Medical Library Assoc.

    Listed in the publication are indexes and abstracts, bibliographies, proceedings of Congress, dictionaries, periodicals, and directories related to such areas as medicine, anatomy, medical education, hospitals, neurology, psychiatry, nursing, nutrition, pediatrics, physical medicine and rehabilitation, psychology, public health research in progress, and sociology. The purpose of the publication, as stated by the editors is "to survey the world's bioscientific, medical, and allied health literature and select and organize from it an annotated list of the major works useful in gaining access to publications or frequently needed data" (p.iii). A supplement compiled by Joy S. Richmond (1975) is available, also.

- Bowker Company (1995). *Medical and Health Care Books and Serials in Print: An Index to Literature in the Health Sciences.* New York: R. R. Bowker Co.

The index covers a wide range of books and serials related to the major health sciences disciplines (e.g., medicine, dentistry, human health, nursing, nutrition, veterinary medicine, psychiatry, psychology, behavioral sciences, and other associated health sciences that are currently available from publishers. This book is a companion to *Books in Print* and *Serials in Print*.

- *Directory of Online Databases.* New York: Cuadra/Elsevier.

This annual directory contains up-to-date lists of the databases available. The directory can be searched online through a number of systems, including CompuServe and EasyLink.

- Enders, A. and Hall, M. (Eds.). (1990). *Assistive Technology Sourcebook.* Washington, D.C.: RESNA Press.

This "doorway to assistive technology resources" (p. xix) is full of information which will help practitioners and researchers obtain the technological support needed for themselves or for clients. Chapters include a list of databases and support groups and ways in which technology can be used with children, at home, at work, in leisure activities, or in mobility. The book is a must for those individuals interested in or working with individuals with disabilities.

- Morton, L. T., and Godholt, S. (Eds.). (1993). *Information Sources in the Medical Sciences.* (4th ed.). London: Bowker-Saur.

As a comprehensive guide to the medical literature, this book provides bibliographical sources for anatomy and physiology, biochemistry, public health, pharmacology, tropical medicine, pathology, microbiology, immunology, clinical medicine, psychiatry, surgery, obstetrics, gynecology, and dentistry. In addition to these specialized areas, the book includes chapters on medical libraries, primary sources of information, general indexes, abstracts, bibliographies and reviews, standard reference sources, and mechanical sources of information retrieval. The chapter on information retrieval systems is particularly helpful as there are very few references available describing these systems. Morton, an editor of the book, is from the National Institute for Medical Research in London, and subsequently, many of the sources of references cited are from Great Britain, in addition to the listed bibliographical sources from the United States.

- Reich, W. T. (Ed.). (1995). *Encyclopedia of Bioethics.* New York: Macmillian Library Reference, Simon and Schuster.

This 5 volume encyclopedia explains terms and concepts related to bioethics. The encyclopedia includes a bibliography and an index.

- Roper, F. W., and Boorkman, J. A. (1994). *Introduction to Reference Sources in the Health Sciences.* (3rd ed.). Methuen, NJ: Scarecrow.

The book contains bibliographic and informational sources of monographs, periodicals, abstracting services, databases, U.S. Government documents and technical reports, conferences, medical and health statistics, and audio-visual reference sources.

- Walters, L., and Kahn, T. J. (Eds.). (1990). *Bibliography of Bioethics* (Vol. 16). Washington, D.C.: Georgetown University, Kennedy Institute.

This bibliography of bioetheical topics is published annually and provides a comprehensive cross-disciplinary listing of journals, newspaper articles, monographs, essays, court decisions, and audiovisual materials. The bibliography is designed for anyone concerned with bioethics, including scientists, health professionals, and legal scholars.

- Welch, J., and King, T. A. (1985). *Searching the Medical Literature: A Guide to Printed and Online Sources*. London: Chapman and Hall.

The authors include valuable information in searching the periodical literature using print and computer online sources. The chapter on online sources includes descriptions of major information retrieval services such as Dialog, BRS, and the Institute for Scientific Information (ISI), among others. Sources of statistical informational are listed also.

5.25 Current Research

Current research not included in computer retrieval systems or annual reviews can be found in the most recently published periodicals. Most university and medical libraries have reading rooms where current scientific journals are placed on open shelves. A perusal of newly published articles is helpful sometimes in gaining an overview of a topic and frequently an up-to-date bibliography of related literature. Key words will often be listed under the abstract. Use of these key words to identify additional literature through databases and indexes may result in additional material. Current journals will also be helpful in locating individuals engaged in ongoing research. It is very useful to request from researchers current reprints of articles, unpublished research, and conference papers. In general, most scholars will be flattered to receive requests by individuals genuinely interested in their work, and they will respond readily. The standard format in requesting reprints is to list the bibliographical citation (i.e., journal, volume, date, and title) as in the example in Figure 5–4.

5.3 Recording Information From Research Articles

The beginning researcher should develop a system for recording, organizing, and storing information related to a content area. It is important to develop this system early in the process by recording bibiographic information from all sources at the time it is being obtained, even if the use of the material is questionable (Englehart, 1972). The reconstruction of bibliographic sources at a later time can be time-consuming and difficult. An effective method of organizing data is to use a letter-size folder for each subject heading or variable in a study. Some investigators photocopy studies from periodicals or newspapers that relate to a specific area. Using information obtained from each of these articles, researchers are able to compile an up-to-date annotated bibliography.

In recording notes from a study, a 3 × 5 index card is helpful in compiling a bibliography, while 5 × 8 index cards may be helpful for more extensive information, such as long quotes or abstracts. An example of a card is shown in Figure 5–5. The card should contain the following information from each study:

```
                                     19524 E. Lewis Avenue
                                     Marketplace, AK  99872
                                     July 15, 1995

Dear Dr. Cutler:

Please send me a reprint of your article: Language and ADHD:
Understanding the bases and treatment of self-regulatory
deficits, which was printed in 1994 in Topics in Language
Disorders, 14(4), 58-76.

                                     Sincerely,



                                     John Walker
```

Figure 5–4.   An example of a request for an article. Notice that the request includes the author, title of article, date of article, journal, and page numbers. If the article is unpublished, the request should state that.

1. A bibliographical notation that includes all information used in a citation (See Chapter 9 for examples of citations)
2. Library call number or ERIC number can be helpful also, as this allows the researcher to find the publication quickly
3. Abstract of study including number of subjects, data collection methodology, test instruments, results, and conclusions
4. Important quotations (including page numbers) that can be cited in literature review
5. Any reactions to the article, such as evaluation of the validity of results or generalizations offered.

By recording this information accurately, the researcher saves time and effort from returning to the library to look up a bibliographical notation or other missing information.

It is important to obtain information from many different types of publications. Although primary sources are used the most, valuable information can be obtained from secondary and tertiary sources. Table 5–4 provides another list of ways to categorize sources of material.

5.4 Evaluating Validity of Research Findings

The finding and citing of research are not the final processes in reviewing literature. A critical analysis is an important task of the investigator. One of the more difficult tasks in a literauture review is the ability to review the articles in an integrated fashion. One cannot evaluate and critique each article separately; rather, the integration of the information must be done by synthesizing the information (Finley, 1989). One outcome of this type of evaluation is that the reader begins to build a conceptual framework, thereby allowing for a more mature evaluation of other literature in the field.

Drager, S., Prior, M., & Sanson, A. (1986). Visual and auditory attention performance in hyperactive children: Competence or compliance. J. of Abnormal Child Psychology, 14(3), 411-424.
Examination of self-control and compliance in attention with children with hyperactivity
Subjects: 16 hyperactive (14 boys, 2 girls), previously diagnosed. Ages between 7-3 and 12-4. IQs in normal range as measured by WISC or PPVT. None on medication. Control group of 16 students w/o behavioral problems, matched for age, gender, and IQ.
Method: Ex. 1: auditory attention, dichotic listening, told to respond to word "dog" by pressing a reaction

Drager, Prior, & Sanson, p.2
button. Reaction time measured. Ex. 2. . . Ex. 3. . .
Results: "There was little evidence for the existence of attention deficits in either auditory or visual modalities in hyperactive children" (p.420). "It can therefore be argued that hyperactive children are capable of performing as well as normal children on quite difficult and tedious monitoring tasks. . ." (p. 420).
Reaction: If children w/ADHD can perform normally, why do they have such difficulty with attending? Was the methodology so different that these children stayed interested?

Figure 5-5. An example of an index card used in collecting information from articles.

The quality of the research and the validity of the conclusions need to be evaluated before the research can be integrated with other results. When contradictory results arising from different studies occur, the investigator should seek to offer an explanation based on the research methodologies. Occasionally investigators reviewing literature cite the results and conclusions of previous research without determining the size of sample, data collection procedures, and measuring instruments used. It should be obvious to the reader that results of studies involving small samples and using tests that have low reliability are not as valid as large scale studies where rigorous methodology and reliable measuring instruments are used. In reporting previous literature, the investigator should consider the following factors in evaluating the validity of the research findings:

Table 5–4   *Categorization of Publications*

Types of Publications	Examples of Publications
Primary data research	Journal articles Dissertations Theses Conference proceedings Government documents
Review of subjects	Journal articles Monographs
Evaluation findings	Joint Commission on Accreditation Results
Conceptual papers	Journal articles Monographs
Position papers	Journal articles Associational and organizational statements Monographs
Learning texts	College texts
Secondary and tertiary information	Popular magazines *Scientific American* Encyclopedias
Reviews of books, tests, self-help devices, software programs	Reference books for test instruments Journal articles reviewing books *PC Computing* or other computer journals
Bibliographic References	*Books in Print* Information retrieval system Directories of reference

- The size of sample, sampling procedure, and representativeness
- Control of extraneous variables that can potentially affect results
- Evidence of research bias in conclusions that are not consistent with results
- Selection of reliable and valid measuring instruments
- Data collection procedures
- Statistical techniques employed.

In addition to these factors, the reader should ask a number of questions about the article. These questions are summarized in Table 5–5.

5.5 Outlining the Literature Review Section

Whether the researcher is reporting results in a journal article or preparing a thesis, he or she must decide how much of the background literature should be cited. *The Publication Manual of the American Psychological Association* (1994) recommends that a writer of a journal article should:

Discuss the literature but do not include an exhaustive historical review. Assume that the reader has knowledge in the field for which you are writing . . . . A scholarly review of earlier work provides an appropriate history and recognizes the priority of the work of

Table 5–5   *Critically Reviewing a Research Article*

Introduction

- Does the introduction state the hypothesis directly and explicitly?
- Has the hypothesis directly related to the literature cited?
- Does the choice of outcome measures appear logical?
- Does the study appear feasible and useful?

Methodology

- Based on the information presented in the study, can the study be replicated?
- Were the subjects and controls chosen in a random manner?
- Are the demographics of the subjects adequately described?
- Were unusual circumstances (e.g., use of medication, time of testing) described?
- Were outcome measures used that had high validity and reliability?
- Were the outcome measures used appropriate for the population and free from external bias?
- Were appropriate statistics used for the number of subjects in the study?

Results and Discussion

- Were the results reported in an understandable and clear manner?
- Are the figures and tables clear and consistent with the text?
- Was the discussion related to the findings, or were there unrelated comments?
- Was there discussion regarding the acceptance or rejection of the null hypothesis?
- Was any mention made of the need for future research or of limitations of the study?

Note. Adapted from material published by Brendan A. Maher (1978).

others. Citation of a specific credit to relevant earlier works is part of the author's scientific and scholarly responsibility. . . .[C]ite and reference only works pertinent to the specific issue and not works of only tangential or general significance. If you summarize earlier works, avoid nonessential details; instead, emphasize pertinent findings, relevant methodological issues, and major conclusions. Refer the reader to general surveys or reviews of the topic if they are available. (p. 11)

In contrast to the journal article, the writer of a master's thesis or dissertation should include extensive background literature, which demonstrates to the reader that the researcher is cognizant of the important findings with which the present study rests. The continuity of findings should be documented by the researcher. The literature review in a master's thesis or doctoral dissertation serves as a vehicle for presenting chronologically the progression of knowledge in a specific area. Thus, the literature review should reflect the development of a problem by first presenting general background findings and then gradually narrowing to the significant variables identified in the title of the study.

A search of the literature will result in identifying literature that is directly related to the topic at hand, literature less directly related but which should be read, and literature that is not related at all. Although it will be important to peruse all of these, only the articles directly related to the topic will be used in a literature review. Locke, Spirduso, and Silverman (1987) suggest that the literature review "is made to serve the reader's query by supporting, explicating, and illuminating the logic now implicit in the proposed investigation" (p. 59). A well-written literature review allows the reader to (a) understand the significance of the research question, (b) validate the connection between previously conducted research directly related to the present research question, and (c) grasp the reasons for the proposed methodology.

The plan for presenting previous literature should include a logical development that incorporates both a chronological sequence and a topical order. By using an outline, the researcher begins to organize the data found in reviewing the literature. The outline is a working tool. It should change to accommodate new ideas and newly found evidence.

One way to develop an outline is by organizing the index cards into groups by topic. This type of organization makes the writing easier for a number of reasons. First, by examining and reviewing the cards, important themes and topics may emerge. Second, because the cards have been organized by subject, the writer does not waste time looking through the articles and other references for related material. Third, by placing the cards into groups, they can be further organized into a logical outline or sequence.

Although actually writing the literature review can be challenging for a number of reasons, the completed product gives the researcher a sense of accomplishment. The literature review section of a study should represent an extensive process that is the basis for implementing the research design. The following worksheet describes this process.

5.6 Worksheet for Literature Review

1. State the research problem in question form.
2. What are the variables identified in the study?
   - Independent Variables:
   - Dependent Variables:
   - Target Populations:
   - Specific Setting for Study (e.g., hospital, clinic):
3. Checklist for locating references (list titles).
   - Information Retrieval Systems:
   - Directories of References:
   - Bibliographical Indexes:
   - Annual Reviews:
   - Abstracting Periodicals:
   - Textbooks:
4. Primary Sources Utilized (list)
   - Journals:
   - Statistical Compendium:
   - Conference Proceedings:
   - Theses and Dissertations:

CHAPTER
6

Research Design and Methodology

The quality of research depends not only upon the adequacy of the research design but also upon the fruitfulness of the data-collection techniques which are employed. The purpose of the various data-collection techniques is simply to produce precise and reliable evidence which is relevant to the research questions being asked. Fulfillment of this purpose, however is rarely simple.—M. Jahoda, M. Deutsch, and S. W. Cook, *Research Methods in Social Relations* (p. 92)

••

Operational Learning Objectives

By the end of this chapter, the reader should be able to

1. state a research hypothesis or guiding question
2. operationally define a research variable
3. identify any assumptions underlying a proposed research study
4. diagram a research study
5. identify the possible methodological limitations in a research study
6. state the theoretical rationale underlying a proposed research study
7. design a procedure for selecting subjects for a study
8. design screening criteria for subject inclusion
9. define and contrast the terms *random sampling, random assignment, convenient sampling, representative sampling*, and *target population*
10. define *test reliability* and *test validity*
11. evaluate the feasibility, reliability, and validity of a published test or measuring instrument
12. compare and contrast the four scales of measurement
13. understand the concept of internal validity
14. design a data collection procedure for a proposed research study
15. understand ethical principles underlying human research
16. outline a research proposal including an informed consent protocol
17. understand the concept of external validity
18. describe the major research designs and methodological limitations of a study

• •

6.1 Proposing a Feasible Research Question

The initial step in research is asking the right questions. Science progresses along the continuum of knowledge by researchers seeking solutions to key problems. Historically, researchers have advanced knowledge by posing feasible questions. For example:

- What are the basic anatomical structures and physiological functions of human beings?
- How are diseases transmitted?
- What chemical substances destroy specific microorganisms that cause diseases?
- How can we detect the presence of trace chemicals in foods and in blood?
- What are the causes of specific diseases?
- What is the effect on the family of having a child with disabilities?
- What are the most effective methods for rehabilitating individuals with traumatic brain injury?

Numerous questions have been raised by scientists that have guided research and led to solutions. In the research design section the investigator raises specific testable or feasible questions that guide the data collection.

In proposing research the investigator considers the following areas:

1. Statements of hypotheses or guiding questions
2. Operational definitions of variables
3. Underlying assumptions of the study

4. Diagrammatical relationship between variables
5. Methodological limitations of the study
6. Overall theoretical rationale guiding the study.

6.2 Statement of Hypothesis

An *hypothesis* is a statement predicting the relationship between variables. In logic it is stated as an *if-then* contingency. For example, consider the hypothesis: There is a positive statistically significant relationship between obesity and heart disease in sedentary workers. In this hypothesis there is a predicted relationship between obesity and heart disease among sedentary workers expressed as *if* obesity (in sedentary workers), *then* heart disease. The hypothesis contains the question and predicts a directional relationship. (A direction could be either positive or inverse.)

How does the investigator arrive at a hypothesis or guiding question? The review of literature as discussed in Chapter 5 serves as the generating force in guiding the hypothesis or guiding question proposed. The relationship between the research question, guiding question, and hypothesis is described in Table 6–1. The hypothesis is a specific statement that can be derived from a research question or guiding question. Table 6–2 shows the relationship between the research model and statement of hypothesis or guiding question.

In all research the investigator needs to state a guiding question or hypothesis that leads to data collection. Once these are stated then the researcher needs to operationally define the variables as stated in the guiding question or hypothesis.

6.3 Operationally Defining a Variable

An *operational definition* makes it possible for researchers to replicate a research study. Many differences arising from inconsistent results among several investigators often can

Table 6–1 *The Relationship Between a Research Question, Guiding Question, and Hypothesis*

	Definition	Purpose	Example
Research Question	Broad inquiry into a general area of investigation	Lead individual into an extensive literature review	What is the relationship between repetitive motion and hand injuries?
Guiding Question	Statement of inquiry that leads to data collection	Identify factors that relate to a specific research question	What factors in repetitive motion injury are related to carpal tunnel syndrome?
Hypothesis	Detailed statement that can be tested through inferential statistics	Evaluate effective or significant relationship between variables	Hypothesis: There is no statistically significant difference in the use of biofeedback vs. splinting in remediating the symptoms of carpal tunnel syndrome.

Table 6–2 *The Relationship Between Research Model and Hypothesis*

Research Models	Statements	Examples of Research Questions
Experimental (Prospective Research Design)	Hypothesis: directional or null	How effective is exercise in treating repetitive motion injuries?
Methodological	Guiding question	What factors must be considered in designing a (specific) instrument or test?
Evaluation	Guiding question	How effective is this organization or facility in relationship to a priori criteria or internal objectives?
Heuristic (Retrospective Research Design)	Guiding question	What risk factors are related to the etiology of multiple sclerosis?
Correlational	Hypothesis directional or null	What is the degree of relationship between perceptual motor abilities and reading?
Clinical Observation (Case Study or Qualitative)	Guiding question	What are the dynamic factors and processes underlying the cause of schizophrenia in a specific individual?
Survey	Guiding question	What are the characteristics of (an identifiable) target population?
Historical	Guiding question	What is the chronology of an event, discovery, or health issue?

be traced to different operational definitions of the same stated conceptual variables. For example, the following variables could become ambiguous unless one specifically describes in detail how they are measured or procedurally defined:

- Cognitive rehabilitation
- Intelligence
- Language disorder
- Muscle strength
- Spasticity
- Sensory-integration therapy
- Visual motor ability
- Work hardening

Research became rigorous when researchers described experimental procedures in detail so that other investigators could duplicate the exact experiment or study. The rigor in operationally defining a variable is associated with *internal validity*. Results cannot be accepted unless it is known how the investigator defined the variables. Conflicts over the effectiveness of treatment techniques, descriptions of target populations, and measurements of outcome are caused by comparing seemingly similar variables, which are, in fact, different because of the way they are measured. How many definitions are there for self-perception, cognitive disability, language therapy, manual dexterity, and work capacity? The conceptualization of variables described by investigators may be entirely different if they are not operationally defined. Ineffectual research is typified by the omission of operational definitions. A further problem is compounded when investigators synthesize findings in an area by "lumping" studies. For example, if intellectual potential is defined operationally through group tests, individual tests, teacher perceptions, and academic achievement, then conflicts will arise when examining the relationship between intelligence and a variable such as social class. A researcher's often fallacious interpretation of the literature and subsequent invalid conclusions are a result of equating variables even though the operational definitions are different.

What factors must be considered in operationally defining a variable? In this process, the investigator should consider the following questions:

- What is the theoretical rationale underlying the definition?
- What is the accepted definition of a variable as stated in a dictionary or encyclopedia?
- How is the variable measured?
- Does the investigator need to establish the screening criteria in defining a target population?
- Is the variable defined by a standardized procedure?
- Can a mathematical formula be employed in the definition?

The following is an example of how government agencies have traditionally operationally defined specific criteria (National Center for Health Studies, 1974).

Example of Operational Definitions Establishing Criteria
Criteria for Classifying Nursing Homes

The criteria for classifying institutions are based on several factors: (a) the number of persons receiving nursing care during the week prior to the day of the survey; (b) administration of medications and treatments in accordance with physician's orders; (c) supervision over medications that may be self-administered; (d) the routine provision of the following criterion of personal services: rub and massage, help with tub bath or shower, help with dressing, correspondence, shopping, walking or getting about, and help with eating; and (e) the employment of registered professional or licensed practical nurses. On the basis of these factors, four types of establishments were distinguished and defined as follows:

1. **Nursing care home.** An establishment is a nursing home if nursing care is the primary and predominant function of the facility. Those meeting the following criteria are classified as nursing care homes in this report: One or more registered nurses or licensed practical nurses are employed, and 50% or more of the residents received care during the week prior to the survey. (*Nursing care* is defined as the provision of one or more of the following services: nasal feeding, catheterization, irrigation, oxygen therapy, full bed bath, enema, hypodermic injection, intravenous injection, temperature-pulse-perspiration, blood pressure, application of dressings or bandages, and bowel and bladder retraining.)
2. **Personal care home with nursing.** An establishment is a personal care home with nursing if personal care is the primary and predominant function of the facility but some nursing care is provided also. If an establishment met either of the following criteria, it was classified as a personal care home with nursing:

- Some, but less than 50%, of the residents received nursing care during the week prior to the survey and there was one registered professional or licensed practical nurse or more on the staff;
- Some of the residents received nursing care during the week prior to the survey, no registered nurses or licensed practical nurses were on the staff, but one or more of the following conditions were met:

  - Medications and treatments were administered in accordance with physician's orders.
  - Supervision over self-administered medications was provided.
  - Three or more personal services were routinely provided.

3. **Personal care home.** An establishment is a personal care home if the primary and predominant function of the facility is personal care and no residents received nursing care during the week prior to the survey. Places in which one or both of the following criteria were met are classified as personal care homes in this report whether or not they employed registered nurses or licensed practical nurses.

  - Medication and treatments were administered in accordance with physician's orders, or supervision over medications that may be self-administered was provided.
  - Three or more of the criteria of personal services were routinely provided.

4. **Domiciliary care home.** A facility is a domiciliary care home if the primary and predominant function of the facility is domiciliary care, but the facility has a responsibility for providing some personal care. If the criteria for a nursing care home or personal care home are not met, but one or two of the criteria of personal services are routinely provided, the establishment is classified as a domiciliary care home in this report.

In the classification process, a criterion was considered as not having been met if the necessary information for that criterion was unknown. For instance, if the type of nursing staff was unknown for a particular place, it was considered as not having met the criteria of having one or more registered nurses or licensed practical nurses on the staff. Establishments indicating that some nursing care was provided but not giving the number of persons to whom this care was provided were considered institutions providing nursing care to some but less than 50% of their patients or residents.

Classification of Hospitals

General medical and surgical hospitals are establishments licensed as hospitals that provide diagnostic and treatment services for patients who have a variety of medical conditions both surgical and nonsurgical. For purposes of this report, a hospital unit of an institution (prison hospital, college infirmary, etc.) is considered a general hospital.

Specialty hospitals are establishments licensed as hospitals that usually limit their admissions to patients with specified illnesses or conditions only. The specialty hospitals discussed in this report are psychiatric, tuberculosis, chronic disease, rehabilitation, maternity, and alcoholic or narcotic. The remaining types of specialty hospitals are grouped together and called "other." This category includes Armed Forces dispensaries; eye, ear, nose and throat hospitals; orthopedic hospitals; and any other type of hospital not already specified. As section B(2) on the hospital questionnaire indicates, there are two categories for the mentally retarded: a hospital unit within a school for individuals with mental retardation and an institution for individuals with mental retardation. Any facility that was one of these two types was removed from the hospital list and placed on the MR portion of the "other health facilities" list.

6.4 Stating Assumptions

A researcher undertaking an investigation may make certain assumptions that are usually unstated. These assumptions can be on a general level, such as:

- All diseases have a cause.
- Intelligence is the result of the interaction between genetic structure and environmental opportunities.
- Obesity is the result of overeating and inactivity.
- Language development is maturational.
- Disengagement from social activity is a learned behavior rather than a biological determinant.
- Learning is a complex variable that is not entirely based on external reinforcement.

Other assumptions can be more subtle such as:

- Rehabilitation of individuals with severe disabilities should have a high priority in a society.
- People with an alcohol dependency should be treated as persons with medical problems rather than as criminals.
- Drug addiction is a social problem rather than a criminal problem.
- Individuals with mental retardation should be integrated into community schools rather than isolated in large institutions.

In designing a research study the investigator should be aware of all the assumptions underlying the study. Whether the assumptions are made explicit in reporting the results is at the discretion of the researcher. However, in preparing a research proposal, it is important that all assumptions be stated.

When distinguishing an assumption from established evidence, it should be clear from the previous examples that assumptions are controversial or inconclusive theory that can also reflect the investigator's values or prejudices. Many assumptions are tacitly implied by an investigator who assumes that all people accept certain beliefs or hold certain opinions. A researcher should try to identify all assumptions being made in the study as an indication of his or her own subjective biases and beliefs. Whenever possible, a reference should be used when stating assumptions. The reference could be either theoretical or supported by research.

6.5 Diagrammatical Relationships Between Variables

In clarifying the research design, it is helpful for the investigator to diagram the study, especially in a proposal, showing the relationship between variables, populations sampled, and operational definitions. For example a researcher is interested in testing two methods of articulation therapy with children with cerebral palsy and dysarthria. The study (which is an experimental model) is diagramed as follows:

In *Experimental Research:*

TWO INDEPENDENT VARIABLES		**DEPENDENT VARIABLE**
• Group 1, cognitive approach • Group 2, behavioral management		• Articulation level as measured by Arizona Test of Articulation

PRETEST:	**INTERVENTION:**	**POSTTEST:**
Test of articulation two groups, 10 subjects in each, randomly assigned	two experimental Independent variables	Test of articulation 3 months after pretest

POPULATION: Children with cerebral palsy: screening criteria include diagnosis, degree of disability, age, gender, intelligence, and SES (socioeconomic status)

GUIDING QUESTION: Is the cognitive approach more effective than behavior management in remediating articulation?

STATISTICAL TESTS: Independent *t* test

A correlational model would be diagramed in a hypothetical study involving coma. The variables are now considered to have an associational or statistical relationship. The independent variable is not experimentally induced.

In *Correlational Research:*

PRESUMED INDEPENDENT VARIABLE	**PRESUMED DEPENDENT VARIABLE**
• Days in coma as measured by the Glasgow Coma Scale (1 hour to 6 weeks)	• Degree of severity of cognitive deficits as measured by the Halstead-Reitan
	Time period, patient tested: 1 month post coma 6 months post coma

TARGET POPULATION: 30 individuals with closed head injury sustained in a motor vehicle accident and in a coma at least 1 hour

VARIABLES TO CONTROL FOR: Age, gender, handedness, treatment facility

GUIDING QUESTION: Is there a statistically significant relationship between the number of days in a coma and the severity of the symptoms?

STATISTICAL TEST: Spearman rank order correlation coefficient

In methodological research (such as in developing a test) the researcher would use the following diagram:

In *Methodological Research*:		
OBJECTIVES	**POPULATION**	**INSTRUMENT**
• measure sensory abilities	• children, birth to 3 years, with typical development	• Individually administered, developmentally appropriate tasks

RELIABILITY: Test–retest (consider maturation)

VALIDITY: Correlate test with an established instrument (concurrent validity)

GUIDING QUESTION: What factors must be considered in devising a test of sensory abilities in children from birth to 3 years old?

STATISTICAL TESTS: Correlation and multivariate tests (e.g., factor analysis)

In evaluation research the investigator would use the following diagram:

In *Evaluation Research*:	
HEALTH CARE SYSTEM OR FACILITY (individuals interviewed)	**CRITERIA FOR EVALUATION** (Examples)
• consumer population • direct service workers • consultants • support staff	• treatment outcome • quality of care • staff-patient ratio • physical plant

GUIDING QUESTION: How effective is the health care system in meeting the internal objectives or a priori criteria?

STATISTICAL TESTS: Descriptive statistics

In *heuristic research* such as in discovering risk factors in a disease, the following diagram is described:

In *Heuristic Research*:		
DISABILITY OR DISEASE	**RISK FACTORS** (OPERATIONALLY DEFINED)	**POPULATION**
Heart Disease (Example)	• age at onset of illness • gender • smoking • alcohol	• patients with post-coronary heart disease • representative sample

(continued)

In *Heuristic Research*: *(continued)*

DISABILITY OR DISEASE	RISK FACTORS (OPERATIONALLY DEFINED)	POPULATION
(Retrospective Research Design)	• dietary habits • use of drugs • blood pressure • personality • socioeconomic status • occupation • activity level	

GUIDING QUESTION: What are the risk factors for heart disease?

STATISTICAL TESTS: Correlation and multiple regression

In *Clinical Observation* (qualitative or ethnological research):

PROCESS OR BEHAVIOR	POPULATION	OBSERVATIONAL METHODS
Childhood Schizophrenia (operationally defined)	• Intact Family	• live with family for six months • record mechanically family interactions

GUIDING QUESTION: What effect does the interaction between the family and the child have on the child's symptoms/illness in childhood schizophrenia?

STATISTICAL TESTS: Descriptive statistics

In the following diagram, the researcher surveys (as an example) the degree of job satisfaction among occupational therapists:

In *Survey (Qualitative) Research:*

	EXAMPLES
TARGET POPULATION:	All registered occupational therapists: 50,000 OTRs in the U.S. (1995)
REPRESENTATIVE SAMPLE (SURVEYED):	10% of OTRs: 5,000 projected
STATISTIC (RESPONDENTS):	50% of sample: 2,500 OTRs

METHOD: Mail questionnaire to subjects

In *Survey (Qualitative) Research: (continued)*

TEST: Reliable and valid test of job satisfaction (qualitative research)

GUIDING QUESTION: What is the level of job satisfaction among OTRs in the U.S.?

STATISTICAL TESTS: Descriptive, frequency distribution table

In *Historical Research:*

TOPIC	**PRIMARY SOURCES**	**OBJECTIVES**
History of rehabilitation movement in the U.S. (Example)	• Conference proceedings • Government documents • Journal articles • Letters • Interviews	• Chronology of events listing individuals who were significant in the growth of rehabilitation and factors in history that influenced society's support

GUIDING QUESTION: What were the factors that led to the rehabilitation movement in the U.S.?

STATISTICS: Tables, figures, and charts that describe the data

6.6 Theoretical Rationale

Theory generates research and research generates theory. Research should be a planned activity based upon a theoretical rationale. Why are variables correlated? Why do we think this treatment will work? Why do we project these results? What factors justify the conclusions proposed? The researcher is not only interested in the questions *Does it work?* or *Is it curative?* but *Why is the treatment effective? Why is there a relationship between causative factors and the onset of illness?* Theories in science are in a continual state of change. As knowledge progresses in an area, theory changes to accommodate the new information. Researchers do not assume that theories and knowledge are static. What is accepted as truth currently may be revised later when new research data are obtained.

The investigator needs to state the underlying theory generating the research design, even if it is meager and incomplete. Research is not justified if we collect meaningless bits of information for future analysis. For example, if a researcher working on techniques to improve language skills in children with severe mental retardation finds a statistically significant difference between behavior modification and a comparable method in motivating the children to learn, but does not explain why behavior modification is effective, the research is incomplete. If, in this example, the group which received behavior modification significantly improved in their language skills more than the control group, the reader is left to speculate the causes for the differences. Was the Hawthorne effect controlled? Are there other explanations? The absence of a theoretical explanation leaves a gap in the research and leaves it open to the reader to speculate why language development was enhanced. Speculations are raised such as:

- Interpersonal relationships influenced learning.
- Treatment stimulated neurological development.
- Traditional training was effective.
- Tests selected were unreliable and inappropriate.

Many speculations can be made in the absence of a theoretical rationale. Research should be guided by theory and explanation and not merely present data describing the relationships between variables.

6.7 Internal Validity

Internal validity is a theoretical concept that refers to the rigor in an experiment or research design. The degree of internal validity depends on the extent to which the investigator has controlled all variables that can potentially affect the results. If an experiment or research design is judged to have good internal validity, then the experimenter has been able to control for factors that could potentially distort the results. High internal validity is demonstrated by:

- Double-blind study where the investigator eliminates researcher bias and subject influence
- Control of the placebo effect where the subject's suggestibility and personal influence are eliminated
- Control group to eliminate the Hawthorne effect
- Matching comparative groups to insure that all groups being compared are not different in variables such as age, gender, degree of disability, intelligence, and socioeconomic status
- Baseline measure of pretest to insure that comparative groups are equivalent
- Posttest measures that are compared to pretest measures
- High reliability and validity of outcome measures or tests to insure that variables are accurately measured
- Regard for maturational factors that could distort results
- Random selection of subjects to reduce bias in samples
- Standardization of administering test and research procedures
- Control for practice effect in test taking to insure that gain in scores is not due to the participant's familiarity with test.

6.8 Methodology Section

The methodology section of a study includes the following components: the method of selecting subjects, location of study, description of tests and apparati used in measuring variables, procedure for collecting data, statistical techniques used for analyzing data, computer use (if applicable), projection of time for completing the study, and the procedure of obtaining informed consent from human subjects. Pragmatic as well as rational considerations guide the investigator in finding the answer to the following questions:

- How many subjects should be included in the study?
- Should subjects be randomly selected, volunteers, or a convenient sample?
- Where should the study take place?
- What tests, diagnostic procedures, questionnaires, or rating scales should be employed in the study?
- What are the procedures and time sequence for data collection?
- What are the costs of the study?

The sequential process for the research methodology is shown in Figure 6–1.

6.9 Selection of Subjects

One prime purpose of research is to discover relationships between variables in sample groups and to generalize these relationships to a larger population. The ability to generalize results establishes the *external validity* of a study. Since research usually involves sample groups from populations rather than the total population, the selection of a representative sample is crucial when generalizing results.

In selecting a sample, the first step is to identify a target population. For example, paraplegics, juvenile offenders, allied health professionals, special education teachers, undergraduate students in dietetics, and administrators of rehabilitation programs are identifiable populations. The target population is narrowed considerably by establishing a screening criteria for subject inclusion. A screening criteria contains both *inclusional* and *exclusional* factors. For example, a researcher interested in cardiac rehabilitation may want to select a specific population within the area of cardiovascular disease. The screening criteria will enable the investigator to identify a specific population and to control the variables that could potentially affect the results. In setting up a screening criteria for cardiac patients, variables such as age, sex, socioeconomic status, occupation, body type (endomorph, ectomorph, and mesomorph), onset of illness, and range of cardiorespiratory function as indicated by pulse rate would be considered.

Refinement of these variables should narrow the population. Middle-class, urban, male coronary patients between the ages of 55 and 65 who are primarily sedentary, and whose resting pulse rates are within the normal range are an example of a research population obtained from a priori criteria. In considering exclusional factors, the researcher specifies variables that are screened out of the study. Exclusional variables could include absence of secondary illnesses (as determined by clinical examination).

The example from a double case study by Kopolow and Jensen (1975) shows the extensiveness of criteria employed in selecting two subjects with quadriplegia. (See Table 6–3.) Screening criteria are identified prior to subject selection. The investigator opera-

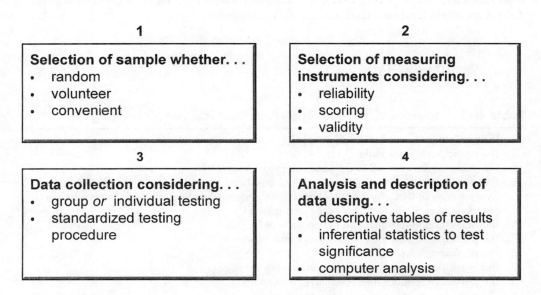

1

Selection of sample whether. . .
- random
- volunteer
- convenient

2

Selection of measuring instruments considering. . .
- reliability
- scoring
- validity

3

Data collection considering. . .
- group *or* individual testing
- standardized testing procedure

4

Analysis and description of data using. . .
- descriptive tables of results
- inferential statistics to test significance
- computer analysis

Figure 6–1. Sequential process of research methodology. Notice that there are four basic steps, and within those steps, questions that must be answered.

tionally defines the variables identified in the criteria. The rigor in specifying the population to be studied within a narrow domain enables other investigators to replicate the research design by isolating specific variables. By specifying the population and operationally defining the variables in the screening criteria, the investigator has identified a target population.

The next step in selecting subjects for the study is to locate all of the units in the target population. Studies of the personality characteristics of allied health professionals, for example, would entail obtaining annual directories of members from professional associations. However, in caution, it is to be noted that not all practicing therapists are members of their professional associations. (See Table 6–4 for a list of professional organizations.) It would be important to estimate the number of individuals of a population who are excluded because of the sampling procedure. Location of populations with disabilities, such as individuals with paraplegia living in the community, could be obtained through consumer organizations that represent geographical areas. By geographically limiting the representativeness of the study, the investigator controls for social and environmental factors that could potentially affect the results. On the other hand, the investigator may want to guide the scope of the study by identifying *stratified samples*, that is, homogeneous subgroups of a population based on variables such as geography, educational level, and treatment setting (community vs. hospital, or disability group). Stratified samples are usually determined by previous evidence implying that the variable identified has a significant effect on a dependent variable. For example, in examining the guiding question *Does exercise affect heart efficiency?* the investigator would control for the variable of smoking because previous evidence has related smoking to heart disease. In using stratified samples the investigator would separate out populations of smokers from nonsmokers.

Participants may also be obtained by contacting members of support groups. Table 6–5 provides a selected list of support groups that may be helpful in obtaining participants. Additional ideas for obtaining participants can be obtained from the following reference, which lists addresses and telephone numbers of approximately 27,000 national and international support groups: C. A. Schwartz, and P. K. Daniels, (1992). *Encyclopedia of Associations* (2nd ed.). Detroit: Gale Research, Inc.

Table 6–3 *Screening Criteria for Study Participant Inclusion (Quadriplegia)*

1. The participants were individuals with C_{5-6} traumatic quadriplegia.
2. The participants were male.
3. The participants were 18 to 26 years of age at onset of injury.
4. The participants had at least a high school education.
5. One participant was engaged in either full- or part-time employment, including student and/or homemaker. One participant was unemployed.
6. The participants were residing in nonmedical facilities.
7. The participants were one to two years post injury.
8. The participants were Caucasian.
9. The participants were native English-speaking Americans.
10. The participants had normal cognitive functioning.
11. The participants' medical records were available.
12. The participants were willing to participate in the study and signed an informed consent form.

Table 6-4 *Addresses of Selected Professional Associations*

- **American Association for Respiratory Care Therapy**
  1720 Regal Row
  Dallas, TX 75235
  (214) 243–2272

- **American Academy of Physician Assistants**
  950 N. Washington St.
  Alexandria, VA 22314
  (703) 836–2272

- **American Association of University Affiliated Programs (AAUAP)**
  8605 Cameron Street, Suite 406
  Silver Spring, MD 20901
  (301) 588–8252

- **American Association on Mental Deficiency (AAMD)**
  1719 Kalorama Road NW
  Washington, DC 20009
  (202) 287–1968

- **American Chiropractic Association**
  1702 Clarendon Blvd.
  Arlington, VA 22209
  (703) 276–8860

- **American Dental Association**
  211 East Chicago Ave.
  Chicago, IL 60611
  (312) 440–2500

- **American Council of the Blind**
  1010 Vermont Avenue NW, Suite 1100
  Washington, DC 20005
  (202) 393–3666

- **American Dietetic Association**
  215 W. Jackson Blvd., Suite 800
  Chicago, IL 60611
  (312) 899–0040

- **American Health Information Management Association (Medical Records)**
  191 N. Michigan Ave., Suite 1400
  Chicago, IL 60690
  (312) 787–2672

- **American Hospital Association**
  840 Lake Shore Dr.
  Chicago, IL 60611
  (312) 280–6000

- **American Medical Association**
  515 N. State St.
  Chicago, IL 60610
  (312) 464–4818

- **American Nurses Association**
  600 Maryland Ave. SW, Suite 100W
  Washington, DC 20013–2571
  (202) 554–4444

- **American Occupational Therapy Association (AOTA)**
  4720 Montgomery Ln.
  P. O. Box 31220
  Bethesda, MD 20824–1220
  (301) 652–2682

- **American Optometric Association**
  243 N. Lindberg Blvd.
  St. Louis, MO 63141
  (314) 991–4100

- **American Orthotic and Prosthetic Association**
  1650 King St., Suite 500
  Alexandria, VA 22314
  (703) 836–7116

- **American Osteopathic Association**
  142 E. Ontario St.
  Chicago, IL 60611
  (312) 280–5800

- **American Pharmaceutical Association**
  2215 Constitution Ave. NW
  Washington, DC 20037
  (202) 628–4410

- **American Physical Therapy Association**
  1111 North Fairfax St.
  Alexandria, VA 22314
  (703) 857–1150

- **American Podiatry Association**
  9312 Old Georgetown Rd.
  Bethesda, MD 20814
  (301) 571–9200

- **American Psychological Association (APA)**
  1200 17th St. NW
  Washington, DC 20036
  1–800–374–2721

- **American Registry of Radiologic Technologists**
  1255 Northland
  Mendota Heights, MN 55120
  (612) 687–0048

- **American Speech–Language–Hearing Association (ASHA)**
  10801 Rockville Pike
  Rockville, MD 20852
  (301) 897–5700

(continued)

Table 6–4 *(continued)*

- **American Society for Medical Technology**
  7910 Woodmont Ave., Suite 1301
  Bethesda, MD 20814
  (301) 657–2768

- **Association and Directory of Acupuncture**
  2 Harrowby Ct., Seymour Place
  London, WI, ENGLAND

- **Council for Exceptional Children (CEC; Special Education)**
  1920 Association Dr.
  Reston, VA 22091–1589
  (703) 264–9948

- **Council for Learning Disabilities (CLD)**
  P. O. Box 40303
  Overland Park, KS 66204
  (913) 492–8755

- **National Association of School Psychologists (NASP)**
  4340 East West Highway, Suite 402
  Bethesda, MD 20814
  (301) 657–0270

- **National Association of Social Workers**
  750 1st St. NE
  Washington, DC 20002
  (202) 408–8600

- **National Rehabilitation Association**
  633 S. Washington St.
  Alexandria, VA 22314
  (703) 836–0850

- **National Therapeutic Recreation Society**
  3101 Park Center Dr., 12th Floor
  Alexandria, VA 22302
  (703) 820–4940

- **RESNA, an Association for the Advancement of Assistive Technology**
  1101 Connecticut Ave. NW, Suite 700
  Washington, DC 20036
  (202) 857–1199

6.9.1 External Validity

External validity refers to the researcher's ability to generalize the results of an experiment from a sample to a total population. In general, researchers seek to generalize the results from an experiment to the population at large. For example, if a researcher found in a clinical study that aerobic exercise is effective in reducing depression, can the results be generalized to all individuals with clinical depression? The extent to which an investigator can with confidence generalize the results of a study depends on the number of subjects in the study and whether the study has been replicated and confirmed previous results. It is not unusual for government agencies to sponsor extensive clinical trials using large numbers of subjects to test the effectiveness of a new vaccine. These type of studies have a high degree of external validity. The example of the development of the polio vaccine demonstrates the ability to obtain external validity from one extensive clinical trial. However, external validity is also dependent on internal validity. In other words, the results of a study cannot be generalized to a population if internal validity is weak.

6.9.2 Random Sampling

Random sampling and *random assignment* are seen by researchers as methodological virtues. If a study includes a random selection of subjects, it is assumed that the investi-

Table 6–5 *Selected List of Support Groups*

- **Alzheimer's Association**
  919 N. Michigan Ave., Suite 1000
  Chicago, IL 60611
  (312) 335–8700

- **American Cancer Society**
  1599 Clifton Rd. NE
  Atlanta, GA 30329
  (404) 320–3333

- **American Heart Association**
  7272 Greenville Ave.
  Dallas, TX 75231–4596
  (214) 373–6300

- **American Lung Association**
  1740 Broadway
  New York, NY 10019–4374
  (212) 315–8700

- **The Arc (Association for Retarded Citizens)**
  500 E. Border St., Suite 300
  Arlington, TX 76010
  (817) 261–6003

- **Arthritis Foundation**
  1314 Spring St. NW
  Atlanta, GA 30309
  (404) 872–7100

- **Association for Children with Retarded Mental Development**
  162 5th Ave. 11th Floor
  New York, NY 10010
  (212) 741–0100

- **Autism Society of America**
  8601 Georgia Ave., Suite 503
  Silver Spring, MD 20410
  (301) 565–0433

- **Brain Injury Association** (formerly National Head Injury Association)
  1776 Massachusetts Av., NW, Suite 100
  Washington, DC 20036
  1–800–444–6443

- **Children with Attention Deficit Disorders (CHADD)**
  1859 North Pine Island Road, Suite 185
  Plantation, FL 33322
  (305) 587–3700

- **Cystic Fibrosis Foundation (CFF)**
  6931 Arlington Road
  Bethesda, MD 20814
  (301) 951–4422 / 1–800–344–4823

- **Epilepsy Foundation of America**
  4351 Garden City Dr., Suite 406
  Landover, MD 20785
  (301) 459–3700

- **Learning Disabilities Association**
  4156 Library Rd.
  Pittsburgh, PA 15234
  (412) 341–1414

- **Multiple Sclerosis Foundation**
  6340 N. Andrew Ave.
  Ft. Lauderdale, FL 33309
  (305) 776–6805

- **Muscular Dystrophy Association**
  3300 E. Sunrise Dr.
  Tucson, AZ 85718
  (602) 529–2000

- **National Alliance for the Mentally Ill**
  2101 Wilson Blvd., Suite. 302
  Arlington, VA 22201
  (702) 542–7600

- **National Association of People with AIDS**
  1413 K St. NW
  Washington, DC 20005
  (202) 848–0414

- **National Easter Seal Society (NESS)**
  2023 West Ogden
  Chicago, IL 60612
  (312) 243–8400

- **National Spinal Cord Injury Association**
  600 W. Cummings Park, Suite 2000
  Woburn, MA 01801
  (617) 935–2732 / 1–800–962–9629

- **Orton Dyslexia Society**
  8600 La Salle Road
  Baltimore, MD 21286–2044
  (410) 296–0232 / 1–800–222–3123

- **Spina Bifida Association of America**
  4590 MacArthur Blvd NW, Suite 250
  Washington, DC 20007
  (202) 944–3285

- **The Association for the Severely Handicapped (TASH)**
  1600 W. Armory Way
  Seattle, WA 98119
  (206) 283–5055

- **United Cerebral Palsy Association**
  1522 K. St. NW, Suite 1112
  Washington, DC, 20005
  (202) 842–1266 / 1–800–872–5827

gator has controlled for researcher bias when selecting a representative sample of the population. The concept of random sampling implies that in a population (which includes all the components, such as all physical therapists, all patients with schizophrenia, all nursing homes) units of subjects or institutions are representative of the total population. Random sampling is a method to select a representative group from the population. Random sampling does not necessarily ensure a representative group; it serves to eliminate researcher bias in selecting a sample. One method used in random sampling is to assign a number to each population unit and select a representative sample by choosing units from a list of random numbers. For example, an investigator wants to randomly select 40 undergraduate programs in physical therapy that are representative of all the programs, totaling approximately 141 in the United States. The investigator would assign a number from 1 to 141 to each school and then from a list of random numbers select 40 schools. Because the schools are dispersed throughout the country, a representative sample of 40 should reflect the geographical distribution. If a check of the 40 schools reveals that the sample is biased in the direction of a single region, then repeated random selections would be obtained until a fair degree of geographical representativeness occurs. At this point, the reader may ask, why bother with obtaining a sample from random numbers? Why not just merely select a school from each geographical region? The reason this is not valid is because the researcher may overtly or inadvertently select schools that are typical of an educational philosophy or teaching model. Random sampling is simply a method to ensure researcher objectivity. In clinical research on human subjects it is sometimes difficult because subjects have the option to participate in the study. Another difficulty is in applying random sampling techniques to potentially large populations of individuals with disabilities situated in a wide geographical area. Is it possible to randomly sample all children with hyperactivity, all patients with coronary disease, all prison inmates, all adolescents who are socially disadvantaged, or all individuals with paraplegia in the United States? The complexities and problems in locating every subject in the population do not warrant the errors that will occur by the very nature of the process. If random sampling of large populations is not practical, are there other objective selection methods that a clinical researcher can use? The answer to this question is yes—if the researcher maintains objectivity by devising systematic methods to obtain subjects and by narrowing the population. By delimiting the population, the investigator can apply random sampling techniques. For example, instead of defining the population as all patients with arthritis in the United States, the researcher delimits the population to all patients with arthritis treated in a specific hospital. The title of the study should describe the population sampled. For example, consider the following titles:

- Survey of Hand Function in the Patient with Arthritis
- Survey of the Hand Function of Individuals with Arthritis in a Boston General Hospital

In the first example the investigator implies that the survey represents all patients with arthritis. In the second example the investigator has delimited the population to those patients with arthritis receiving treatment in a specific hospital. For most investigators it is almost impossible to feasibly sample a nationwide population of patients with arthritis. The difficulty in locating every member of the population, the cost of the survey, and the extensive time involved in collecting data are practical considerations that would hinder such a study.

6.9.3 Convenient Sample and Volunteers

On the other hand, it is valid to randomly sample from a *convenient population* (i.e., a population readily available to a researcher), as long as the researcher does not generalize the results to that portion of the population that was not sampled. In selecting a random sampling of patients with arthritis from an identified population, the researcher would consider the following factors:

- Diagnosis of arthritis operationalized by physician evaluation, or anatomical/physiological evidence
- Age groupings separated into designated units
- Differentiation of sex
- Occupational groupings, such as professional, skilled, unskilled
- Socioeconomic status
- Educational level
- Age of onset
- Presence of stress
- Other relevant variables that could potentially affect the onset and course of arthritis, such as personality, obesity, and geographical area.

The variables above can be used to establish screening criteria for subject inclusion in the study or in setting up striated groups that can later be statistically analyzed for differences.

Another method to counteract researcher bias in selecting subjects is *random assignment*. For instance, an investigator is interested in comparing simultaneously two treatment methods for patients with stroke. Random assignment would be applied after a population of patients with stroke in a specific rehabilitation center is identified by screening criteria. The investigator would establish two samples by randomly assigning subjects to each group from a list of random numbers. In this hypothetical example, the selection of the specific rehabilitation center where the patients with stroke were being treated actually provides a convenient population.

Another frequently used method of obtaining subjects in clinical research is the use of *volunteers*. The limitation of using volunteers is that they are a self-selected group who may not be representative of a population. The use of screening criteria with volunteers is one method to determine if the volunteers are a representative group in a target population. In many studies volunteers are used to assess normal physiological function. In these studies it is important that the investigator establish criteria for normality excluding individuals with above or below average vital capacities. In combination with an objective screening procedure, volunteers are acceptable samples in selected studies.

The relationship between the target population and representative sample and statistic is shown below:

TARGET POPULATION	REPRESENTATIVE SAMPLE	STATISTIC
|	|	|
All units in a group with common characteristics (parameters)	Units of a target population selected for a study	Single unit included in the results of a study

A statistic is the actual subject included in a study. Subjects can be lost in a study through attrition, such as death, change of residence, or voluntarily dropping out of the study. The characteristics of a population such as physiological capacities, personality factors, and demographic information, (i.e., social and personal data) are parameters. These values are usually estimated or unknown because most populations are too large to measure in their entirety.

6.10 Size of Sample

Researchers are constantly plagued by the question, How many subjects should I include in the study? The often repeated response is as many as possible because the higher percentage of subjects from a population, the more the likelihood that the sample is a true representation. The problem of the sample size can also be analyzed from the statistical point of view, which takes into account statistical significance at a confidence level. If one is familiar with statistical tables for t test, analysis of variance, and correlation coefficient, then it will become clear that in arriving at a statistically significant result, the number of subjects affect significance, because the degrees of freedom are derived from the number of subjects in a study. For example, in applying the Pearson correlation coefficient to a study, small rs of .20 can be statistically significant at the .05 level with samples sizes over 100. On the other hand, the researcher needs an r of .58 for a sample size (of 10 subjects in order to obtain statistical significance at the .05 level. In summary, if an investigator is interested in using statistics to derive an adequate sample size, he or she must take into consideration the critical values needed at specific levels of statistical significance, such as the .05 or .01 levels and the difference between means of groups that will be accepted as clinically significant.

Another consideration in determining sample size are the problems of the time length for the study and the resources available to collect data from subjects. If the researcher assumes that he or she needs as many subjects as possible, then he or she should analyze the time and costs for the collecting of data for each subject. Many times these pragmatic considerations are the sole criteria for determining sample size.

6.11 Selection of Measuring Instrument

6.11.1 Selecting a Specific Test for a Research Study

The decision whether to select a test from a published source or to construct a new test is a frequent dilemma for the researcher. Figure 6–2 describes this process.

The conceptual definition of a variable should lead the investigator to a specific test that is the most appropriate one in operationally defining a variable. In clinical research it is crucial that the investigator select a measuring instrument that has a high reliability and is a valid measure of outcome. Measuring improvement in such areas as personality, physical capacity, cognitive functions, vocational skills, and perceptual–motor abilities depends directly on the adequacy and sensitivity of the instrument to measure changes. A crude measuring device that does not have the capacity to detect subtle changes in an individual's functioning or behavior is either of limited or no value to the researcher.

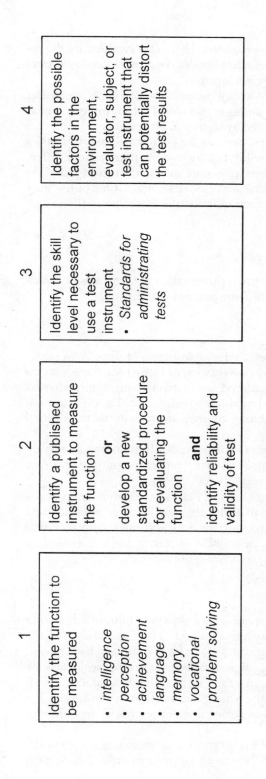

1

Identify the function to be measured

- *intelligence*
- *perception*
- *achievement*
- *language*
- *memory*
- *vocational*
- *problem solving*

2

Identify a published instrument to measure the function

or

develop a new standardized procedure for evaluating the function

and

identify reliability and validity of test

3

Identify the skill level necessary to use a test instrument

- *Standards for administrating tests*

4

Identify the possible factors in the environment, evaluator, subject, or test instrument that can potentially distort the test results

5

Identify the target population for which the test is intended and for which norms have been established

- *infant*
- *child*
- *adolescent*
- *adult*

6

Strictly follow the directions and procedures for administering and scoring the test or modifying the test procedure to enable the client with disabilities to perform at a maximum level

7

Interpret the results for client performance or competence based on

- *norm-referenced data*

or

- *criterion-referenced data*

Figure 6–2. Steps in choosing a test instrument; the process of deciding what to use as the outcome measure. The researcher must decide whether to construct a new test or use a previously published test based on a number of factors.

195

6.11.2 Concept of Measurement and Numbers: Data

Data in statistics are derived from empirical observations. These observations are the result of a standardized measurement procedure such as simple counting, interviews, psychometrics, or machine monitoring of physiological functions.

Measurement is the assignment of numbers to objects, persons, or events according to rules. Measurement transforms certain attributes of the world into numbers, which can then be summarized, organized, and analyzed by statistical procedures.

The properties or characteristics of objects, persons, or events are called *variables* (e.g., height, weight, intelligence). A variable will typically assume two or more different values, reflecting the fact that objects, persons, or events vary in characteristics. This concept of *individual differences* is central to most scientific disciplines. One of the purposes of statistics is to reflect and summarize such individual differences in the values of variables.

6.11.3 Measurement Scales

Measurement scales are a system for the numerical representation of the values of a variable. Four basic types of measurement scales are distinguished in statistics:

Nominal Scale Data

Nominal scale measurement is the most discrete and simplest level of data. With nominal scale data, observations are arranged into various classes or categories. Observations falling into the same class or category are considered qualitatively equivalent, whereas observations in different classes are considered qualitatively different. The classification of eye color, for example, into blue, brown, hazel, or grey, is an example of nominal scale data.

Numbers are assigned usually to each class or category, but these numbers merely reflect differences between the classes. The numbers do not reflect magnitude or order; they only distinguish one class or category from another.

With nominal scale measurement, categories and classes are determined and a count is made of the number of observations in each category. Because nominal data constitute the most elementary level of measurement, the only arithmetic operation that can be performed on the numbers is counting the number of observations in a category and then analyzing proportional differences between categories.

Ordinal Scale Data

Ordinal scale data is the next level of measurement where objects or individuals are not only distinguished from one another, but they are arranged in order or rank. The numerical values of a variable are arranged in a meaningful order to indicate a hierarchy of the levels of the variable or to show relative position. Examples of ordinal scale data are birth order among siblings, the order of finish in a race, or the relative academic standing of university students in a class. The numbers assigned in the above examples not only distinguish between individuals, but also indicate the order or rank of the individuals relative to one another.

The major limitation of ordinal scales is the inability to make inferences about the degree of difference between values on the scale. Numbers assigned in ordinal scale measurement have the properties of both distinctness and order, but the difference between the numbers may not be equal. For example, the difference between 1st and 3rd place in a race may not be equivalent to the difference between 25th and 27th place in the race. There may be wide or narrow differences between each rank. With ordinal scale data, it is only possible to state that one individual or object ranks above or below another.

Interval Scale Data

Interval scale measurement extends ordinal scales by adding the principle that equal differences between scale values have equal meaning. Thus, the difference between each variable score is equivalent. With interval measurement, numbers serve two purposes: (a) to convey the order of the observations, and (b) to indicate the distance or degree of differences between observations. Numbers are assigned so that equal differences in the numbers correspond to equal differences in the property or attribute being measured. However, the zero point of the interval scale can be placed arbitrarily and does not indicate absence of the property measured.

Examples of interval scale data are calendar years and the temperature scales of Celsius and Fahrenheit. In a temperature scale the difference between 10 and 15 °C is the same quantitative difference as between 20 and 25 °C. But 20 °C is not twice as warm as 10 °C because there is no true zero point.

Interval scales are very important in social science research. Many human characteristics and attributes, such as intelligence scores and personality traits, are scales with approximately equal intervals (e.g., IQ scores). As well, more sophisticated statistical procedures may be performed with interval scale data compared to the lower level nominal and ordinal data.

Ratio Scale Data

Ratio scale data is the highest level of measurement and includes the maximum amount of information. The ratio scale is named as such because the ratio of numbers on the scale is meaningful. Because there is a genuine zero point, equal ratios between scale values have equal meaning (i.e., the ratio 40:20 is equivalent to 100:50 or 120:60). The zero point on a ratio scale indicates total absence of the property measured. With ratio scale data, all arithmetic operations (addition, subtraction, multiplication, and division) are possible. Measurement of such variables as height, weight, muscle strength, and range of motion are all ratio scaled. Figure 6–3 illustrates the differences between the four basic types of measurement scales, while Table 6–6 illustrates their characteristics and properties.

Progress in scientific research gained momentum with the design of tests and instruments that measured and recorded human functioning accurately. The measuring instrument is the sine qua non of research. Without an adequate measuring instrument a problem remains unresearchable. The adequacy of a measuring instrument is determined by its reliability (i.e., consistency in measurement) and validity, (i.e., soundness in measurement).

Various examples of measurable variables in health and education research are described in Table 6–7. "In its broadest sense, measurement is the assignment of numerals to objects or parts according to rule" (Stevens, 1951, p. 1).

In the foregoing example (Table 6–6) of measurable variables, numbers can be assigned to indicate the degree of improvement, strength, perceptual ability, and quality of nutrition. Rating scales can also be devised using a continuum of measurement, equal intervals, or item ranking. Likert-type scales using descriptor adjectives is another alter-

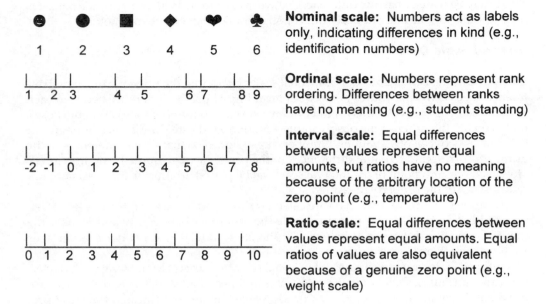

Nominal scale: Numbers act as labels only, indicating differences in kind (e.g., identification numbers)

Ordinal scale: Numbers represent rank ordering. Differences between ranks have no meaning (e.g., student standing)

Interval scale: Equal differences between values represent equal amounts, but ratios have no meaning because of the arbitrary location of the zero point (e.g., temperature)

Ratio scale: Equal differences between values represent equal amounts. Equal ratios of values are also equivalent because of a genuine zero point (e.g., weight scale)

Figure 6–3. Differences between the four measurement scales.

Table 6–6 *Classification of Scales of Measurement*

Measurement Scale	Type of Variable	Researcher Application	Tasks Purpose	Examples
Nominal	Discrete	Sorting of items	Establishing mutually exclusive groups	Occupations, Diagnostic groups
Ordinal	Discrete	Rank ordering of items	Determination of greater or lesser	Patient improvement, Clinical Performance of students
Interval	Continuous	Equal ordering of items	Establishing equal intervals on a continuum	Intelligence, Perceptual-motor abilities, Work capacities
Ratio	Continuous	Equal ordering of items with an absolute zero point	Establishing continuous measurement with zero point	Range of motion, Muscle strength, Weight, Height, Auditory and visual acuity

native. In this scale, it is not assumed that there are equal intervals between numbers, (e.g., 1 to 2 is not assumed to be the same distance as 2 to 3), or that there is an absolute zero. However, measurement at this level is an improvement over a clinician subjectively stating, on the basis of treatment, that the patient has either improved or not improved. Measurement enables the clinical researcher to operationally define and objectively evaluate an outcome variable. Without objective measurement, clinicians have no criteria or standards to compare the effects of various treatment modalities.

For example, an investigator is interested in comparing two methods of increasing cardiac efficiency in patients with post myocardial infarction. After establishing two groups on the basis of screening criteria and random assignment, the researcher operationally defines cardiac efficiency, such as increasing the range of heart rate. The operational definition includes the test and procedure in measuring the dependent variable, *cardiac efficiency*. In another example involving retrospective research, an investigator is interested in correlating the relationship between disengagement in social decision making and choice of housing for individuals who are older (e.g., nursing home care or independent community living). The presumed independent variables, *housing arrangements*, are hypothesized to affect social decision making. Screening criteria are established in operationally defining the two housing arrangements. The researcher would then select the settings, and subjects would be randomly selected from each institution. The crux of the research is in operationally defining the concept of social decision making by selecting an objective standardized test.

In selecting a measuring instrument the researcher is faced with two basic questions:

1. Does the instrument measure a variable consistently?
2. Is the instrument a true measure of the variable?

The first question seeks a reliability index and the second question raises the issues of validity.

Table 6–7 *Measurement Variables*

Variable to Be Tested	Examples of Measuring Instruments
Hand strength	Dynamometer
Range of motion	Goniometer
Cardiovascular functioning	Electrocardiogram
Attitudes towards individuals with disabilities	Attitudes Towards Disabilities Scale
Clinical performance of students	Burks' Behavior Rating Scale
Psychological improvement	Tennessee Test of Self Concept
Social values and life goals	Life Satisfaction Index
Stress management	Stress Management Questionnaire
Activities of daily living	Barthel Scale
Cognitive functioning	Allen's Cognitive Level
Intelligence	Wechsler Scales of Intelligence
Developmental levels	Miller Assessment Profile
Eye-hand coordination	Developmental Test of Visual–Motor Integration
Perceptual ability	Test of Visual Perceptual Scales
Reading achievement	Woodcock Reading Mastery Test–Revised
Handwriting	Jebsen Test of Hand Function

6.11.4 Reliability

If one assumes that a specific stable characteristic of an individual remains stable over time, then a reliable measuring instrument should reflect the stable characteristics through repeated trials. For example, an electron microscope, sensitive enough to enlarge chromosomes so that a researcher can perceive them, maintains a consistency in measurement. In the physical sciences, where comparison dictates the foundation of measurement, the reliability of instruments has evolved progressively. However, the individual using a sensitive measuring instrument can affect what is being measured. For example, astronomers observed that the individual's reaction time in viewing the movement of stars affects the calculation in determining distances between the stars. In response to this human factor, astronomers developed automatic means to record distances between celestial objects. The control of the personal equation in measurement is an important factor to consider in every research study where there is an interaction between the object observed and the investigator. This is especially true in qualitative research, such as in interviewing subjects.

Researchers strive to reduce the error factor in measurement by increasing the reliability of an objective test or instrument and reducing the variability of extraneous factors in the individual. Instruments, such as the electrocardiograph (EKG or ECG), electroencephalograph (EEG), X-Ray, electromyograph (EMG), positron emission tomography (PET scan), magnetic resonance imaging (MRI), and single-photon emission computed tomography (SPECT) are usually reliable indicators of bodily functions. On the other hand questionnaires, surveys, rating scales, attitude inventories, interest tests, and objective psychological tests may be less reliable. The very nature of the test affects the reliability index. Automatic instruments that record bodily functions need to be mechanically sound or calibrated to be reliable. In devising a reliable instrument the investigator is concerned with eliminating items that are ambiguous or can be answered in more than one way. However, reliability is not a simple concept that merely reflects the consistency of the instrument. In any test administered to subjects, individual differences, such as level of reading ability, need to conform, desire to please the examiner, motivation, and test anxiety, are important factors that could potentially increase the error variance and decrease the consistency of response. Since human beings are constantly reacting to internal and external factors, reliability must be interpreted in a relative degree when considering psychological tests, questionnaires, and attitude scales. Most researchers with human subjects accept a reliability coefficient of approximately $r = .80$ or above to be an acceptable level of a test's consistency in measuring a variable.

Techniques for Measuring Test Reliability

Test reliability is usually measured by correlating two sets of scores and arriving at a correlation coefficient. For example, an investigator is interested in devising a test of perceptual–motor ability with school-age children 8 to 11 years old. In the process of devising the test, the investigator constructs 50 items that measure perceptual–motor ability. The items are screened for clarity in a pilot study with 24 children as subjects. The investigator is interested in determining split half reliability and test–retest reliability. In split half reliability the test is broken into two equal parts (in this example 25 items each) and correlated with each other. In test–retest reliability a test is given twice within a short period of time (usually within two weeks) and the scores on the two tests are correlated.

In the following hypothetical example (Table 6–8) there is a perfect positive correlation (+1.00) between the scores on the first and second tests. The scores reflect also a practice effect, which is typical of test–retest reliability. A practice effect exists when scores increase consistently as a function of the subject's being familiar with the content of the test and feeling less anxious.

6.11.5 Item Analysis

A researcher in devising a test or in assessing students may be interested in the effectiveness of individual test items that differentiate between high and low achievers. The researcher may also be interested in eliminating those items that are ambiguous and have a low discriminative level. Item analysis is a method of gauging the difficulty value and ambiguity of each item. In item analysis the percentage of passes and failures are calculated for each item. For example, if items 1, 2, and 3 are passed respectively by 80, 60, and 40% of the subjects, we can infer that item 3 is either more difficult or more ambiguous than item 1 or 2. Another method is analyzing items to determine which items were passed by high scorers and failed by low scorers. This analysis will enable the researcher to separate out those items that have discriminative value. Items that are passed in all cases have little discriminative value, but may indicate the level at which all members of the group are functioning. This may be particularly important in criterion-reference tests where the test administrator is most concerned with issues related to competency.

Table 6–8 *Hypothetical Data for Testing Reliability*

Subject	Test–Retest Test 1	Reliability Test 2
01	69	72
02	34	37
03	71	74
04	20	23
05	95	98
06	10	13
07	99	102
08	81	84
09	92	95
10	49	52
11	97	100
12	63	66
13	86	89
14	9	12
15	96	99
16	81	84
17	20	23
18	69	72
19	81	84
20	24	27
21	97	100
22	55	58
23	54	57
24	97	100
25	68	71

6.11.6 Validity

Validity reflects the authenticity of a test. Does the test measure what it purports to measure? A test may measure a concept consistently but it may not, in fact, measure what the researcher identifies as the intent of the test. Psychological tests purporting to measure general intelligence, self-image, body defensiveness, and attitude toward individuals with disabilities may be measuring other concepts. The degree to which a test is valid is the degree of empirical evidence that corroborates the results of a test. Tests or instruments that collect primary data, such as an EMG, X-Ray, goniometer, ergometer, and MRI are easily verified and corroborated. However, tests that collect secondary data derived from multiple factors in the individual, such as personality characteristics, are more difficult to validate. Personality, attitude, values, and interests are complex variables derived from many facets of the individual's life, related to genetic, social learning, cultural identification, and physiological factors. The researcher seeking to validate a personality test is limited by the ability to corroborate the findings. Traditionally, validity is established on the following bases:

- *Content or face validity*: the degree to which the test appears to measure a concept by a logical analysis of the items.
- *Concurrent validity*: the degree of correlation with another standardized instrument. A new test may be derived because it is less time consuming and less expensive than another established validated instrument.
- *Predictive validity*: the degree to which a test can predict success or accuracy over a period of time (longitudinally). For example, a test devised to predict success in an undergraduate program for physical therapists or success in a rehabilitation program for patients with stroke are examples of predictive validity. In the examples, follow-up data from longitudinal studies would determine the correlation between the initial test predictor score and subsequent success in a program. Predictive validity is perhaps the best type of substantiating evidence in psychological tests.
- *Construct validity*: considered to be the highest form of empirical evidence that is most sought after by scientific researchers. Construct validity assumes a theoretical rationale underlying the test instrument. In testing an instrument for construct validity the researcher seeks behavioral data to substantiate the position that the test is in fact measuring a defined variable. For example, an investigator devising a test to measure self-image would first construct a theory that underlies the concept. The theory would include developmental factors, relationships with other variables, and behavioral observations supporting the evidence for construct validity. In another example, the electroencephalogram, which records brain waves and is used indirectly for diagnosing brain damage, can be checked for construct validity through dissection of an animal brain or through post mortem examination.

6.12 Ethical Principles Guiding Human Research

Below are examples of documents related to ethical issues guiding clinical research.

6.12.1 Declaration of Helsinki[1]

DECLARATION OF HELSINKI

World Medical Association

1964, revised 1975, 1983, 1989

The Declaration of Helsinki, which offers recommendations for conducting experiments using human subjects, was adopted in 1962 and revised by the 18th World Medical Assembly, Helsinki, Finland, in 1964. Subsequent revisions were approved in Tokyo (1975), Venice (1983), and Hong Kong (1989). The 1989 version is reprinted below . . . .

Introduction. It is the mission of the doctor to safeguard the health of the people. His or her knowledge and conscience are dedicated to the fulfillment of this mission.

The Declaration of Geneva of The World Medical Association binds the physician with the words: "The health of my patient will be my first consideration" and the International Code of Medical Ethics which declares that "A physician shall act only in the patient's interest when providing medical care which might have the effect of weakening the physical and mental condition of the patient."

The purpose of biomedical research involving human subjects must be to improve diagnostic, therapeutic and prophylactic procedures and the understanding of the aetiology and pathogenesis of the disease.

In current medical practice most diagnostic, therapeutic or prophylactic procedures involve hazards. This applies especially to biomedical research.

In the field of biomedical research a fundamental distinction must be recognized between medical research in which the aim is essentially diagnostic or therapeutic for a patient, and medical research, the essential object of which is purely scientific and without implying direct diagnostic or therapeutic value to the person subjected to the research.

Special caution must be exercised in the conduct of research which may affect the environment, and the welfare of animals used for research must be respected.

Because it is essential that the results of laboratory experiments be applied to human beings to further scientific knowledge and to help suffering humanity, the World Medical Association has prepared the following recommendations as a guide to every physician in biomedical research involving human subjects. They should be kept under review in the future. It must be stressed that the standards as drafted are only a guide to physicians all over the world. Physicians are not relieved from criminal, civil and ethical responsibilities under the laws of their own countries.

I. **Basic Principles**

1. Biomedical research involving human subjects must conform to generally accepted scientific principles that justify medical research and should be based on adequately performed laboratory and animal experimentation and a thorough knowledge of the scientific literature.

2. The design and performance of each experimental procedure involving human subjects should be clearly formulated in an experimental protocol which should be transmitted for consideration, comment and guidance to a specially appointed committee independent of the investigator and the sponsor, provided that this independent committee is in conformity with the laws and regulations of the country in which the research experiment is performed.

3. Biomedical research involving human subjects should be conducted only by scientifically qualified persons and under the supervision of a clinically competent medical person. The responsibility for the human subject must always

---

[1] Printed in the *World Medical Association, Handbook of Declarations*, 1993.

rest with a medically qualified person and never rest on the subject of the research, even though the subject has given his or her consent.

4. Biomedical research cannot legitimately be carried out unless the importance of the objective is in proportion to the inherent risk to the subject.

5. Every biomedical research project involving human subjects should be preceded by careful assessment of predictable risks in comparison to foreseeable benefits to the subject or to others. Concern for the interests of the subject must always prevail over the interests of science and society.

6. The right of the research subject to safeguard his or her integrity must always be respected. Every precaution should be taken to respect the privacy of the subject and to minimize the impact of the study on the subject's physical and mental integrity and on the personality of the subject.

7. Physicians should abstain from engaging in research projects involving human subjects unless they are satisfied that the hazards involved are believed to be predictable. Physicians should cease any investigation if the hazards are found to outweigh the potential benefits.

8. In publication of the results of his or her research, the physician is obligated to preserve the accuracy of the results. Reports of experimentation not in accordance with the principles laid down in this Declaration should not be accepted for publication.

9. In any research on human beings, each potential subject must be adequately informed of the aims, methods, anticipated benefits and potential hazards of the study and the discomfort it may entail. He or she should be informed that he or she is at liberty to abstain from participation in the study and that he or she is free to withdraw his or her consent to participation at any time. The physician should then obtain the subject's freely-given informed consent, preferably in writing.

10. When obtaining informed consent for the research project, the physician should be particularly cautious if the subject is in a dependent relationship to him or her or may consent under duress. In that case the informed consent should be obtained by a physician who is not engaged in the investigation and who is completely independent of this official relationship.

11. In case of legal incompetence, informed consent should be obtained from the legal guardian in accordance with national legislation. Where physical or mental incapacity makes it impossible to obtain informed consent, or when the subject is a minor, permission form the responsible relative replaces that of the subject in accordance with national legislation. Whenever the minor child is in fact able to give a consent, the minor's consent must be obtained in addition to the consent of the minor's legal guardian.

12. The research protocol should always contain a statement of the ethical considerations involved and should indicate that the principles enunciated in the present Declaration are complied with.

II. Medical Research Combined with Professional Care (clinical research)

1. In the treatment of the sick person, the physician must be free to use a new diagnostic and therapeutic measure, if in his or her judgment it offers hope of saving life, reestablishing health, or alleviating suffering.

2. The potential benefits, hazards and discomfort of a new method should be weighed against the advantages of the best current diagnostic and therapeutic methods.

3. In any medical study, every patient—including those of a control group, if any—should be assured of the best proven diagnostic and therapeutic method.

4. The refusal of the patient to participate in a study must never interfere with the physician- patient relationship.

5. If the physician considers it essential not to obtain informed consent, the specific reasons for this proposal should be stated in the experimental protocol for transmission to the independent committee (1, 2).

6. The physician can combine medical research with professional care, the objective being the acquisition of new medical knowledge, only to the extent that medical research is justified by its potential diagnostic or therapeutic value for the patient.

III. Non–Therapeutic Biomedical Research Involving Human Subjects (Nonclinical biomedical research)

1. In the purely scientific application of clinical research carried out on a human being, it is the duty of the physician to remain the protector of the life and health of that person on whom biomedical research is being carried out.

2. The subjects should be volunteers—either healthy persons or patients for whom the experimental design is not related to the patient's illness.

3. The investigator or the investigating team should discontinue the research if in his/her or their judgement it may, if continued, be harmful to the individual.

4. In research on man, the interest of science and society should never take precedence over considerations related to the well-being of the subject.

6.12.2 Harvard University Health Services: Rules Governing the Participation of Healthy Human Beings as Subjects in Research

The following rules and procedures, formulated by the University Health Services, were adopted by the President and Fellows on April 1,1963. They will apply hereafter to all parts of the University except the Medical School. These rules are not intended to cover research on sick patients.

Statement of Policy

1. In considering the participation of human beings as research subjects, the guiding principle is that no one, whether students or other persons, should be exposed to unreasonable risk to health or well-being.

2. All persons involved in initiating, approving, or conducting research involving human subjects shall be aware of a joint responsibility for the welfare of the individuals who serve as subjects.

3. It shall be the responsibility of the individual investigator to decide when he does not have adequate knowledge of the possible consequences of his research, or of research done under his direction. When he is in doubt, he must obtain the advice of others who do have the requisite or relevant knowledge.

4. Any hazards to health of each research procedure must be first investigated through animal research, whenever such be possible and relevant.

5. Whenever medication or physical intervention is used, or whenever the subject's environment is altered beyond the limits of normality, the research must be performed under medical protection and supervision.

6. The purpose of the research, the procedures to be followed, and the possible risks involved must be carefully and fully explained to the subject; the investigator must be satisfied that the explanation has been understood by the subject; and the consent of the subject must be obtained in writing without duress or deception.

Where unreasonable risks to the subject are not involved, and a full account of purpose and procedure in advance might bias the results, as in some psychological and social research, such an account may be postponed to a later appropriate time or may be omitted—as for example in public opinion research, or observation of children in educational or play situations, provided there is no ethical problem.

7. A research project shall not be represented to potential research subjects as being sponsored by Harvard University or by a given department of the University except by explicit arrangements with appropriate administrative authorities. It is appropriate for the researcher to make known his position at Harvard. It is the subject's right to know, if he so desires, the source of support for the research in which he is being asked to participate.

8. The individual's personal privacy and the confidentiality of information received from him must be protected.

9. An individual's time should not be invaded to the extent that it creates conflicts with his other obligations; whenever possible the research project should contribute to the subject's knowledge of himself and/or his knowledge of the topic under investigation.

10. Remuneration may be offered to an individual for the time involved in a study provided the investigator is satisfied that under the circumstances the remuneration is not so large as to constitute an improper inducement.

11. Any individual may request termination of his participation in an experiment at any time, and this request will be honored promptly and without prejudice.

Procedure

The responsibility of the Dean of each faculty to the Corporation should be that research involving healthy human subjects by members of his faculty is conducted with care and propriety. The procedures used in the Faculty of Medicine are described in a statement, dated January 1, 1958. All other Faculties will observe the following procedures. The Deans may delegate this responsibility to department chairmen who may in turn delegate it to other responsible members of their department.

1. All officers of the University shall evaluate research using human subjects, to be conducted or directed by them, in terms of ethical and legal standards as well as according to scientific criteria, keeping in mind that the acceptance of individual responsibility for one's actions constitutes the foundation of the trust that the individual enjoys as a member of the University.

2. All research must comply with all requirements in the statement of policy listed above.

3. The following list is illustrative of the types of research procedures that are likely to involve consequences beyond the ability of many investigators to evaluate adequately, and will, therefore, make it necessary that the investigator in any such research refer his proposal to other responsible persons for further consideration. In such cases the University Health Services through Environmental Health & Safety are prepared to provide advice and to evaluate and approve procedures. The list is not intended to be inclusive.

   a. Injection, ingestion or inhalation of any potentially toxic material, including all drugs, or any usually ingested or inhaled material in excess of, or in less than, normal amounts.

   b. Physical stimuli, in abnormal amounts, such as:

Noise	Ionizing radiation
Vibration	Non-ionizing radiation
Electric shock	Ultra violet
Heat and/or humidity	Visible light
Cold and/or wind	Infra-red radiations
Magnetic fields	Microwaves
Gravitational fields	Ambient pressure

    c.   Sensory deprivation

    d.   Sleep deprivation

    e.   Special diets that vary appreciably from generally accepted standards.

    f.   Psychological experiments using hypnosis, deception, or mental stresses.

4.   A department whose members may need advice may appoint a committee to assist the investigator in obtaining the advice he requires. When such a committee exists, it will ordinarily be the first group to which the investigator turns and shall have power to require that the investigator obtain approval from the University Health Services, through Environmental Health and Safety, before going ahead to recruit subjects for his research.

5.   In cases where the departmental committee learns informally of a proposed research project that it believes should be referred to it, it will be appropriate for the committee to request that the proposal be submitted to it for evaluation.

6.   It shall be the prerogative of both the department committee and the University Health Services to require for projects referred to them that parental consent be obtained before individuals under the age of 21 may participate in a research project.

7.   For those cases in which it has been determined that approval by Environmental Health and Safety is required, the proposed research will be presented in proper form to that body. Approval of the use of human beings as research subjects in such cases will be valid only for a specific project and for a maximum of one year. If further time or change in protocol is necessary, application for re-approval will be necessary. It is recommended, in order to prevent delay of the investigation, that sufficient time be allowed before the start of the project for review by Environmental Health and Safety and other responsible parties.

8.   In all cases where it has been determined that a proposal is one requiring approval of the division of Environmental Health and Safety or another administrative body, no action to recruit individuals will be taken until written approval from this body has been received. The principal investigator, the departmental committee, and the Student Employment Office will receive notification of the action taken on a proposal.

9.   The investigator will report immediately to the University Health Services any significant observations of change in the behavior or health of any subject during or following an experiment, and the investigator will terminate that experiment.

10.   Whether a specific project has been cleared or not, the investigator should feel free to seek advice from the University Health Service at any time during a study.

11.   These regulations shall be circulated to the members of the departments concerned at the beginning of each academic year.

Dana L. Farnsworth, M.D., Director

6.12.3 Children's Hospital Guidelines: Clinical Research

Clinical research is an investigation involving the biological, behavioral, or psychological study of a person, his body or his surroundings. This includes but is not limited to any medical or surgical procedure, any withdrawal or removal of body tissue or fluid, any administration of a chemical substance, any deviation from normal diet or daily regimen, and any manipulation or observation of bodily processes, behavior or environment. Clinical research comprises four categories of activity:

1.   Studies that conform to established and accepted medical practice with respect to diagnosis or treatment of an illness.

2.   Studies that represent a deviation from accepted practice but are specifically aimed at improved diagnosis, prevention, or treatment of a specific illness in a patient.

3. Studies that are related to a patient's disease but from which he or she will not necessarily receive any direct benefit.

4. Investigative, non-therapeutic research in which there is no intent or expectation of treating an illness from which the patient is suffering, or in which the subject is a "normal control" who is not suffering from an illness but who volunteers to participate for the potential benefit of others. It is important to emphasize that "non-therapeutic" is not to be understood as meaning "harmful." Understanding of normal processes is essential; it is a prerequisite, in many instances, to the recognition of those deviations from normal which define disease. Important knowledge can be gained through such studies of normal processes. Although such research might not in any way benefit the subjects from whom the data are obtained, neither does it necessarily harm them. Patients participating in studies identified in (1) above are not considered to be at special risk, by virtue of participating in research activity. When patients or subjects are involved in procedures identified in (2), (3), or (4) above, they are considered to be "at risk." Excluded from this definition are studies in which the risk is negotiable, such as research requiring only, for example, the recording of height and weight, collecting excreta, or analyzing hair, deciduous teeth or nail clippings. Some studies that appear to involve negligible physical risk might, however, have psychological, sociological or legal implications that are significant. In that event, the subjects are in fact "at risk" and appropriate procedures for review of these activities shall be applied.

6.12.4 The University of Wisconsin-Milwaukee Human Subjects Review Protocol (HSRP)

THE UNIVERSITY OF WISCONSIN-MILWAUKEE
HUMAN SUBJECTS REVIEW PROTOCOL (HSRP)

PART ONE

This form is submitted for:

☐ ORIGINAL SUBMISSION ☐ PROTOCOL MODIFICATION

☐ CONTINUATION/or DUPLICATE SUBMISSION
(see protocol #_____)

I. Principal Investigator_____Rank_____

Dept_____

Phone_____

Co-Investigator_____Rank_____

Dept_____

Phone_____

UWM Proposal No. (if appropriate)_____

Total Project Period:_____to_____

Application Deadline or Date of Transmittal:_____

☐ Federal Agency_____ ☐ Non-Federal Agency_____

☐ None (i..e., Thesis or Dissertation)

☐ Other (please specify)_____

Project Title:_____

II. Description or Abstract of project (attach); stress nature of human subject involvement (no more than 1 page).

III. Protected Populations and Sensitive Subjects

Human subjects would be involved in the proposed activity as either:

☐ Minors ☐ Fetuses ☐ Mentally Retarded ☐ Prisoners

☐ Abortuses ☐ Pregnant Women ☐ Mentally Disabled ☐ Illegal Behavior

☐ Test subjects for new drugs or clinical devices

If you checked any of the boxes above, IRB review is required. Contact compliance specialist; obtain and completed Part Two of HSRP. Submit completed protocol directly to IRB.

IV. Determination of Risk: "Minimal risk" means that the risk of harm anticipated in the proposed research is not greater, considering probability and magnitude, than those risks normally encountered in daily life or during the performance of routine physical or psychological examinations or tests. If more than minimal risk is involved, or deception is involved, or if federal money is requested and research is not exempt, a complete protocol must be filed with the IRB.

	PI	Decentralized Comm.	IRB
This project poses *minimal risk* as defined above:	☐	☐	☐
This project involves *significant risk* or deception:	☐	☐	☐
Determination of Exemption from Human Subjects Review:			
This project is exempt from HS review per guidelines: (cite specific form exemption in Project Description)	☐	☐	☐
This project is not exempt from HS review per guidelines	☐	☐	☐
IRB review required:			
This project does not require IRB review:	☐	☐	☐
This project requires IRB review:	☐	☐	☐
		For Committee Use Only	

If Project requires IRB review, contact compliance specialist at Graduate School (X6012); obtain and complete Part Two of HSRP, submit completed protocol directly to IRB.

V. Principal Investigator Assurance

I have read the statement of UWM research ethics, including the responsibility to obtain informed consent from Subjects and will comply. Signed:

_____   _____

Principal Investigator   (date)

_____   _____

Faculty Advisor (for students only)   (date)

Disposition

DECENTRALIZED COMMITTEE: NOTE

Approved to proceed ☐   Needs IRB review ☐   Approval is valid for one calendar year only.

_____   _____

Signature   (date)

  IRB

  Approved ☐   Disapproved ☐

_____   _____

Signature   (date)

THE UNIVERSITY OF WISCONSIN-MILWAUKEE
HUMAN SUBJECTS REVIEW PROTOCOL

PART TWO

Instructions

Describe the subject population and summarize procedures to be used according to the following outline. It is not requested that the entire project design be included, but that procedures involving human subjects be fully described. More detail is required for any procedure that could potentially be harmful, such as the use of electric shock, hypnosis, unusual stress, drugs, or the imposition of demeaning and dehumanizing conditions.

PLEASE RESTATE THE OUTLINE HEADING

AND POINT TO WHICH YOU ARE RESPONDING

I. SUBJECTS

    A. Describe the pool(s) of human subjects you will be using:

        1. Sex, race or ethnic group, age range, etc.;

        2. Affiliation of subjects, e.g., institutions, hospitals, general public, etc.

        3. Subject's general state of health (mental and physical)

    B. If human subjects are children, mentally incompetent, or legally restricted groups, give explanation as to:

        1. The necessity for using these particular groups;

        2. Why adult "normal" groups cannot be used.

II. PROCEDURES

    A. Describe information to be gathered and means for collection and recording

    B. Describe personnel interacting with the subject

    C. Will deception be used in gathering data: If so, describe and justify

    D. At what location will the human subject involvement occur?

III. RISKS

    A. Describe in detail any physical, psychological, social, legal, economic or other risks you can foresee, both immediate and long range:

        1. Immediate risks;

        2. Long range;

        3. Rationale for the necessity of such risks;

        4. Alternatives that were or will be considered;

        5. Why alternative may not be feasible.

B. "Non-Beneficial Research" is designed as research involving investigators of a person, his or her body, life, or surroundings, which is devoid of benefit to that person. If you plan to conduct this type of research and feel that there are no other methods available for obtaining the information needed, please describe:

1. What other methods were or will be explored;

2. The extent of the risks (physical, psychological, social, legal and other);

3. The importance of the knowledge to be gained;

4. Why you feel that the value of the information to be gained outweighs the risks.

IV. SAFEGUARDING SUBJECTS' IDENTITY

A. What uses will be made of the information obtained from the subjects? What elements of your project might be openly accessible to other agencies or appear in publications?

B. What precautions will be taken to safeguard identifiable records or individuals? These questions also apply to secondary sources of data.

1. Long range use of data (by you and others);

2. Immediate use of data (by you and others);

3. Describe specific procedures to be used to provide confidentiality of data.

V. INFORMED CONSENT

(Use the sample informed consent format. It includes material in addition to what is described below.)

A. Describe procedure for obtaining informed consent. Informed consent must include:

1. A fair explanation of the procedures to be followed and their purposes, including identification of any procedures that are experimental;
2. A description of any attendant discomfort and risks reasonably to be expected;
3. A description of any benefits reasonably to be expected;
4. A disclosure of any appropriate alternative procedures that might be advantageous for the subject;
5. A description of the safeguards to be used for confidentiality;
6. An offer to answer any inquiries concerning the procedures;
7. An instruction that the person is free to withdraw consent and to discontinue participating in the project or activity at any time without prejudice to the subject;
8. A statement that the information collected from the subject up to the point of withdrawal would be destroyed if the subject so desired.

B. In addition, it should be stated that the subject in no way diminishes the quality of care otherwise available to him or her by not participating.

C. The agreement, written or oral, entered into by the subject, should include no exculpatory language through which the subject is made to waive or to appear to waive, any of his or her legal rights, or to release the institution or its agents from liability for negligence.

D. Informed consent must be documented. A copy of the signed informed consent form must be obtained from each subject for the principal investigator's files and a copy should be given to each subject (or legal representative). The subject's copy should include the name, address and telephone number of the person to whom requests for information or results may be addressed. The subject's copy must include the name, address and telephone number of the person to whom complaints may be addressed:

Institutional Review Board for the Protection of Human Subjects
Graduate School
University of Wisconsin-Milwaukee
PO Box 413
Milwaukee, Wisconsin 53201

INFORMED CONSENT FORMS LACKING THIS REFERENCE WILL NOT BE APPROVED.

A statement regarding the confidentiality of the subjects' complaints is needed.

E. For questionnaires, informed consent is usually obtained by including an explanation of all the elements at the beginning with a statement that completion of the questionnaire constituted informed consent.

Contact The Graduate School for sample informed consent forms.

VI. COOPERATING INSTITUTIONS (Use the Consortia Agreement Sample)

Protocols for projects involving cooperating institutions must be accompanied by evidence of a contractual agreement with each agency that (1) specifies the management of responsibility for the activities to be performed and (2) identifies the supervisory personnel in the agency.

RE: CONSORTIA AGREEMENT

When the Principal Investigator has returned the Consortia agreement with the appropriate contracting agency signature, someone from The Graduate School with signature authority for UWM will sign on behalf of the Board of Regents of the University of Wisconsin-Milwaukee.

The signature of the principal investigator is not appropriate. Contact Graduate School for sample Consortia Agreement forms.

6.13 Data Collection Procedures

The time schedule for collecting data, the costs of the study, the setting for administering group or individual tests, a cover letter to prospective subjects explaining the nature of the study, an individual data collection sheet recording descriptive information and test scores, an informed consent agreement between the researcher and subject, and the statistical techniques used to analyze the data are all factors for the investigator to consider in the prospectus for the study.

The checklist in Table 6–9 should guide the investigator in preparing a data collection procedure. The reader should review this frequently to insure that all parts of the data collection have been considered.

6.13.1 Informed Consent and Forms

The informed consent is a legal document that informs the subject about the procedures that are to occur, the place in which the data collection will occur, the amount of time required for participation, and the potential risks or hazards of the study. Informed consent must be documented. A copy of the signed informed consent form must be obtained from each subject for the principal investigator's files and a copy should be given to each subject (or legal representative). The subject's copy should include the name, address, and telephone number of the person to whom requests for information or results may be addressed. It must also include the name, address, and telephone number of the person to whom complaints may be addressed.

The following is described in detail in the informed consent form:

1. a procedure for obtaining informed consent
2. a brief statement regarding the objectives of the study
3. the amount of time in which each subject will participate
4. the compensation, remuneration, or other awards, if any, to be received by the subject

Table 6–9   *Questions Guiding Methodology*

Time Schedule
- Have you determined the length of time needed for administering individual or group testing?
- Have you considered travel time and time for test preparation?
- Have you determined the length of time for scoring tests?

Informed Consent
- Have you prepared a form describing to the subject the procedure, tests, information, and length of time involved?
- Have you informed the participant that he/she may decline from the study without any implied penalty?
- Does the participant have a signed form in his/her possession?

Data Collection Sheet
- Have you prepared a data collection sheet for each subject, coding the name to guarantee anonymity and providing room for every datum item collected?

Computer Analysis
- Have you considered using computer time in analyzing the data?

Statistical Techniques
- Does the study meet the assumptions of a parametric statistic?
- If not, what specific nonparametric statistics will be used to analyze the data?
- Have you done a statistical analysis of the hypothetical data?

Cost Analysis
- Have you considered costs for purchasing tests or instruments?
- Have you considered costs for address labels and mailings?
- Have you considered costs for analyzing data?

5. a description of any expected benefits that may be obtained by the participant
6. a description of the procedures and methods to be used in the study
7. the identification of potential risks or hazards which mighty occur during the study
8. the procedures that will minimize any risks or hazards identified in #7
9. the procedures that will insure confidentiality of the participants.

6.13.2 Example of Informed Consent Form

Following is an example of an informed consent form.

CONSENT FORM FOR PARENTS

I understand that my child has been invited to participate voluntarily in a study which will examine students' ability to plan and carry out a complex task. This study will also examine the way that emotions affect children's planning abilities. I understand that if my child agrees to participate, he or she will be given a number of tests. These will include tests that examine planning abilities, how well he or she can remember information, and a questionnaire about feelings. If my student has not had an intelligence test within the last two years, an intelligence test will be given. I understand that some of these tests will be audiotape-recorded.

I understand that these tests will be given during the school day. The tests will take approximately 2 hours. I realize that there may be no direct benefit to my child; however, indirectly my child may benefit because the information obtained will allow the teachers and school professionals to gain new information about teaching students the planning process for carrying out complex tasks.

I understand that if I allow my child to participate in this study, I will be contacted by Ms. Susan K. Cutler in order to complete a questionnaire about my child's behavior.

I understand that my child's participation is voluntary and that he or she will be asked for consent. My child can choose not to participate or may want to stop at any time during the testing session without any penalty.

I give my consent for my child, _____,
to participate in the study. I give permission for Susan K. Cutler to examine my child's educational records to obtain previously administered intelligence and achievement tests. I give permission for my child to be audiotaped.

I UNDERSTAND THAT BY SIGNING THIS FORM, I AM GIVING MY CONSENT FOR MY CHILD TO PARTICIPATE IN THE STUDY.

I have received two copies of this consent form, one for me to keep and one to return to the investigator, Susan K. Cutler.

_____   _____
Signature of Parent   Date

_____   _____
Signature of Investigator   Date

PERMISSION FORM FOR STUDENTS

You are being asked to take part in an activity that will help me understand more about how you solve problems. I hope to learn how you plan and organize your school assignments and how well you remember information. Your participation is voluntary. If you begin and decide that you don't want to continue, you may withdraw from the study. There will be no penalty if you decide that you don't want to participate.

If you participate, you will be given different tasks to find out how well you can solve problems and remember information. You will also be asked to answer a questionnaire that talks about your feelings. These tasks will take between 1 and 2 hours to complete all of the tasks. They will be given at a time when it is convenient to you and your teacher. Some of these tasks will be audiotaped. The only people who will listen to these tapes are me and my assistant. Your name will not be used in the study, but how you do will be used to find out how students solve problems. No one will know your name. You will be identified by a special code. The tape recordings will also be identified by this code.

I will answer any questions about these tasks after you have finished. I will also talk with you about any feelings which you may have had after doing the questionnaire.

You will be given a copy of this permission form for your records.

YOU ARE MAKING A DECISION WHETHER OR NOT TO PARTICIPATE IN THE STUDY DESCRIBED ABOVE. YOUR SIGNATURE INDICATES THAT YOU HAVE DECIDED TO TAKE PART IN THE STUDY.

_____   _____
Signature of Student   Date

_____   _____
Signature of Investigator   Date

6.14 Methodological Limitations of a Study

Researchers can assume that most studies have limitations in selecting a sample, using a measuring instrument, collecting data, or analyzing results. A section devoted to the limitations of a study is an objective means for discussing flaws in research methods. This section is not meant to be an excuse or rationalization for not obtaining acceptable results or confirming predicted hypotheses, but rather an unbiased analysis of shortcomings in the research. These flaws in methodology do not necessarily mean that the research is worthless or inadequate; on the contrary, it serves to guide future researchers in avoiding the same mistakes when the research is replicated or another research design is proposed. Research, many times, involves trial and error methods with factors of risk and uncertainty. Results are significant if the researcher has been objective and unbiased. The honesty and integrity of the researcher are enhanced when both the merits and deficiencies of a study are objectively reported. The limitations of a study can serve as the basis for recommending further research.

Methodological Limitations of a Study

CHAPTER
7

Data Analysis and Statistics

Statistical interpretation depends not only on statistical ideas, but also on "ordinary" thinking. Clear thinking is not only indispensable in interpreting statistics, but is often sufficient even in the absence of specific statistical knowledge.—W. A. Wallis and H. V. Roberts, *The Nature of Statistics* (p. 29)

••

Operational Learning Objectives

At the end of this chapter, the reader will be able to

1. define statistics
2. describe the importance of statistics in contemporary society
3. understand the difference between descriptive and inferential statistics
4. understand the concept of measurement and data
5. understand the difference between discrete and continuous data
6. identify seven statistical models for analyzing clinical research data
7. distinguish between parametric and nonparametric statistical tests
8. understand when to apply specific statistical tests to clinical research designs

7.1 Definition and Meaning of Statistics

Statistics, as a practical discipline, is defined as the application of statistical tests and procedures for organizing, analyzing, and interpreting results or data according to mathematical formulas. Statistics is taught in almost every university and college in the United States. Although statistics is derived from mathematics, it is taught in many academic departments with application to economics, agriculture, medicine, natural, physical and social sciences, nursing, the allied health professions, and education. The rapid evolution of main frame and personal computers has expanded the role of statistics to almost every aspect of our life such as banking, retailing, education, manufacturing, farming, politics, communication, transportation, and health care. Through the availability of modems and electronic mail, statistical programs and databases are easily accessible by researchers. Computer programs using sophisticated statistical models have enabled pollsters to predict election results based on representative sampling procedures and insurance companies to set up actuarial tables based on the presence or absence of risk factors for morbidity and mortality.

Statistics is also an essential component of clinical research, enabling the investigator to objectively describe and infer logical conclusions from the results. In general, statistical analysis of the data strengthens the impact of the results and allows the investigator to compare current findings with previous research. The researcher in the health professions should have a basic understanding of descriptive statistics and the most frequently used inferential statistical tests and procedures. Inferential statistics include *t* test and analysis of variance, for comparing sample means; Pearson correlation coefficient and Spearman rank order correlation, for testing relationships between variables; and Chi-square, for testing the differences between observed and expected frequencies. The researcher should be able to calculate the incidence (initial occurrences) and prevalence (prevailing rates) of diseases and to be able to read and interpret vital statistics related to morbidity and mortality. Quantifiable or measurable data are counted as statistics. For example, the total number of individuals with a spinal cord injury, number of workers with disabilities, or the number of occupational therapists working in public schools are identifiable statistics.

Historically, the earliest statistics amassed by local authorities were census counts. Statistical occurrences also replaced subjective descriptions of populations, such as "abundant," "flourishing," and "enormous" to describe epidemics and population density. The first use of statistics recorded factual information, such as the annual rate of births, deaths, and marriages. During periods of epidemics, such as the "black death" (bubonic plague) in London during the sixteenth and seventeenth centuries, statistics were used to tabulate the number of deaths and their presumed causes. Also, statistics were used in Europe before the Middle Ages by tax collectors who used data to assess wealth and agricultural holdings. In the latter half of the eighteenth century, census taking became a systematic governmental function. In the U.S. Constitution of 1790, provision was made for a regular population census every 10 years. The application of probability theory to the prediction of death rates (actuarial tables among populations) and the use of sampling procedures advanced the science of statistics. In the mid-nineteenth century, statistical societies were founded (e.g., the American Statistical Association was organized in Boston in 1839). Vital statistics became more accurate and methods were developed to analyze health data and correlate injuries and diseases with occupation and social class. The emergence of modern statistics based on probability theory led to the application of statistical methods in laboratory and clinical research. R. A. Fisher, a geneticist, extended statistics from small samples where inferences were made to large populations. The work of Fisher and his colleagues in the early part of the 1900s led the way to quantifiable analysis of research data in the biological, physical, and social sciences. Currently hundreds of textbooks are published on the application and theory of statistics in a wide range of professional disciplines. In spite of this, the field of statistics is as much of an art as an empirical science. There are many points of disagreement on the correctness of applying specific statistical tests to research data. The student learning and applying statistics must decide which statistical tests are most appropriate for analyzing the results. How the variable is measured (e.g., continuous or discrete), the probability level required, and the direction of the hypothesis stated will help the researcher to select a specific statistical test. The material presented in this chapter is organized to aid the student to read and understand statistics presented in research articles and to follow a step-by-step procedure in calculating statistical results. Each step of the process of deciding upon the statistical test to be employed, the analysis of the raw data, and the interpretation of the statistical results should be carried through in a problem-solving, reflective manner.

7.2 Relationship of Statistics to Clinical Practice

Statistics as a methodology enables the researcher to organize, analyze, and interpret data. In the context of a research design, statistical application does not change the quality of the data, nor influence the validity of the results. In conducting research, the investigator should have an overall concept of the meaning of the projected results and how a statistical test will be used to accept or reject a hypothesis. For example, an investigator wishes to compare attitudes of health professionals and non-health professionals toward individuals with disabilities, utilizing a survey questionnaire. He or she has hypothesized that health professionals will have more positive, realistic attitudes toward those individuals with disabilities than non-health professionals. Then the researcher would apply a statistical test, such as an analysis of variance, to accept or reject the hypothesis.

The process of statistical analysis and its relationship to clinical practice is illustrated in Figure 7–1. In this example a clinician proposes to test the effectiveness of a specific treatment method.

Six stages may be distinguished in this process:

1. A hypothesis is conceived.
2. A research plan is devised to study the effects of a treatment method or procedure traditionally used by clinicians.
3. Quantifiable data are collected from a patient group.
4. The data are statistically processed and analyzed.
5. The results are interpreted.
6. Conclusions are drawn and the information is disseminated back to the scientific community and clinical practitioners.

The cycle continues with new treatment methods introduced and ineffective methods discarded. Hopefully, the process leads to the evolution of clinical efficacy.

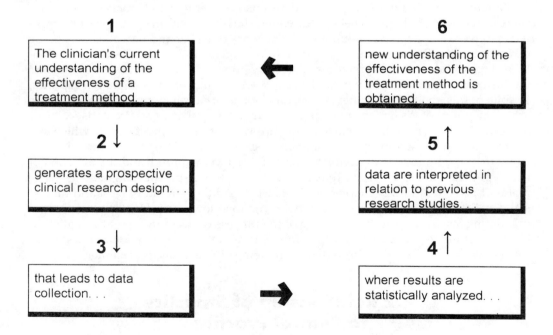

1
The clinician's current understanding of the effectiveness of a treatment method. . .

6
new understanding of the effectiveness of the treatment method is obtained. . .

2 ↓
generates a prospective clinical research design. . .

5 ↑
data are interpreted in relation to previous research studies. . .

3 ↓
that leads to data collection. . .

4 ↑
where results are statistically analyzed. . .

Figure 7–1.   Relationship between research and clinical practice. Notice that the relationship is continuous; the completion of Step 6 leads back to Step 1. A clinician should be continually involved in practices that lead to research that can be applied to clinical practice.

This example demonstrates the importance of statistics to clinical research. What are the most common statistical procedures employed in clinical research?

Statistical procedures employed in clinical research are based on descriptive and inferential statistics. Figure 7–2 outlines the specific descriptive and inferential statistical tests.

Descriptive statistics are procedures for reducing, summarizing and describing results or data. In descriptive statistics, for example, a large set of data are reduced to summary values, graphs, frequency polygons and scatter diagrams, measures of central tendency (mode, median, and mean), measures of variability (range, standard deviation, and variance), and incidence and prevalence rates.

Inferential statistics are methods for generalizing data collected from a representative sample to a larger target population that includes all subjects or observations. The essence of inferential statistics is to sample a representative portion of a population in order to infer information representative of the whole population. Inferential statistics are applied for two main purposes: (a) to estimate the characteristics of a population (parameters), and (b) to test hypotheses about populations. In inferential statistics a sample is drawn from the target population, the characteristics of this sample are measured, and inferences or estimates about the corresponding characteristics are made to the population at large.

A *parameter* is a descriptive value assigned to a condition or population. Parameters are constant—like the characteristics of a specified population. For example, in the population of individuals with paraplegia in North America, the parameter value of age would be inferred or estimated since it would be almost impossible to survey all individuals who have paraplegia within North America. The parameter value is usu-

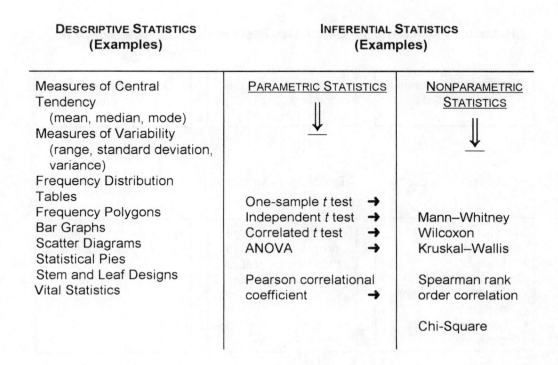

DESCRIPTIVE STATISTICS (Examples)	INFERENTIAL STATISTICS (Examples)	
	PARAMETRIC STATISTICS ⇓	NONPARAMETRIC STATISTICS ⇓
Measures of Central Tendency (mean, median, mode) Measures of Variability (range, standard deviation, variance) Frequency Distribution Tables Frequency Polygons Bar Graphs Scatter Diagrams Statistical Pies Stem and Leaf Designs Vital Statistics	One-sample *t* test → Independent *t* test → Correlated *t* test → ANOVA → Pearson correlational coefficient →	Mann–Whitney Wilcoxon Kruskal–Wallis Spearman rank order correlation Chi-Square

Figure 7–2. Statistical procedures and tests used in the analysis of data.

ally estimated through descriptive studies of representative samples in more than one geographical area. The data from a representative sample are extrapolated to the target population. The reliability of the estimate increases with the number of descriptive studies that show concurrence.

A *statistic* is a quantitative measure of a sample. For example, the average heart rate of a sample of college students is 72 beats per minute. This is a statistic with a summary value representing the average heart rate in the sample. When a total population is available and every individual is measured, a parameter value may be computed directly. Population data usually are not available, so that researchers use a representative sample drawn from a population to compute a statistic and employ inferential statistics to estimate or extrapolate parameter values. Vital statistics are used to estimate the incidence or prevalence rates of a specific disability in a population. For example, if an investigator is interested in determining the number of individuals with a diagnosis of muscular dystrophy in the United States, he or she can carry out epidemiological studies with representative samples in specified geographical areas such as in the Midwestern States. Frequently, epidemiological studies are replicated in other geographical areas to test the validity of previous results and to monitor trends in the incidence and prevalence rates of specific diseases.

The Process of Statistical Analysis

The important steps for the researcher are to develop a hypothesis, select the appropriate statistical test, calculate the results, and finally interpret the data. Diagrammatically the decision process in applying statistics and interpreting the results is shown in Figure 7–3.

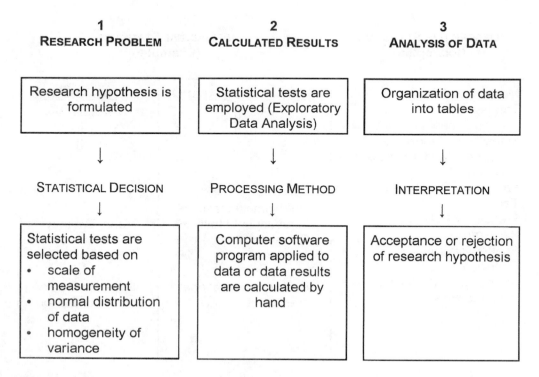

Figure 7–3.   The process of statistical analysis.

7.3 Key Definitions of Statistical Concepts

The first step in understanding statistics is to understand the definitions of statistical terms. With a conceptual understanding of statistics one can critically understand published studies that use statistical designs. The bases on which hypotheses are substantiated or rejected and conclusions generated are derived from a statistical analysis of the results. The following definitions are essential to understand statistics. They are listed alphabetically and are intended to be used as a reference aid.

Continuous variables are examples of *interval* or *ratio scale measurement*. Weight, height, age, muscle strength, blood pressure, and hearing acuity are all examples of continuous variables. It is assumed that in measuring continuous variables there are infinite degrees of values between each score.

Data are the numerical results of a study. In a descriptive study of a population, data are enumerated totals, such as the number of emergency patients in a hospital clinic or the number of health care workers in a rural area. Descriptive averages of population, such as the mean and median, are data. In small sample research in which inferential (probability) statistics are used, data represent comparative results derived from the research. These results are the bases of discussion and interpretation. The singular of data is datum or statistic.

Degrees of freedom (df) is a mathematically derived value used in reading statistical tables. It is *usually* calculated by subtracting 1 from the total number (N) of subjects in a group. It is defined as the number of observations in the calculation of a statistic that are free to vary.

Dichotomous variables contain only two subsets such as gender, improvement or no improvement, experimental and control group, or any other two variable sets created by the investigator or found naturally.

Discrete variables identify separate categories such as diagnostic groups, allied health professions, occupations, vitamins, pharmaceutical drugs, and treatment methods. Discrete variables belong to a set of objects sharing some trait or characteristic. They are examples of nominal scale measurements.

A *directional hypothesis* predicts:

a.   there will be a statistically significant difference between two groups after applying a treatment in experimental research, or
b.   there will be a statistically significant relationship between two variables.

Frequency is the number of times that a result occurs. A frequency distribution table of results describes the number of times a variable falls into a discrete category.

Measures of central tendency are descriptive statistics such as the mean, median, and mode.

Measures of dispersion or variability are descriptive statistics that indicate the spread of results in a distribution of scores. The range, variance, and standard deviation are measures of dispersion. Factors such as the difference between the highest and lowest scores and the number of scores that deviate from the mean influence measures of dispersion.

Nonparametric statistics are sometimes referred to as "distribution-free" statistical tests because they are applied to data for which no assumptions are made regarding the normal distribution of the population and interval scale measurement. The advantages of nonparametric statistics are that they can be applied to small sample data without having to meet the stringent assumptions of parametric statistics. Examples of nonparametric tests include Chi-square, Spearman rho, Mann–Whitney test, Wilcoxon test for correlated samples, and Kruskal–Wallis test.

The *normal curve or bell-shaped distribution* represents a theoretical distribution that approximates the range and frequency of many normal human functions and anatomical descriptions, such as blood pressure, lung capacity, height, and weight. The major assumption underlying the concept of a normal curve is that variables are distributed along a continuum with the greatest frequency in the middle and the least frequency at the outer edges of the distribution. Figure 7–4 indicates the percentage of cases found within each area of the normal curve. For example, 68% of cases are distributed towards the center of the curve in a symmetrical pattern. The basis of inferential parametric statistics rests on the assumption that the sample data are derived from a population that is normally distributed.

A *null hypothesis* predicts that there will be no statistically significant difference or correlation between two or more specified groups, that is, after experimentally manipulating a variable or when testing the relationships between variables.

Parametric statistics are applied to data where certain underlying assumptions have been made. These are:

a.   The variables measured approximate a normal distribution curve in the target population sampled.
b.   The sample is a random selection or is representative of the target population.
c.   The variables are measured by an interval scale; that is, there is equal arithmetical distance between each value or scores.
d.   The variance, such as the standard deviation, within the groups being compared are approximately the same.

Examples of parametric statistics are *t* test, analysis of variance (ANOVA) and Pearson product–moment correlation coefficient.

A *research hypothesis* is a prediction of results.

Standard deviation is a statistical measure of the variability of scores from the mean.

Standard error of measurement (SEM) is a statistical value that indicates the band of error surrounding a test score. For example, a raw score of 90 with a SEM of 4 represents a score ranging from 86 to 94.

Statistical assumptions are preconditions that are required before a specific statistical test can be applied. These assumptions usually involve the following factors:

a.   The variable distributed in a population approximates the normal curve. For example, muscle strength, intelligence, systolic blood pressure, and

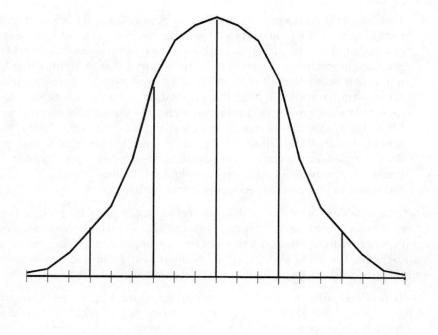

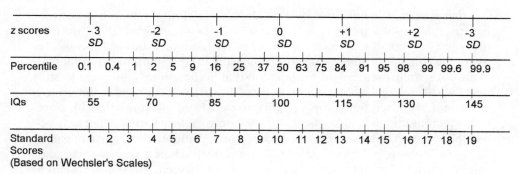

z scores	- 3 SD		-2 SD		-1 SD		0 SD		+1 SD		+2 SD		-3 SD

Percentile	0.1	0.4	1	2	5	9	16	25	37	50	63	75	84	91	95	98	99	99.6	99.9

IQs	55	70	85	100	115	130	145

Standard Scores
(Based on Wechsler's Scales)

1	2	3	4	5	6	7	8	9	10	11	12	13	14	15	16	17	18	19

Figure 7–4. The bell-shaped curve, which illustrates the percentage of population at each level. Included in this figure are the relationships between the standard deviations (z scores), percentiles, IQ scores, and standard scores (based on Wechsler's scaled scores).

height are variables that are assumed to approximate a normal curve in a standard population.

b. The data collected are measurable. Some statistical tests require interval scale data whereas other tests allow for ordinal or nominal scale data.

c. There is a homogeneity of variance within the group scores. Large differences in standard deviations of two groups present some difficulty. However, it is unclear what constitutes a large difference. Some statisticians (Welkowitz, Ewen, & Cohen, 1971) say to ignore this assumption if the two sample sizes are equal (and there are not vast differences between the standard deviations) when applying the t test.

d. The sample is randomly selected from a population. The object of random sampling is to obtain an unbiased sample that is to be truly representative of a population. The difficulty in obtaining a true random sample when applied to clinical research is that it is almost impossible to identify and locate a population, such as all individuals diagnosed with diabetes, arthritis, or schizophrenia, and then from this population select a random sample. The most prevalent sample in clinical research is the convenient sample accessible to the researcher, such as in a teaching hospital, university, public school, or outpatient clinic. On the other hand it is possible to assign random samples from a convenient population, such as hospital patients, who can be randomly assigned to experimental and control groups.

e. The groups compared are independent of each other.

Statistical tables contain critical levels and values of probability for accepting or rejecting a hypothesis. By using a statistical table the investigator determines whether the statistical value obtained is significant as compared to the critical value. In using statistical tables the investigator decides the level of significance, such as .05 or .01.

Statistically significant results means that there are differences between two or more groups that are not due to chance. In every statistically significant result there is a comparison between the effects on two or more groups.

Experimental Clinical Research: Traditionally, in clinical research statistically significant results are accepted at the .05 level or .01 level, which means that the results are not due to chance in 95 out of 100 cases or 99 out of 100 cases. In using the concept of statistical significance, the investigator, in experimental clinical research, assumes an explanation that is sometimes confusing to students who think that statistics is an exact science that can be used to determine cause and effect relationships. Conclusive cause and effect relationships are only meaningful when an investigator can control every variable that may affect the results. The closest that medical research comes to the control of extraneous variables is in experimental animal research where environmental and sometimes genetic factors can be rigorously controlled. In clinical research with human subjects it is almost impossible to attain results that are 100% conclusive because of the interactional effects between the therapist, patient, treatment method, and environment. It is also important to bear in mind that inferential statistics, which are based on probability theory, are applied to data derived from samples of populations, so that everyone in a population is not tested or measured. Samples per se indicate inconclusive data and an uncertainty even if a representative sample has been selected. In summary, a statistically significant result in experimental clinical research implies that:

a. Probability theory is assumed in interpreting the data.
b. A sample of population is used rather than the entire population.
c. There is an allowance for error based on a researcher's inability to control all variables that may possibly influence the results.
d. Conclusiveness of results is not assumed, and the investigator can only suggest that a cause–effect relationship exists.

Test of statistical significance based on the characteristics of the normal curve and probability theory imply the following:

a. *Two-tailed tests of statistical significance* are used in analyzing data if the researcher has stated the hypothesis in a null form.

b. *One-tailed tests of statistical significance* imply that the researcher has predicted a directional hypothesis and there is prior evidence, either through a literature review or clinical observation, that there will be a statistically significant difference between the groups or a statistically positive correlation between variables.

Variables are factors that can be operationally defined, categorized, and measured. Variables can be homogeneous groups, such as undergraduate university students, patients with hemiplegia, or hospital administrators. Variables are also conditions or behavior such as group therapy, cardiovascular disease, or ADL training. In experimental research, the *independent variable*, which is manipulated by the investigator, is the direct cause of the *dependent variable*, which is the resultant effect. Variables can be discrete, dichotomous, rank order, or continuous. (Also refer to Chapter 6, Research Design and Methodology, for further discussion about variables.)

Variance is a measure of the average of each score's deviation from the mean. Variance is an intermediate value used in calculating the standard deviation.

Universal Symbols Used in Statistics

$\propto$ alpha, usually associated with hypothesis testing (Type I error)

β beta, usually associated with hypothesis testing (Type II error)

χ^2 Chi-square statistical test

df   degrees of freedom

f   frequency of cases in a distribution

F   statistic associated with analysis of variance (ANOVA)

H_0 null hypothesis (no statistically significant difference; $\bar{x}_1 = \bar{x}_2$)

H_1 alternative hypothesis (opposite of null hypothesis; $\bar{x}_1 \neq \bar{x}_2$)

μ mu, the population or parameter mean; oftentimes, this value is unknown and estimated by $\bar{x}$

n   number of subjects within a designated sample

N   total of number of subjects in a group or population

p   probability, such as $p < .05$ (the level of error accepted in the study)

r   the Pearson product–moment correlation coefficient indicating the degree of relationship between two variables

s   the standard deviation of a sample (*SD*)

r_s the Spearman rank order correlation for ordinal data (formerly rho [ρ])

σ lowercase sigma, the standard deviation of a population, usually estimated

Σ uppercase sigma, sum of an arithmetic calculation

t   *t* test statistic

t_{obs} *t* observed, *t* value derived from the *t* test

t_{crit} *t* critical, the value derived from a statistical table of values

$\bar{x}$ the mean value of a sample

z   standard score measured in standard deviation units

$\neq$ not equal to

$\geq$ more than or equal to

$\leq$ less than or equal to

7.4 Seven Statistical Models for Clinical Research

Seven statistical models for analyzing data are outlined in Table 7–1. These models represent the most frequently used statistical tests for clinical researchers. The format in presenting each model is to define the model and the statistical tests which the models represent, analyze an example of the statistical test from the literature, outline sequential steps in calculating the statistical results, and follow through with a hypothetical stepwise example. Many statistical tests are not covered in these models. References to textbooks on statistics are provided throughout the chapter as a guide for those researchers inspired to look further into the world of statistics. As one becomes adept in using statistical software programs for personal computers, the options for selecting statistical tests broaden. However, first it is important for the clinical researcher to understand the concepts underlying the statistical applications. Doing statistical tests with a hand calculator and doing exploratory data analysis aids the researcher to better understand statistical processes that are later done through computer software programs.

Model I: Descriptive Statistics

In this model the researcher calculates descriptive statistics based on data collected from a representative sample or the total population. The statistical procedures include:

- Frequency Distribution Tables
- Frequency Polygons
- Histograms and Bar Graphs
- Scatter Diagrams
- Statistical Pies
- Stem and Leaf
- Measures of Central Tendency
- Measures of Variability
- Vital Statistics

Model II: One-Sample Problems

The purpose of this statistical model is to compare data collected from a representative sample of a population and to compare this value with a parameter value that already exists. Examples include comparing air samples from a metropolitan area to a standard accepted for clean air. The research question answered by this model is whether the mean of the representative sample and the established parameter mean value are statistically significantly different. The statistical procedure for this model is the one-sample t test.

Model III: Two Independent Samples

The purpose of this statistical model is to test whether the means for two representative samples are statistically significantly different. An example in clinical research is determining whether one treatment method (such as sensory integration therapy) is more effective in reducing hyperactivity than another comparable treatment method (such as relaxation therapy) in two independent groups. The statistical test (indepen-

Table 7-1 *Seven Statistical Models*

Statistical Model	Purpose	Examples of Statistical Tests or Procedures
I. **Descriptive Statistics**	describe the statistical characteristics in samples or populations	Measures of central tendency (mean, mode, median), measures of variability (range, standard deviation, variance), frequency distribution table, frequency graph, scatter diagram, statistical pie, stem and leaf, vital statistics
Inferential Statistics		
II. One–Sample	test the difference between a sample mean and a parameter mean	One–sample *t* test
III. Two Independent Samples	test the differences between sample means from two independent groups	Independent *t* test (parametric statistic) Mann–Whitney *U* test (nonparametric statistic)
IV. Paired–Data Sample	test the differences between two conditions (means) in the same sample	Correlated *t* test (parametric statistic) Wilcoxon signed rank test (nonparametric statistic)
V. k–Independent Samples	test the differences between means from two or more independent groups	ANOVA (parametric statistic) Kruskal–Wallis (nonparametric statistic)
VI. Correlation	test the relationship between two variables	Spearman rank order (nonparametric statistic), Pearson correlation coefficient (parametric statistic), regression line, correlation matrix
VII. Observed Frequencies	test the differences between observed minus expected frequencies	Chi–square (nonparametric statistic)

Note. Adapted from *Statistics for the Allied Health Sciences* by R. J. Larson, 1975, Merrill Publishing.

dent *t* test) is applied to determine whether there is a statistically significant difference between the two treatment methods. The *Mann–Whitney* nonparametric statistical test is another example used to evaluate data using this model.

Model IV: Paired-Data Sample

The primary purpose of this statistical model is to examine the difference between mean values in one sample group with two data points, such as pretest and posttest. This statistical model employs the correlated *t* test to test whether there will be a statistically significant difference between the means in two conditions. This statistical model is frequently used in clinical research to determine if a treatment method is effective when compared to a baseline measure of a dependent variable. The *Wilcoxon* nonparametric statistical test is an alternative to the parametric one-sample correlated *t* test.

Model V: Independent Samples

If the researcher is comparing the means of more than two independent samples, then the researcher applies an analysis of variance (ANOVA). The ANOVA is similar to the independent test when two independent samples are being compared. If the results of the ANOVA are statistically significant, then the researcher employs post hoc tests to determine which groups are statistically different from each other. These post hoc tests (similar to *t* tests) include the Scheffé, Duncan multiple analysis, or Tukey tests. The nonparametric alternative to ANOVA is the *Kruskal–Wallis* statistical test.

Model VI: Correlational Sample

In this statistical model the researcher measures the degree of relationship between two variables, such as in a study examining the relationship between perceptual motor skills and reading achievement. The relationship can range from zero, indicating that the two variables are completely independent and do not affect each other, to 1.00, indicating a perfect relationship between two variables. An example of a perfect correlation is the effect of temperature on the expansion of the chemical element mercury. As the temperature goes up mercury expands, and as the temperature goes down mercury contracts. A perfect correlation can be positive (+1.00), when both variables change in the same direction, or negative/inverse (−1.00) when the variables change in inverse directions, so that as one variable goes up, the other variable goes down. An example of an inverse relationship is the presence of serotonin, a neurotransmitter, and symptoms of depression. As serotonin is depleted in the blood, the symptoms of depression increase.

The relationship between two variables can be described in a scatter diagram. The Pearson correlation coefficient for interval scale data and the Spearman rank order correlation for ordinal scale data are applied to evaluate the degree of relationship (*r*) between two variables. A regression line can be calculated when there is a high correlation between two variables. The regression line is calculated by using the results of the Pearson correlation coefficient and plugging the values into a formula for the regression line. In this formula, variable values are estimated from known *X* variable values. This is illustrated in Figure 7–5.

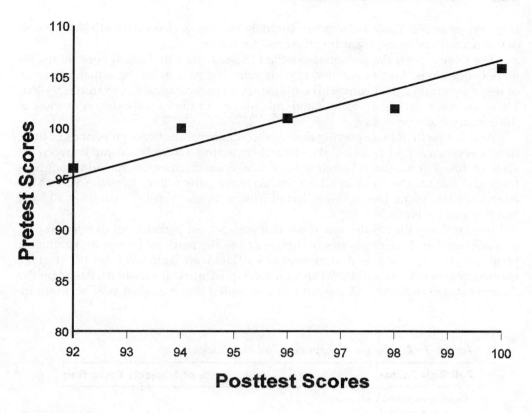

Figure 7–5.   Example of a scattergram, showing the relationship between two variables. When the value of *X* is known, then the value of *Y* can be predicted by the use of the regression line.

Model VII: Observed Minus Expected Frequencies

In this model the investigator compares groups or conditions on the basis of frequency or nominal data. Chi-square is the statistical test used when comparing the differences between observed frequencies and expected frequencies based on probability. Chi-square is used frequently, for example, in drug research to compare the differences in the number of patients who have improved with an experimental drug as compared to the number of patients taking a placebo who have improved.

7.5 Model I: Descriptive Statistics: Organization and Tabulation of Descriptive Data

7.5.1 Percentage Table

Statistical analysis begins with organizing data into summary tables and diagrams. In descriptive studies like in survey research, tabular summaries of data provide the results. For example, Table 7–2 summarizes data from interviews with 115 elderly residents in a nursing home, regarding their risk for falling.

The table reports the percentage of the 115 residents who replied "yes" to the interview questions. An alternative way of describing data is to list the actual frequency of responses rather than convert the frequency to percentages. For example, 96% or 110 of the residents use eyeglasses and only 6% or 7 of the subjects always or most of the time are dizzy on arising.

Another method of displaying data is to compare results between periods of time, distances or events. In Table 7–3 the researchers examine the relationship between the stage of illness at diagnosis (whether the cancer is localized or has spread throughout the body) and the distances in kilometers (k) that a patient lives from the Three Mile Island Nuclear plant. Data were collected from a review of patient charts at all local and regional hospitals.

In examining the results, one notes that pre vs. post percentages of selected cancers are listed at three categories of distance from the patients' homes to the nuclear plant, (i.e., 0–6 k, 6–12 k, and more than 12 k). Data were collected from 1975 to 1979 (pre-nuclear accident) and 1979 through 1985 (post-nuclear accident). Based on the data presented in Table 7–3, the authors concluded that a modest post-accident in-

Table 7–2 *Subjects' Reported Fall Risk Factors*

Fall Risk Factor	% of Subjects Reporting
Health compared with peers	
Excellent	7
Good	57
Fair	28
Poor	8
Use eyeglasses	96
Always/Most of the time	55
Use walking aid	38
Always/Most of the time	20
Dizzy on arising	31
Always/Most of the time	6
Pain in muscles, bones, joints	80
Always/Most of the time	45
Hold on for support	30
Always/Most of the time	13
Difficult to get in and out of bed	16
Always/Most of the time	4
Use prescription medication	80
Use alcohol	43
One a week or more	7
Stand on chair to reach	56
Have grab bars in bathroom	85
Breathless	54
Always/Most of the time	23

Note. From "Falls and Fear of Falling among Elderly Persons Living in the Community" by J. E. Walker and J. Howland, 1991, *American Journal of Occupational Therapy, 45,* p. 120. Copyright 1991 by *American Journal of Occupational Therapy.* Reprinted with permission.

crease in cancer was observed. The reader will note that of the 36 possible results (12 cancer sites × 3 distance categories) there were 21 increased percentages from pre to post, while 15 of the results showed decreased percentages from pre- to post-accident.

The above examples demonstrate the importance of descriptive statistics in summarizing results from a research study. A number of methods can be used to describe data. The most frequently used descriptive methods for organizing data are discussed in the section below.

7.5.2 Frequency Distribution Table

A *frequency distribution table* is organized into columns of data that include the number or frequency of cases (and the equivalent percentages) that fall into a designated category. In the research study in Table 7–4, a frequency distribution table describes the age and sex of the population sampled in the study.

The first column of a frequency distribution table includes the class intervals (in this example, age group by years). It could also represent data such as range of motion in degrees, scores on perceptual tests, or diastolic blood pressure. The class intervals are separated into equal 10-year intervals in the above example (e.g., 15–24 and 25–34). The second column of a frequency distribution includes the number of classes tallied within the class interval, as with 36 males between the ages of 5 and 14. The third column includes the percentage of cases within a class interval. For example, there are 52 females in the class interval of 25–34, which represents 52 over a total of 228 females in the study or 22.8%, which is rounded to 23%. We can also determine the *cumulative frequency* of each class interval and the *cumulative relative frequency* with the data provid-

Table 7–3 *Example of a Frequency Distribution*

Stage at Diagnosis	0–6 k pre vs. post		> 6–12 k pre vs. post		> 12 k pre vs. post	
Breast Cancer						
Local	39.3	40.4	39.4	51.8	46.0	48.5
Regional	52.6	42.5	31.3	30.7	32.2	36.5
Distant	8.2	17.0	29.1	17.8	21.7	15
Prostate Cancer						
Local	62.2	41.7	56.1	59.8	53.3	60.9
Regional	9.0	13.5	20.2	10.7	17.7	15.6
Distant	29.8	44.9	23.7	29.5	29.0	23.5
Lung Cancer						
Local	30.7	36.9	37.5	24.0	23.6	26.7
Regional	23.9	16.9	13.6	26.2	29.4	25.5
Distant	45.4	46.4	48.9	49.8	47.0	47.9
Colon Cancer						
Local	29.7	39.3	30.9	29.1	27.0	30.8
Regional	43.9	29.9	31.7	34.7	35.9	36.2
Distant	26.4	30.8	37.4	36.2	37.1	33.0

Note: From "Cancer Rates after the Three Mile Island Nuclear Accident and Proximity of Residents to the Plant" by M. C. Hatch, S. Wallenstein, J. Beyen, J. W. Nieves, and M. Susser, 1991, *American Journal of Public Health, 81,* p. 723. Copyright 1991 by *American Journal of Public Health.* Reprinted with permission.

Table 7-4   *Age and Sex Distribution of Migrant Survey Population*

Age Group (Years)	Male No.	Male (%)	Female No.	Female (%)	Total No.	Total (%)
5–14	36	6	31	14	67	8
15–24	147	24	75	33	222	26
25–34	200	33	52	23	252	30
35–44	105	17	29	13	134	16
45–54	60	10	24	11	84	10
55–64	41	7	10	4	51	6
65 +	21	3	6	3	27	3
Unknown	4	0	1	0	5	0
Total	**614**	**100**	**228**	**(101)***	**842**	**99**

*Totals differ from 100% due to rounding.

Note. From "Tuberculosis Risk among Migrant Farm Workers on the Relmarva Peninsula" by M. L. Jacobson, M. A. Mercer, L. K. Miller, and T. W. Simpson, 1987, *American Journal of Public Health, 77,* p. 30. Copyright 1987 by *American Journal of Public Health.* Reprinted with permission.

ed in the study. The following data are reorganized into a frequency distribution table to include relative frequency and cumulative relative frequency for males only:

Frequency Distribution Table for Males

Class Interval	Frequency (*F*)	Relative *F* (%)	Cumulative *F*	Cumulative *rf*%
5–14	36	6	36	6
15–24	147	24	183	30
25–34	200	33	383	63
35–44	105	17	488	80
45–54	60	10	548	90
55–64	41	7	589	97
>65	21	3	610	100
Unknown	4	.006	614	100
Total	**614**	**100%**	**614**	**100%**

In summary:

Class interval is the category of score values in a distribution. The number of class intervals is determined by the number of subjects in the study and the range of values or scores.

Frequency of cases include the total number of cases within an assigned class interval.

Relative frequency or *percentage* is the percentage of cases falling within the class interval and is calculated by dividing the number of cases within the class interval by the total number of cases in the distribution.

Cumulative frequency represents the total number of scores within a class interval that is added cumulatively from the lowest to the highest class interval. The grand total of the cumulative frequency equals the total number of scores or cases in the distribution.

Cumulative relative frequency or *cumulative percentage* is the percentage of cases added from the lowest class interval through the highest class interval. The percentage should total to 100%.

Constructing a Frequency Distribution Table

The table below displays hypothetical ungrouped raw scores on resting heart rate for 50 healthy young adults.

Step 1. Record raw scores from ungrouped data.

Subject	Score	Subject	Score	Subject	Score	Subject	Score
01	54	14	67	27	54	40	79
02	72	15	74	28	73	41	85
03	80	16	76	29	72	42	52
04	53	17	79	30	78	43	56
05	75	18	77	31	78	44	67
06	53	19	48	32	56	45	55
07	78	20	76	33	80	46	79
08	47	21	47	34	84	47	81
09	72	22	50	35	72	48	72
10	54	23	65	36	68	49	67
11	66	24	83	37	57	50	71
12	68	25	55	38	57		
13	68	26	76	39	63		

Step 2. Identify the highest and lowest values in the distribution. Subjects 08 and 21 have heart rate scores of 47 (lowest score). Subject 41 has a heart rate score of 85 (highest score).

Step 3. Calculate the range (highest score to lowest score). In our example, the range is 85 − 47 = 38.

Step 4. Determine the number of class intervals. The determination of the number of class intervals depends upon the number of scores in the frequency distribution and the range of scores. Too many or too few class intervals may not give adequate information to describe the distribution. Determining the number of class intervals is a trial and error process. For example, let us compare three frequency distributions using the same scores, but with class intervals of too many, too few, and approximately correct. This data is shown in Table 7–5. Most researchers constructing frequency distributions establish 6 to 15 class intervals as a general rule.

Step 5. Determine the size of a class interval. The size of the class interval is determined through estimation by dividing the range of scores by the number of class intervals. Using the same example, the range of 38 is divided by 13 (the number of class intervals) to yield a class interval size of 3. It is recommended that an odd number be selected for the class interval so that the midpoint of the class interval is a whole number. For example, the midpoint of the class interval of 83–85 is 84. Later, in calculating

Table 7–5 *Intervals for Class Data*

Too Many (20 CI)	Too Few (4 CI)	Approximate Correct (13 CI)
84–85	75–85	83–85
82–83	65–74	80–82
80–81	55–64	77–79
78–79	45–54	74–76
76–77		71–73
74–75		68–70
72–73		65–67
70–71		62–64
68–69		59–61
66–67		56–58
64–65		53–55
62–63		50–52
60–61		47–49
58–59		
56–57		
54–55		
52–53		
50–51		
48–49		
46–47		

Number of Class Intervals (CI)

group means from a frequency distribution table, the reader will find that it is easier to work with whole numbers than with fractions in calculating values.

On the other hand, if we determine that the size of a class interval in the above example is 5, how many class intervals would be established? In this case the range of scores (38) is divided by the size of the class intervals (5) to arrive at 8 class intervals.

CI	Midpoint
81–85	83
76–80	78
71–75	73
66–70	68
61–65	63
56–60	58
51–55	53
46–50	48

Step 6. Tally the number of scores within each class interval. Check to determine if the number of tallies total up to the number of scores in the frequency distribution.

Class Interval	Real Limits*	Midpoint	Tally	f	cf
83–85	82.5–85.5	84	III	3	3
80–82	79.5–82.5	81	III	3	6
77–79	76.5–79.5	78	IIIIIII	7	13
74–76	73.5–76.5	75	IIIII	5	18
71–73	70.5–73.5	72	IIIIIII	7	25
68–70	67.5–70.5	69	II	2	27
65–67	64.5–67.5	66	IIIIII	6	33
62–64	61.5–64.5	63	I	1	34
59–61	58.5–61.5	6	0	0	34
56–58	55.5–58.5	57	IIII	4	38
53–55	52.5–55.5	54	IIIIIII	7	45
50–52	49.5–52.5	51	II	2	47
47–49	46.5–49.5	48	III	3	50
	Total		**50**		**50**

*Defining the upper and lower real limits of the class intervals is described below.

The upper real limit of a class interval is the highest value contained in the interval. Conversely the lower real limit of a class interval is the lowest value contained in the interval. In dealing with numbers with at least two decimals, round the number up, in order to include it in the nearest class interval. For example, 82.50 or above would be tallied in the class interval 83–85. On the other hand, 82.44 would be tallied into the class interval 80–82 as shown in the example.

Step 7. Determine the relative frequency or percentage. Calculate the relative frequency of the scores in each class interval by dividing the number of cases or scores in the class interval by the number of cases in the frequency distribution. This is illustrated in Table 7–6.

$$\text{Percentage} = \frac{\text{Frequency of cases in the class interval}}{\text{Total cases in the frequency distribution}}$$

Step 8. Determine cumulative frequency. Calculate the cumulative frequency by adding the total frequency in each class interval consecutively from the highest class interval to the lowest. In the above example, the number of cases in the class interval 83–85 is 3. This number is added to the number of cases in the class interval 80–82 which is also 3, giving a cumulative frequency of 6. The completed frequency distribution table is shown in Table 7–7.

Summary of Construction of Frequency Distribution Table

1. Organize raw scores from ungrouped data by arranging values from the lowest to the highest scores.
2. Identify the lowest and highest scores in the distribution.
3. Calculate the range, which is the difference or distance from the lowest to the highest scores in the distribution.
4. Determine the number of class intervals, using the rule of thumb of selecting within a range of six to fifteen categories of intervals.
5. Determine the size of each class interval. First estimate the size of class intervals by dividing the range by the number of class intervals. Try to select

Table 7–6 *Calculation of Cumulative Frequency*

Class Interval	Frequency	Percentage	Cumulative Percentage
84	3	3/50 = 6%	6%
81	3	3/50 = 6%	12%
78	7	7/50 = 14%	26%
75	5	5/50 = 10%	36%
72	7	7/50 = 14%	50%
69	2	2/50 = 4%	54%
66	6	6/50 = 12%	66%
63	1	1/50 = 2%	68%
60	0	0/50 = 0%	68%
57	4	4/50 = 8%	76%
54	7	7/50 = 14%	90%
51	2	2/50 = 4%	94%
48	3	3/50 = 6%	100%
TOTAL	**50**	**50/50 =100%**	**100%**

Table 7–7 *Frequency Distribution of Heart Rate Scores for Hypothetical Population*

CI	Midpoint	f	cf	rf	crf
83–85	84	3	3	6%	6%
80–82	81	3	6	6%	12%
77–79	78	7	13	14%	26%
74–76	75	5	18	10%	36%
71–73	72	7	25	14%	50%
68–70	69	2	27	4%	54%
65–67	66	6	33	12%	66%
62–64	63	1	34	2%	68%
59–61	60	0	34	0%	68%
56–58	57	4	38	8%	76%
53–55	54	7	45	14%	90%
50–52	51	2	47	4%	94%
47–49	48	3	50	6%	100%

an odd number so that the midpoint of the class interval will be a whole number.

6. Count or tally the number of scores within each class interval.
7. Calculate the relative frequency or percentage of scores in each class interval.
8. Calculate the cumulative frequency by adding in succession the frequencies in each class interval. Check that the number of cases counted in succession is equal to the total number of cases or scores in the distribution.
9. Determine the cumulative relative frequency, which is the percentage of cumulative frequency sitting in each class interval. It is customary to start from the lowest class interval when calculating cumulative values.

Graphs and Other Pictorial Representations

In addition to presenting data in tables, many researchers use pictorial presentations to display results and describe data. These presentations can be in the form of frequency polygons, histograms, bar graphs, pie graphs, and stem and leaf.

7.5.3 Frequency Polygon

A frequency polygon is a line graph displaying the frequency of data by categories. The categories compared are on the horizontal axis (abscissa) and the frequencies of occurrences are on the vertical axis (ordinate).

The frequency polygon in Figure 7–6 shows the number of coronary artery bypass surgeries performed in Ontario for the years 1979, 1981, 1983, and 1985. The age group categories are listed on the X axis, the abscissa. Note that usually the midpoint of the category is used as a reference point for plotting the frequencies within each category.

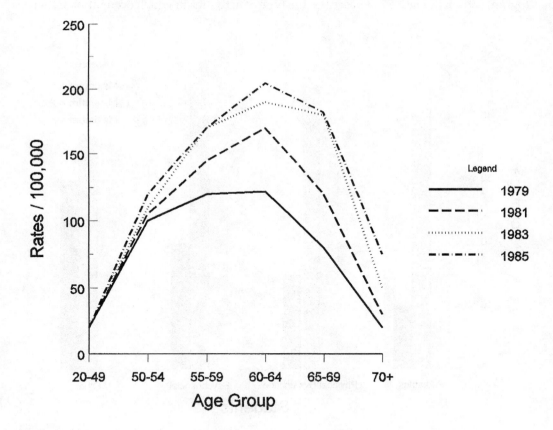

Figure 7–6.   Age-specific rates of coronary artery bypass surgery illustrated in a frequency polygon. (From "Monitoring the Diffusion of Technology: Coronary Artery Bypass Surgery in Ontario" by G. M. Anderson and J. L. Lomas, 1988, *American Journal of Public Health, 78*, p. 252. Copyright 1988 by *American Journal of Public Health*. Reprinted with permission.)

In this example the age categories range from 20 to 49, through 70 and above. The age groups of 50–54, 55–59, 60–64, and 65–69 have an interval of five years and the first age grouping includes those from 20 to 49, an interval of thirty years. The investigators collapsed the data for this age group because so few bypass surgeries were performed on persons of age 20 through 49 years. Surgeries were also infrequent for those age 70 and above. The frequency of cases is shown on the ordinate, or Y axis. In this example the investigators transformed the actual numbers into rates per 100,000 of the population. For example, in the age group 55–59, 150 per 100,000 of this population in Ontario had artery bypass surgery in 1981. Equal intervals of 50 per 100,000 were selected by researchers to indicate categories of frequency.

7.5.4 Histograms and Bar Graphs

Histograms and bar graphs are often used by investigators to display frequency of data within categories, similar to frequency polygons. In histograms the bars are attached to each other, as in Figure 7–7, whereas in bar graphs, each bar is detached from one another. The distinction sometimes is based on aesthetic reasons. The histogram shown in Figure 7–7 describes the type of activities in which occupational ther-

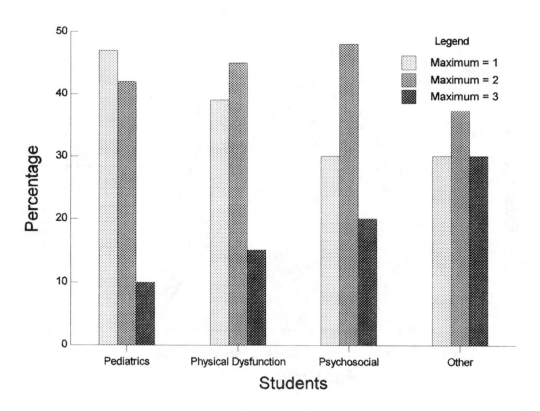

Figure 7–7.   Example of a histogram depicting the maximum number of Level 1 field work students supervised at one time in each type of facility. (From "The Level 1 Field Work Process" by L. D. Shalik, 1990, *American Journal of Occupational Therapy, 44*, p. 702. Copyright 1990, *American Journal of Occupational Therapy*. Reprinted with permission.)

apy students participated while completing their level 1 fieldwork experiences. On the abscissa is the type of fieldwork experience and on the ordinate, the relative frequency or percentage of time spent in a specific activity, such as passive observer, is plotted.

Constructing a Frequency Polygon, Histogram, or Bar Graph

A frequency polygon, histogram, and bar graph graphically depict the data provided in a frequency distribution table. The data provided in the *Frequency Distribution of Heart Rate Scores* in Table 7–7 will be used in the following examples.

Step 1. Identify the X axis (abscissa) and the Y axis (ordinate). This is illustrated in Figure 7–8.

Step 2. Label the abscissa descriptively. In the example in Table 7–7, the heart rate values range from the lowest score of 47 to the highest of 85. The midpoints of each class interval are located on the abscissa (Figure 7–9.) The class intervals are extended on both ends of the class intervals to include zero frequency intervals. The lowest class interval with zero frequency is 44–46 with a midpoint of 45. The highest class interval with zero frequency is 86–88 with a midpoint of 87. There are now 15 class intervals including the zero frequency intervals.

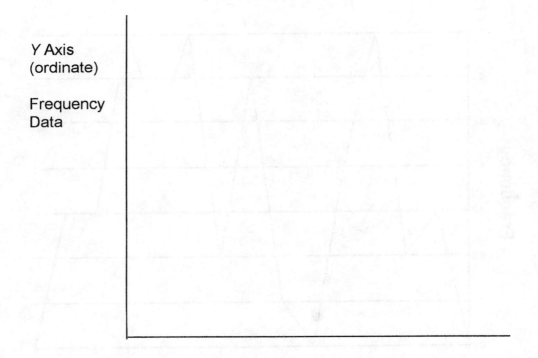

Figure 7–8.   Parts of a frequency polygon, histograph, or bar graph. The frequency data are plotted along the vertical axis or ordinate (Y axis), while the class intervals or time data are plotted along the horizontal axis of abscissa (X).

Step 3. Organize the ordinate into frequency of occurrence. In the above example frequencies of occurrence range from 0 to 7. As a rule of thumb the number of class intervals for frequency should be between 8 and 15. In this case there will be 8 class intervals including 0.

The frequency polygon is depicted in Figure 7–9 with the data from Table 7–7. The histogram is depicted in Figure 7–10 with the exact same data used in constructing the frequency polygon. Bar graphs are similar to histograms with the only difference being that the bars are detached (McCall, 1986).

7.5.5 Cumulative Frequency Distribution Polygon

A cumulative frequency distribution polygon is a line graph that shows the total number of observations or cases up to the upper real limit of a given class interval. For example, in Step 8, determining cumulative frequency (Section 7.5.2), the data for the heart rates for 50 subjects are displayed. In Figure 7–11, the cumulative frequency distribution polygon is constructed from the previous table of hypothetical heart rate values (Table 7–7).

Cumulative frequency curves are useful in specifying the individual subject's relative position or standing in a total distribution of scores. For example, someone with a heart rate of 80 in the above distribution is in the 94th percentile or upper 6% of the

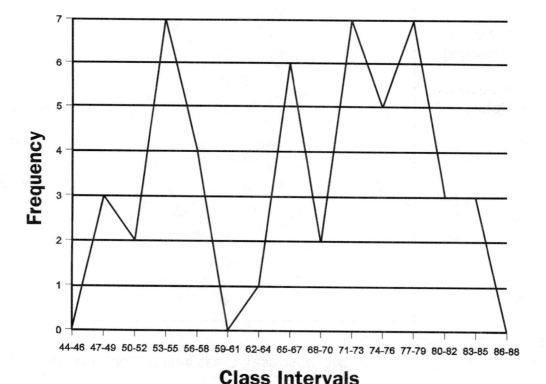

Figure 7–9. Frequency distribution polygon illustrating the frequencies of heart rate scores for a hypothetical population. The data used to plot this polygon are from Table 7–7.

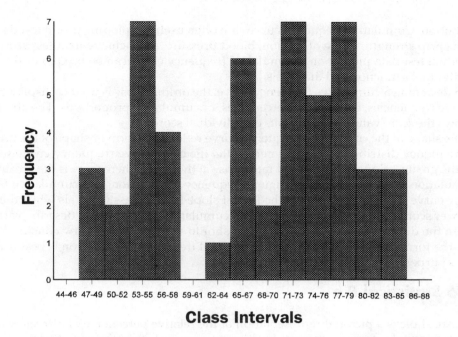

Figure 7–10. Histogram of heart scores in a hypothetical population. The data from Table 7–7 and depicted in Figure 7–9 in a frequency polygon are depicted in a histogram here.

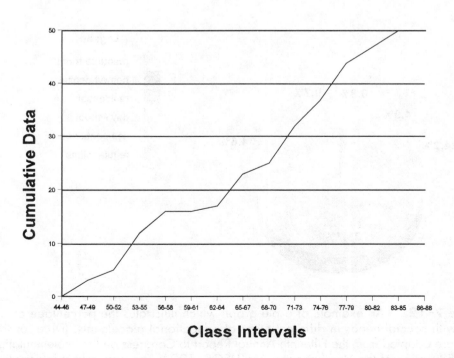

Figure 7–11. Cumulative frequency distribution polygon using data from Table 7–7.

distribution. Cumulative frequency curves are often useful in plotting group test data, such as grip strength, range of motion, blood pressure, and achievement test scores. Individual test data plotted on a cumulative frequency curve can be used to evaluate an individual's function and diagnosis.

In designing a cumulative frequency curve, the ordinate axis is used to display cumulative frequencies, cumulative percentages, or cumulative proportions. The abscissa shows the score values as midpoints or individual scores.

The shape of the cumulative frequency curve reflects the form or shape of the original frequency distribution. As a general rule, the cumulative frequency curve will have the greatest slope or most rapid rate of rise at the point where there is the greatest accumulation of the scores in the original frequency distribution. The cumulative frequency curve levels off and shows the lowest slope for the class intervals when there are fewer scores. It is important to note that cumulative curves do not describe variations in the data as well as histograms and should not be used to draw conclusions about the form or shape of the data. The original frequency distribution is best used for this purpose.

7.5.6 Statistical Pie

A statistical pie is a pictorial representation of the relative percentage of discrete variables or nominal categories, such as health professions, distributions of disease, occupational role functions, types of work injuries, or treatment techniques applied. It is particularly useful to quickly assess the relative percentage of each category. In Figure 7–12, the percentage of placement of students with special needs in each type of educational placement is graphically displayed in a statistical pie.

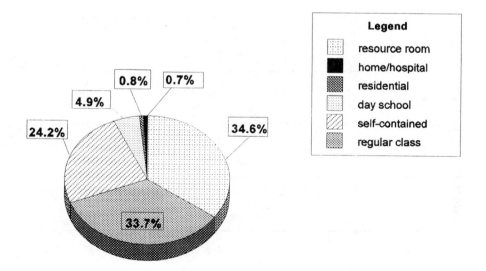

Figure 7–12. An example of a pie graph which illustrates the percentage of students with special needs in different types of educational placements. (Data for this graph are adapted from the Fifteenth Annual Report to Congress on the Implementation of the Education of the Handicapped Act, USOE, 1993. The data reflect information collected in 1990.)

Constructing a Statistical Pie

Step 1. Make sure the statistical pie is relevant for describing data. The statistical pie is appropriate when there are between 3 and 10 discrete categories. If there are more than 10 categories, the data will be better presented in a frequency distribution table. The data collected should be categorical and inclusive. For example, data collected regarding the cause of death should include all major causes for a designated population and should add up to 100%. Unknown causes should be included in the statistical pie.

Step 2. First organize data into a frequency distribution table deriving relative percentages for each category. In the hypothetical example below, specialty areas for female physicians are described. A sample of 250 female physicians were surveyed.

Medical Specialty	Frequency	Relative Percent
Pediatrics	84	33.6
Psychiatry and Neurology	34	13.7
Internal Medicine	25	10.0
Anesthesiology	23	9.1
Pathology	22	8.6
General Surgery	04	1.6
Other	58	23.4
Totals	**250**	**100.0**

Step 3. Transform relative percent into the degrees of a circle, which is the proportion of 360 degrees. The relative percent is multiplied by 360 degrees.

Relative Percent		Relative Degrees
33.6		121
13.7		49
10.0	Relative Percent	36
9.1	× 360 =	33
8.6	Relative Degree	31
1.6		6
23.4		84
Total 100.0		**360**

Step 4. Use a protractor and compass to construct the statistical pie. Divide the statistical pie with a protractor into seven segments running clockwise starting with the largest category at 12 o'clock, which in this example, is pediatrics (33.6% or 121°), other (23.4% or 84°), psychiatry and neurology (13.7% or 49°). Continue with the other specialty areas in completing the 360°.

Step 5. Label each segment category with the relative percent rather than the degrees of arc. The completed statistical pie is shown in Figure 7–13.

7.5.7 Scatter Diagram

A scatter diagram is a graphic representation of the relationship between two variables. In this example the researchers graphically depict the relationship between age

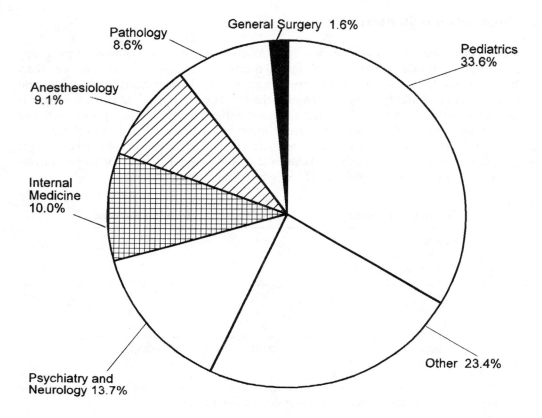

Figure 7–13.   Statistical pie illustrating data from the hypothetical data of women physicians.

(presumed independent variable) and heart rate (presumed dependent variable) in boys and girls between the ages of 2 and 18. (Figure 7–14.) The size of the class interval for age is two years and the size of the class interval for heart rate is 10 beats per minute with a range of 60 to 110. The highest heart rate score observed in the sample of 24 subjects was approximately 105, and the lowest was 60. Note that the researcher set up the graph with break line (//) on the ordinate to indicate that there were no heart rate scores below 60. This is a convenient way of preparing scatter diagrams where ranges begin way above zero.

The points located on the scatter diagrams are coordinates where the two variables intersect. For example, the 10-year-old boy had a heart rate of approximately 70 beats per minute. Each use of the coordinate points indicates the relationship between the two variables for each subject.

Visual examination of the scatter diagram (Figure 7–14) often reveals a trend. In this example heart rate scores became lower as the age increased from 2 to 17. There are also gender differences, which are noted starting at age 10.

Constructing a Scatter Diagram

In a hypothetical example a researcher collects the following data, examining the relationship between grip strength as measured by a Jamar dynamometer and Functional

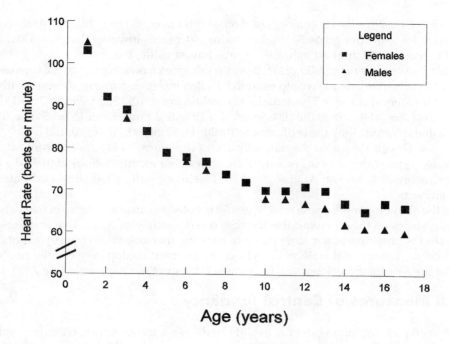

Figure 7–14. Age differences in heart rate. (From "Pulse Rate, Respiratory Rate and Body Temperature of Children Between Two Months and Eighteen Years of Age" by A. Iliff & V. A. Lee, 1952, *Child Development, 23,* 237–245. Copyright 1952 by the *Child Development.* Reprinted with permission.)

Activities of Daily Living scores as measured by the Klein–Bell test for patients with muscular dystrophy.

Step 1. Record raw data for hypothetical example of grip strength and ADL scores in patients with muscular dystrophy.

Subject	Grip Strength (abscissa)	ADL Score (ordinate)
01	15	20
02	40	95
03	30	50
04	30	80
05	10	20
06	25	15
07	10	15
08	20	42
09	20	15
10	15	75
11	40	70
12	30	60
13	20	45
14	10	30
15	40	85

Step 2. Determine the range along the abscissa (grip strength) and ordinate (ADL scores). The range for grip strength is 30 (highest value, 40, minus lowest value, 10). The range for ADL scores is 80 (highest value, 95, minus lowest value, 15).

Step 3. Determine the number of the class intervals for each variable. Using the convention of 6 to 15 class intervals we would establish 8 class intervals for grip strength with the size of the interval being 5. The actual score values are 5, 10, 15, 20, 25, 30, 35, 40 along the abscissa. For ADL scores the class interval is 10 with a range from 15 to 95. The actual score values plotted along the ordinate are 10, 20, 30, 40, 50, 60, 70, 80, 90, 100.

Step 4. Design the scatter diagram (illustrated in Figure 7–15) with the score value on the abscissa (grip strength) and ordinate (ADL scores). For example, Subject 01 had a grip strength score of 15 and an ADL score of 20. The investigator plots the coordinates for all 15 subjects.

In the above example a *positive relationship* is noted because as scores on one variable increase, scores on the other variable increase correspondingly. A negative or inverse relationship is obtained when scores on one variable increase while the corresponding scores on the other variable decrease. The degree of relationship between the two variables of the *correlation coefficient* will be discussed later in this chapter (Section 7.11).

7.5.8 Measures of Central Tendency

The first step in organizing data is usually to design a frequency distribution table or graph. The table or graph provides information concerning the form of the data. The

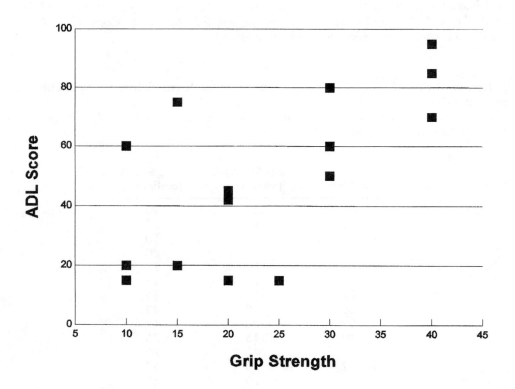

Figure 7–15.   Example of a scattergram. Hypothetical example showing the relationship between grip strength and ADL scores in patients with muscular dystropy.

properties of a set of data can be further described by calculating a summary statistic such as a measure of central tendency. Measures of central tendency describe "typical" or "average" values in a distribution of data. An index of central tendency provides one value that best captures the distribution as a whole. There are generally three ways to do this:

1. The most frequent score in a distribution *(mode)*.
2. The point halfway between the top and bottom halves of a distribution (50th percentile) *(median)*.
3. The arithmetic average of all the scores *(mean)*.

7.5.8.1 Mode

The mode is the easiest measure of central tendency to compute and the simplest to interpret. It may be used to describe any distribution, whether the data is nominal, ordinal, interval, or ratio.

Definition. The mode is the most frequent score (raw or ungrouped data) or the midpoint of the interval containing the most scores (grouped data). In a frequency distribution graph, the mode is the highest peak in the graph. Figure 7–16 illustrates the mode using the following data on a distribution of scores in which there is only one mode:

Score (X)	Frequency of Score (f)	
3	1	
4	2	
5	2	
6	4	Mode = 6
7	2	
8	3	
9	2	

There is no mode in a distribution of scores if all the scores occur with the same frequency (Figure 7–17). For example:

Score (X)	Frequency of Score (f)
1	2
2	2
3	2
4	2

When two adjacent scores have the same frequency, and this frequency is higher than any other scores in the distribution, the mode is the average of the two adjacent scores (Figure 7–18). For example:

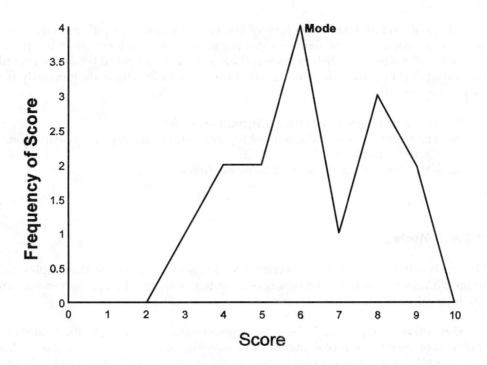

Figure 7-16. Illustration of a mode. The highest point is the mode.

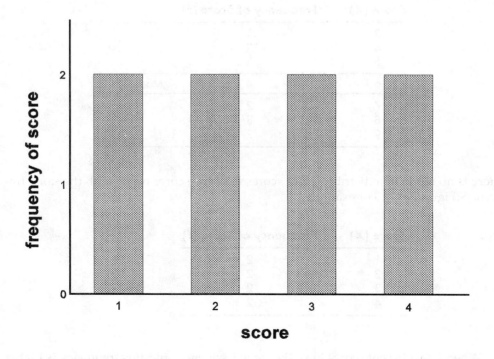

Figure 7-17. Example of data where there is no mode. Note that the frequency of each score is the same.

Score (*X*)	Frequency of score (*f*)	
1	1	
2	2	
3	4	
		Mode = 3.5
4	4	
5	2	
6	1	

For grouped data it is necessary to first calculate the midpoint of each class interval before computing the mode. The mode is then the midpoint of the interval containing the most scores (Figure 7–19).

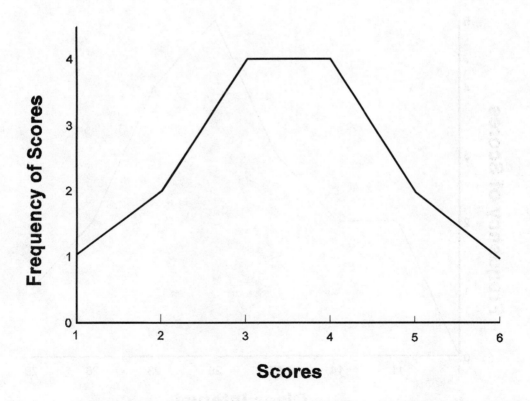

Figure 7–18. Example illustrating the mode when the data has two adjacent numbers with the same frequencies. In this case, the mode is equal to the average of the two adjacent numbers.

Class Interval	Midpoint	Frequency of Scores (f)	
10–12	11	2	
13–15	14	2	
16–18	17	3	
19–21	20	5	Mode = 20
22–24	23	4	
25–27	26	2	
28–30	29	1	

The mode is the simplest measure of central tendency and it has a number of limitations:

1. Frequency distributions may have more than one mode, such as a bimodal or even trimodal distribution. In this case there may be ambiguity about which mode to report, especially if the two (or more) peaks in the distribution are nearly equal. Often one mode is reported as the *primary* or major mode (slightly higher peak) and the other peak reported as the *secondary* or minor mode (Figure 7–20).

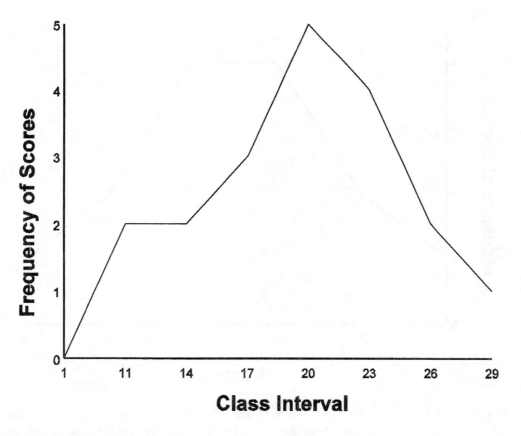

Figure 7–19. Example of a mode when grouped data are used.

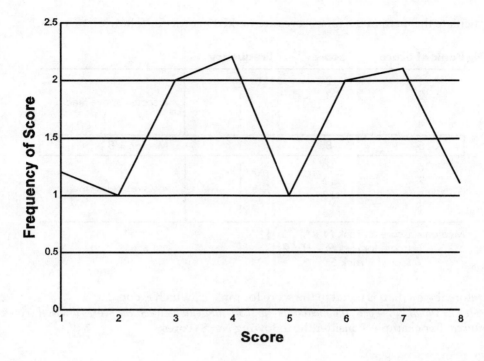

Figure 7–20.   Example of scores with an ambiguous mode. The slightly higher peak is considered the primary or major mode, while the next highest peak is considered the secondary or minor mode.

2. When data are grouped, the mode is very sensitive to the size and number of class intervals. By changing the class intervals for a distribution the mode will change, sometimes drastically.

7.5.8.2 Median

A second and more sophisticated measure of central tendency is the median. The median is appropriate as a measure of central tendency for ordinal, interval, or ratio data, but not for nominal or categorical data from which the mode is the only measure of central tendency that can be calculated.

Definition.   The median is the 50th percentile in a group of scores, that is, the point in an array of scores that has 50% of the cases below it and 50% of the cases above it. The median divides the ranked scores into halves, with one half of the scores below the median and one half of the scores above the median.

The calculation of the median is a simple procedure for raw or ungrouped data:

Step 1. When the number of cases, N, is odd, the median is the score of case (N+1)/2 after scores are ranked (either in ascending or descending order). For example, consider the following array of nine scores:

6, 2, 17, 5, 11, 8, 3, 13, 10

To calculate the median the nine scores are ranked in order as follows:

Rank of Score	Score	Frequency	
1	2	1	
2	3	1	4 scores above median
3	5	1	
4	6	1	
5	8	1	Median = 8
6	10	1	
7	11	1	4 scores below median
8	13	1	
9	17	1	

Median = (score for rank N + 1) / 2
= (score for rank 9 + 1) / 2
= score for rank 5.

Therefore the median is equal to the score for rank #5, which is equal to 8.

Step 2. When N is even, the median is the score midway between the scores after all scores are ranked. For example, consider the following $N = 8$ scores:

2, 1, 10, 7, 0, 15, 8, 5

The first step in calculating the median is again to rank order the scores.

Rank of Score	Score	Frequency of Score	
1	0	1	
2	1	1	3 scores above median
3	2	1	
4	5	1	Median = 6
5	7	1	midpoint of 5 and 7
6	8	1	
7	10	1	3 scores above median
8	15	1	

For grouped data, the median is the point in a distribution at or below which exactly 50% of the cases fall. The median is calculated by constructing a cumulative frequency distribution. The median is then calculated from the cumulative frequency distribution with the following formula:

$$\text{Median} = LL + w_i \{ [(N / 2) - cf] / f_i \}$$

where LL = lower real limit of the median interval

w_i = width of class interval

N = number of cases

cf = cumulative frequency up to the median interval

f_i = frequency within the median interval

The first stage in calculating the median is to construct a cumulative frequency distribution beginning with the lowest class interval and proceeding in ascending order to the highest class interval. The next step is to locate the interval that contains the 50th percentile or the median by examining the cumulative frequency column. For example:

Class Interval	Real Limits	f	cf	Cumulative Percentile	
12–14	11.5–14.5	2	2	10	
15–17	14.5–17.5	4	6	20	
18–20	17.5–20.5	3	9	45	
21–23	20.5–23.5	5	14	70	The median is in the class interval where the 50th percentile rests
24–26	23.5–26. 5	3	17	85	
27–29	26.5–29.5	2	19	95	
30–32	30.5–32.5	1	20	100	

Inspection of the above cumulative frequency distribution shows that the median or 50th percentile must fall in the class interval of 21–23 since the previous interval of 18–20 has cumulated only 9 of the 20 total cases, that is, 45% or 45th percentile.

LL = lower real limit of median interval = 20.5

w_i = width of class interval = 3

N = total number of cases in the frequency distribution = 20

cf = cumulative frequency *up* to median interval = 9 (starting from the lowest to the highest score)

f_i = frequency within median interval = 5

Therefore, Median = $LL + w_i \{ [(N / 2) - cf] / f_i \}$

$= 20.5 + (3)\{ [(20 / 2) - 9] / 5 \}$

$= 20.5 + 3 (1 / 5)$

$= 20.5 + 3 (.20)$

$= 20.5 + .6$

$= 21.1$

The above formula can be used to calculate the median for any grouped frequency distribution as well as for ungrouped distributions (with or without tied scores).

Calculation of the Raw Score from the Percentile Rank.   A modification of the formula allows a generalized method for calculating raw scores corresponding to a given percentile rank (PR).

$$\text{Score at PR} = LL + w_i \frac{[(PR) (N) / 100] - cf}{f_i}$$

where LL = lower real limit of the interval containing the given raw score, that is, (PR) (N) / 100

> w_i = width of the class interval
>
> PR = percentile rank
>
> N = number of cases in the distribution
>
> cf = cumulative frequency up to the given class interval containing the raw score
>
> f_i = number of cases within the class interval containing the raw score

In the above example, what is the raw score corresponding to the 90th percentile rank (using data from the previous example)?

$$\text{Raw score } (rs) \text{ at 90th percentile rank} = LL + w_i \frac{[\,(90)\,(N)\,/\,100\,] - cf}{f_i}$$

where LL = 26.5   cf = 17
     w_i = 3 f_i = 2
     N = 20   PR = 90

$$rs = 26.5 + (3) \frac{[\,(90)\,(20)\,/\,100\,] - 17}{2}$$

$$rs = 26.5 + (3)\,\{\,[\,(180\,/\,100\,) - 17\,]\,/\,2\,\}$$

$$rs = 26.5 + 3\,[\,(18 - 17\,)\,/\,2\,]$$

$$rs = 26.5 + 3\,(1\,/\,2\,)$$

$$rs = 26.5 + 1.5$$

Therefore, a percentile rank of 90 corresponds to a raw score of 28.

7.5.8.2.1 Calculation of the Percentile Rank (PR) From the Raw Score.

A researcher may also want to calculate the PR from the raw score. For example, given a raw score of 19 in a group distribution (see above data), what is the PR?

$$PR = \{\,f_i\,(rs - LL) + [\,(w_i\,)\,(cf\,)\,]\,\}\,/\,[\,(N)\,(w_i\,)\,]$$

where f_i = 3 w_i = 3
     rs = 19   cf = 6
     LL = 17.5   N = 20

$$PR = \{\,3\,(19 - 17.5) + [\,(3)\,(6)\,]\,\}\,/\,[\,(20)\,(3)\,]$$

$$= (\,4.5 + 18)\,/\,60$$

$$= 22.5\,/\,60$$

$$= 37.5\%$$

Therefore, a raw score of 19 equals a percentile rank of 37.5.

7.5.8.3 Mean

The mean is the most widely used and familiar index of central tendency. The mean is the arithmetic average of all the scores in a distribution and is calculated by summing all scores and dividing by the total number of scores.

The general formula for the mean ($\bar{x}$) is:

$$\bar{x} = [\, X_1 + X_2 + X_3 + \ldots X_n \,] / N$$

$$\bar{x} = \Sigma X / N$$

where X_1 = first raw score X_n = nth raw score
          X_2 = second raw score Σ = summation or sum of
          X_3 = third raw score N = number of subjects in the distribution

The mean may be conceptualized as a "center of gravity" or "balance point" in which the scores or "weights" on one side exactly balance the scores or weights on the other side. Each weight represents a score from a distribution of scores. The arithmetic mean of all the scores or weights is the center of gravity or balance point. The deviation of scores in one direction exactly equals the deviation of scores in the other direction.

Calculating the Mean with Raw or Ungrouped Data.   The mean is readily calculated for a distribution of raw scores in which each score occurs only once. The mean is simply the sum of the raw scores divided by the number of scores. For example, consider the following distribution of eight scores:

$$3, 6, 7, 8, 11, 15, 16, 22$$
$$\Sigma X = 88$$
$$N = 8$$
$$\bar{x} = \Sigma X / N$$
$$\bar{x} = [\, 3 + 6 + 7 + 8 + 11 + 15 + 16 + 22 \,] / 8$$
$$= 88 / 8$$
$$= 11.0$$

The mean or average value is calculated as 11.0.

When some scores occur several times, the above procedure may be used to calculate the mean. Alternatively, a frequency distribution may be set up. Then the mean is calculated from the frequency distribution table by multiplying each score by the frequency of occurrence and summing the total across all scores, before dividing by the total number of scores.

In the following example several scores occur more than once:

2, 3, 3, 4, 5, 5, 6, 6, 6, 7, 8, 8, 9, 9, 9

Step 1. The first stage in computing the mean is to form a frequency distribution table.

X	f	fX
2	1	2
3	2	6
4	1	4
5	2	10
6	3	18
7	1	7
8	2	16
9	3	27
		$\Sigma (fX) = 90$

The number in the third column is obtained by multiplying each each raw score by the frequency of occurrence. The symbol fX represents the product of the scores multiplied by the frequency of scores. This column is then summed and divided by the total number of scores, in this example, 15 scores.

$$\bar{x} = \Sigma fX / N$$
$$\Sigma fX = 90$$
$$N = 15$$
$$\bar{x} = 90 / 15$$
$$= 6.0$$

Calculating the Mean for Grouped Data.   When working with grouped data, first find the midpoint of each score interval before calculating the mean. The general formula to determine the mean for grouped data is:

$$\bar{x} = \Sigma fX / N$$

As an example, consider the following scores grouped into six class intervals:

Class Interval	Midpoint (X)	f	fX
3–5	4	2	8
6–8	7	1	7
9–11	10	4	40
12–14	13	6	78
15–17	16	3	48
18–20	19	4	76
		$\Sigma f = 20$	$\Sigma fX = 257$

Therefore, the $\bar{x} = 257 / 20$

$\bar{x} = 12.85$

In the above example, the midpoint of each class interval (X) was multiplied by the frequency in each interval. This product was summed over all the class intervals to give a value equal to 257. This value (ΣfX) is then divided by the total number of scores or the sum of the frequencies (i.e., $\Sigma f = 20$) to yield the final calculated mean of 12.85.

It is important to note that the mean calculated from a grouped frequency distribution will differ slightly from the mean calculated from raw scores. When scores are grouped, information is lost and a certain amount of inaccuracy introduced. As a general rule, the coarser the grouping of scores, the more the grouped mean will differ from the raw score mean. However, for most situations in which 10 to 20 class intervals are typically used, the agreement is close enough between the two calculated means.

7.5.8.4 Comparing the Mode, Median, and Mean

1. As a measure of central tendency, the mean takes into account all the scores of distribution and is affected by each single value. One extreme score or "outlier" can influence the mean to a very large degree, especially with small samples. For example, in the following distribution of ten scores both the mean and median have a value of 6.0 but when an extreme score of 50 is added as the eleventh score, the mean dramatically increases to 10.0, while the median changes only to 7.0:

    > Scores: 2, 3, 4, 4, 5, 7, 8, 8, 9, 10
    > Mean = 6.0   Median = 6.0

    The mean is changed when an extreme score of 50 is added:

    > Scores: 2, 3, 4, 4, 5, 7, 8, 8, 9, 10, 50
    > Mean = 10.0   Median = 7.0

    Therefore, when extreme scores or outliers are present in a frequency distribution of scores, the median may be a more appropriate measure of central tendency than the mean.
2. In distributions that are symmetrical in shape, the mean equals the median and both are equal to the mode if the distribution is unimodal. This is illustrated in the Figure 7–21.
3. In distributions that are symmetrical but not unimodal, it is important to report the mode, mean, and median to provide a clearer picture of the shape and central tendency of the distribution. In Figure 7–22, which depicts a bimodal distribution, there are two modes (at 28 and 40) that should be noted. Note also that the mean equals the median and both equal 34.
4. In distributions that are skewed to the left or right, the mode, median, and mean will have different values. Note that the mean is pulled either to the right or to the left by the outliers or extreme scores on one end of the skewed distribution. The median is the preferred measure of central tendency for skewed distributions, especially when the degree of skewness increases. Figures 7–23 and 7–24 illustrate the locations of the three measures of central tendency for a right and left skewed distribution.

7.5.9 Measures of Variability

Measures of variability are descriptive statistics that indicate how scores in a distribution differ from each other and from the mean. For example, in a distribution with the scores

7, 7, 7, 7,

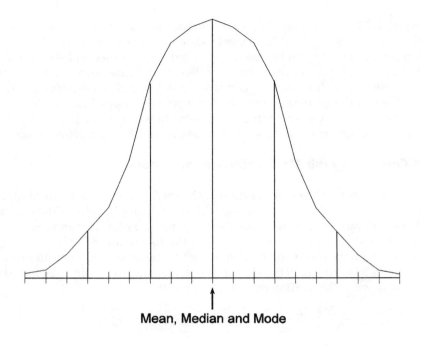

Mean, Median and Mode

Figure 7–21. The normal unimodal curve depicting the mean, median, and mode. All three fall at the same place on a bell-shaped curve.

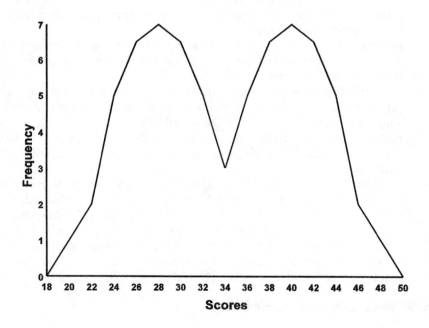

Figure 7–22. Comparison of mean, median, and mode in a bimodal distribution. The two modes have the value of 28 and 38. The median and the mean have the same value, 34.

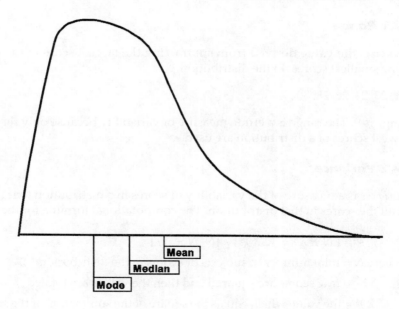

Figure 7–23.   A positively skewed distribution. Notice that the figure is pulled to the left, indicating that the scores with the largest frequencies are at the lower end of the distribution.

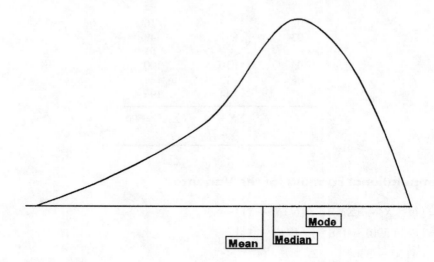

Figure 7–24.   A negatively skewed distribution. The figure is pulled to the right, indicating that the scores with the largest frequencies are at the upper end of the distribution.

the measure of variability is 0, because the scores do not differ from each other and from the mean of 7. The measure of variability increases from zero as the scores vary from each other and from the mean. The *measures of variability* are the range, variance, and standard deviation.

7.5.9.1 Range

The *range* is the value derived from subtracting the largest score in the distribution from the smallest scores. In the distribution

21, 23, 24, 26, 28, 30

the range is 9. The range is a crude measure of variability because only the highest and the lowest scores of a distribution are used.

7.5.9.2 Variance

The *variance* is a measure of the variability of scores in a distribution that takes into account all the scores in that distribution. The computational formula for the variance is:

$$s^2 = [N \Sigma X^2 - (\Sigma X)^2] / [N (N - 1)]$$

where N = total number of subjects or scores in the distribution

ΣX^2 = raw scores are squared and then the values are totaled

$(\Sigma X)^2$ = the value which equals the square of the summation of the scores.

Example of Calculating the Variance.

Subject	Score (X)	X^2
01	2	4
02	4	16
03	7	49
04	9	81
05	10	100
06	12	144
07	14	196
	$\Sigma X = 58$	$\Sigma X^2 = 590$
	$N = 7$	

Computational Formula for the Variance.

$s^2 = [N \Sigma X^2 - (\Sigma X)^2] / [N (N - 1)]$

$s^2 = [(7) (590) - (58)^2] / [7 (7 - 1)]$

$s^2 = [4130 - 3364] / 42$

$s^2 = 766 / 42$

$s^2 = 18.23$

7.5.9.3 Standard Deviation

The *standard deviation* is the square root of the variance. In the example above, the variance equals 18.23. Therefore, the standard deviation equals 4.27. The standard deviation is an important value that is analogous to the mean. It is used in inferential statistics such as with the *t* test.

7.5.10 Stem and Leaf

Stem and leaf is a method of displaying data developed by Tukey (1977) and is an alternative to the frequency distribution. It derives its name because of the display: Any given number is divided into two parts, a stem and a leaf. The first part, the stem, represents a large class into which the number falls, while the second number, the leaf, designates the actual placement in the larger class. For example, the number 15 can be divided into 1 (the stem) and 5 (the leaf), while the number 216 can be divided into 2 or 21 (the stem) and 16 or 6 (the leaf). When the stem and leaves are displayed in a column, the researcher can easily visualize the organization of the data. The researcher is able to identify the specific scores obtained as well as the frequency of the class of scores. Once the data has been organized into a stem and leaf display, a graph is drawn, allowing the researcher to visualize the structure of the data.

An example of unpublished data help the explain the concept. Pre- and posttest data were collected to determine the change in understanding of collaboration techniques. The pre- and posttest scores, as well as the ranks for each of the scores, are reproduced in Table 7–8.

Table 7–8   *Pretest and Posttest Scores on Collaboration Data*

Subject	Pretest		Posttest	
	Score	**Rank**	**Score**	**Rank**
1	118	13	102	11.5
2	59	1	94	8
3	140	16	114	13
4	99	9	96	9
5	96	8	102	11.5
6	63	2	159	16
7	100	10	71	3
8	15	136	76	4
9	152	18	186	18
10	133	14	198	19
11	92	6	65	2
12	62	3	63	1
13	82	5	148	15
14	192	19	222	20
15	106	11	87	7
16	71	4	82	5
17	—	—	101	10
18	108	12	175	17
19	151	17	140	14
20	95	7	84	6

Note. From S. K. Cutler, D. W. Keyes, and M. Urquhart, 1993, unpublished raw data.

The stem and leaf display is as follows:

Pretest Scores	Pretest Leaf	Stem	Posttest Leaf	Posttest Scores
59	9	5*		
63, 65	35	6	53	65, 63
71	1	7	16	61, 76
82	2	8	724	87, 82, 84
99, 96, 92, 95	9625	9	46	94, 96
106, 108, 118, 136, 133, 140	06,08,18,36,33,40	1**	02,02,01,14,48,40	102, 102, 101, 114, 148, 140
152, 151, 192	52,51,92	1	59,75,86,98	159, 175, 186, 198
222		2	22	

The asterisks that follow the number in the stem indicate the number of digits that are included in each leaf. For example, 1** means there are two digits that are to be added to the stem. Although commas are not necessary between the leaves, we have chosen to use them. Notice that the number of digits in the leaf can change within a single display. Notice also that in this display the pretest leaves are displayed on the left, and the posttest leaves are displayed on the right. The stem is placed in the center with the leaves on either side. This allows the researcher to compare sets of data easily. For the reader's convenience, the pre- and posttest scores have been listed.

This system has advantages. First, the leaves do not have to be placed sequentially beside the stems. When the numbers are ranked later (necessary for the graph), the researcher will want to put them in sequential order, however. Second, not only is the researcher able to tell the shape of the data, but he or she can obtain the specific scores. This is not possible in a frequency distribution graph.

When building a stem-and-leaf display, the number of stems is only limited by the data. The researcher does not want to use so many stems that the data are too spread out, or too few lines so that the data are too crowded. Trial and error may be necessary to determine the appropriate number of stems. In general, the last digit of a given number becomes the leaf, while the first digit(s) will be used as the stem. Sometimes, when there are too many leaves on one stem, the stem may be split into parts. By splitting the stem, the leaves may be divided. An example of a split stem can be seen by the repetition of the digit 1.

Once a stem and leaf display has been produced, the researcher needs to make a graph. The graph is called a box and whisker plot because of the way in which it is drawn. The graph consists of a box which has lines connected to either side (the whiskers). A box and whisker plot makes use of the ranks of median or middle score, the ranks of the extremes, and the ranks of the hinges. An examination of Table 7–8 shows the median for the pretest to be 100 (rank of 10) and the median of the posttest to be 101.5 (rank of 10.5). The extremes are the ranks of the highest and lowest scores. The pretest extremes are 59 and 192, ranked at 1 and 19. The posttest extremes are 63 and 222, ranked at 1 and 20. The hinges or quartile ranks lie halfway between the median and the extremes. They are obtained by the following formula:

Lower hinge = 1/2 (lower extreme + median).
Upper hinge = 1/2 (upper extreme + median).

When the rank of a median is not a whole number, drop the decimal (e.g., 11.5 becomes 11). The upper and lower hinges become the upper and lower limits of the box.

The whisker is a line that connects the hinges to the extremes. An example of this is seen in Figure 7–25. An examination of the two box plots in this figure reveals that there is little difference between the two scores. Although the upper extreme and the upper hinge is higher on the posttest, the medians, lower extreme, and lower hinge are similar. There is more variability on the posttest.

Construction of a Stem and Leaf Display and Box Plot

Step 1. Make a stem and leaf display. The following scores have been collected from posttests. As the scores are between 75 and 96, both the stem and leaf will consist of a single digit. Because of the number of scores that fall between 80 and 89, the stem will be divided into two.

Scores: 88, 82, 75, 93, 96, 81, 83, 82, 97, 96, 87, 88, 72, 75, 95, 82, 80, 87, 89, 88

Stem	Leaf	Cumulative Rank	Scores repeated	No. of leaves
7*	535	3	75, 73, 75	3
8	213220	9	82,81,83,82,82,80	6
8	878798	15	88, 87, 88, 87, 89, 88	6
9	36765	20	93, 96, 97, 96, 95	5

The asterisk is placed after the 7 to denote that only one digit is used in the leaf.

2. Find the median score. Because there are 20 scores, the median rank will be 10.5. The score that falls at this rank is 87.

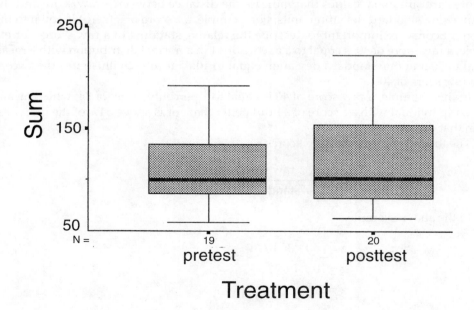

Figure 7–25.   An example of a box and whisker plot using the data from Table 7–8. (The data are taken from an unpublished study by Cutler, Keyes, and Urquhart, 1993.)

3. Find the extremes. The extremes are the ranks of the highest and lowest scores or, in this case, those scores with a rank of 1 and 20. The scores for rank 1 and rank 20 are 73 and 97, respectively.

4. Calculate the hinges. The hinges or quartile ranks lie halfway between the median and the extremes. They are obtained by adding the rank of the extremes to the rank of the median and dividing by 2. When the median rank has a decimal, drop the decimal.

Lower hinge = (1 + 10) / 2 = 11 / 2 = 5.5. The rank for the lower hinge is at 5.5. The score that would fall at this rank is 81.5, obtained by finding the halfway point between the scores that rank at 5 and 6, respectively (e.g., 81, 82).

Upper hinge = (20 + 10) / 2 = 15. The score at this rank is 89.

Step 5. Draw a box using the lower and upper hinges as the outer limits of the box and connect the extremes to the box with a solid line. Notice that the box can be drawn horizontally or vertically.

Lower Extreme	Lower Hinge		Median 87	Upper Hinge	Upper Hinge
73	81.5			89	97

An examination of this box plot suggests that the scores are positively skewed; that is, more scores are at the upper end of the distribution than the lower end.

Reference: J. W. Tukey, (1977). *Exploratory Data Analysis.* Reading, MA: Addison-Wesley Publishing Company.

7.5.11 z Scores and the Normal Curve

z Scores are summary values that indicate the distance between a raw score and the mean, using standard deviation units. For example, a z score of 0 (zero) is equal to the mean. z Scores are important to describe the relative standing of a raw score. For example, a raw score of 40 is equal to a z score of +1 in a normal distribution with a mean equal to 30 and one standard deviation equal to 10. Figure 7–26 illustrates the z score for a raw score of 40.

In this example, a raw score of 40 is equal to a percentile rank of 84, which means that an individual with a z score of +1 did better than, or is above 84% of the individuals in that distribution.

The formula for calculating z scores is:

$$z = \frac{\text{raw score} - \text{mean}}{\text{standard deviation}}$$

In the above example:

$$z = [\, 40 - 30\,] / 10$$
$$z = 10 / 10$$
$$z = +1$$

z Scores can be positive or negative depending on whether the raw score is above or below the mean. z Scores are widely used in psychometric testing and are helpful in interpreting raw scores.

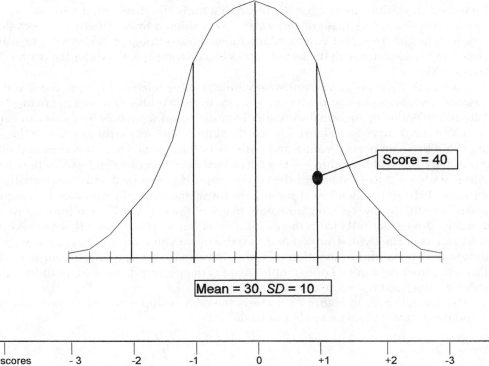

z scores	- 3	-2	-1	0	+1	+2	-3	
	SD	*SD*	*SD*	*SD*	*SD*	*SD*	*SD*	

Percentile	0.1	0.4	1	2	5	9	16	25	37	50	63	75	84	91	95	98	99	99.6	99.9

Figure 7–26. Normal curve depicting raw score of 40, mean of 30, *SD* of 10. Notice that a raw score of 40 lies one standard deviation above the mean (e.g., *z* score of +1) and at a percentile of 84.

Normality and the Normal Curve

For the health practitioner and special educator one of the most difficult decisions is to decide whether a physiological or psychological function is within normal limits. What is normal blood pressure, heart rate, muscle strength, height, reading achievement, or intelligence? Is normality a function of personality or behavior, or it is a statistical value?

When an individual goes to a physician for a physical examination, the physiological and neurological functions are tested to determine whether they are within normal limits. Predetermined values are used by the physician to compare with the patient's results. Individual differences within a range of normality are accepted by the physician to determine whether a function is abnormal. The same judgments are made by the occupational therapist and physical therapist in testing range of motion in a specific joint or evaluating muscle strength.

On the other hand, the statistician's definition of normality and abnormality will depend upon the frequency of occurrences within designated class intervals. Abnormality is interpreted by the statistician as a variance from the mean value, such as 1 or

2 standard deviations units from the mean of a normally distributed variable. In research, scores or values that are abnormal are considered to be outliers or scores that vary widely from expected values. Many times those outliers or abnormal scores are considered at variance with the test of values in a distribution. Consider the scatter diagram in Figure 7–27.

Four of the five scores are consistent with a positive relationship with the X and Y variables. However, one coordinate (50, 5) seems to be an outlier and does not fit into the pattern. The outlier or abnormal score should be discussed separately by the researcher.

The normal curve (see Figure 7–22) is the statistician's guide for examining the relationship between normal values and outliers. In the normal curve it is expected that 68% of the cases will lie within −1 to +1 standard deviation units and 98% of the cases will lie within −2 to +2 standard deviations units. If we know that a characteristic is normally distributed, then by calculating the mean and standard deviation of a population, we will be able to determine how many of the cases will be within −2 to +2 standard deviation units from the mean. For example, if we know that the resting heart rate is normally distributed and that the mean value for adults is 72 beats per minute with a standard deviation of 5, then we can determine the percentile ranks (PR) from the raw scores. For example, what is the percentile rank of an individual with a resting heart rate score of 78?

The normal curve in Figure 7–28 shows the relationship between the raw score of 78 and the normal values for resting heart rate.

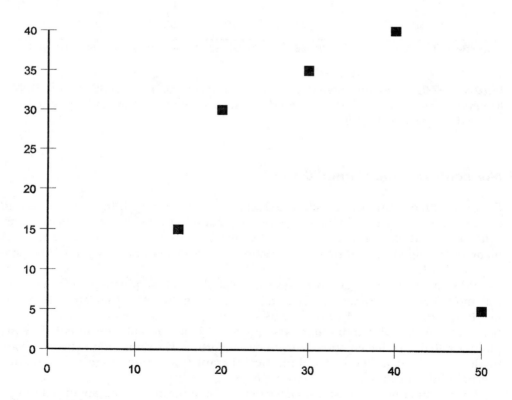

Figure 7–27.   Scattergram showing an outliner at the coordinates of 50, 5. The outliner is the score which appears to be significantly different from the other scores.

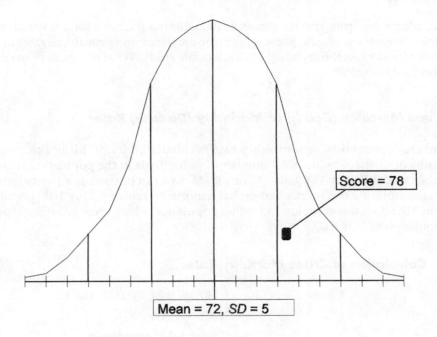

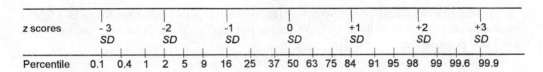

Figure 7–28. Normal curve depicting the relationship between the heart beat rate of 78 when the mean is 72 and the standard deviation is 5. What is the z score of this heart rate? Is it above or below normal?

We estimate that based on the diagram the PR for a raw score of 78 will be slightly above the 84th PR.

Calculation of PR. First calculate z scores from raw scores:

$$z = (rs - \bar{x}) / SD$$
$$z = (78 - 72) / 5$$
$$z = 6/5 = 1.2$$
$$z = 1.2$$

Look up the percentile rank from the statistical table for the z score of 1.2. Note that in Table C–2 in the Appendix, a z score of 1.2 is equal to the percentile rank of .8849.

7.5.12 Vital Statistics

The quality of a health care system in a country is usually described by vital statistics such as the infant mortality rate, rates of illnesses and diseases, life expectancy, and mortality rates from specific diseases. In justifying the need for a research study in a clinical area, the researcher first reports the incidence and prevalence rates of a disability or illness to establish the significance of the study. What are some of the most common vital statistics?

Crude Mortality (Death) or Morbidity (Disease) Rates

The crude mortality or morbidity rate is calculated by dividing the frequency of deaths or illnesses by the total number of individuals in the population. This number is then multiplied by 1,000, 10,000, or 100,000 so it can be used as a comparative figure. For example, if a certain population has a mortality rate of 9.3 per 1000 population per year, how does this compare to another population where there are 180,000 deaths in a population of 24,000,000?

Calculation of Crude Mortality Rate.

$$\text{Crude death rate} = (180,000 / 24,000,000) (1,000)$$
$$= .0075 \times 1,000$$
$$= 7.5 \text{ per } 1,000 \text{ population.}$$

In this hypothetical case, the investigator would conclude that there is a lesser mortality rate in the sample of 180,000 deaths per 24,000,000 population than in the 9.3 per 1,000 population.

Prevalence and Incidence Rates of Disability or Disease

How do we determine the incidence rate of a disease? For example, in 1991, there were 43,000 new cases of individuals with AIDS in the United States. At that time the total population was about 240,000,000. What is the incidence rate of AIDS per 100,000 population for 1991?

Calculation of Incidence Rate.

$$\text{incidence rate} = (43,000 / 240,000,000) (100,000)$$
$$= (.0001791) (100,000)$$
$$= 17.91 \text{ per } 100,000 \text{ population.}$$

Adjusted Rate

Researchers are also interested in obtaining statistics for specific populations. In these examples, the calculation of rates are adjusted. For example, an investigator is interested in comparing infant mortality rates adjusted for gender. In a hypothetical population there are 40,000 births of males and 35,000 births of females. In this population 150 males and 180 females die at birth. What are the adjusted infant mortality rates for females as compared to the total crude rates per 1,000 population?

Calculation of Crude Rate.

$$\text{crude rate} = [\, (\, 150 + 180) \, / \, (\, 40{,}000 + 35{,}000 \,) \,] \, (\, 1{,}000 \,)$$
$$= (\, 330 \, / \, 75{,}000 \,) \, (\, 1{,}000 \,)$$
$$= (\, .0044 \,) \, (\, 1{,}000 \,)$$
$$= 4.4 \text{ per } 1{,}000 \text{ (for both males and females)}$$

Adjusted Rate—Females.

$$\text{adjusted rate} = (\, 180 \, / \, 35{,}000 \,) \, (\, 1{,}000 \,)$$
$$= .0051 \times 1000$$
$$= 5.14 \text{ per } 1{,}000$$

For this hypothetical example, it appears that the infant mortality rate is higher in females as compared to the total population.

7.6 Inferential Statistics and Testing a Hypothesis

7.6.1 Probability and Clinical Research

When an investigator predicts a statistically significant relationship between two variables, it is assumed that the relationship will be greater than by chance alone. In other words, the researcher is predicting that X factor is related to Y factor, or the independent variable, whether manipulated or not, is related to the dependent variable. However, in clinical research it is very difficult to control for all possible factors that could affect the dependent variable. For example, if a researcher discovers through a thorough search of the literature that arthritis is a psychophysiological disorder, then a set of research investigations would be generated based on this assumption. For example in a retrospective correlational study the researcher could select a group of patients with arthritis and investigate personality relationships and the incidence of arthritis. If a statistically significant relationship is found between the incidence of arthritis and personality relationships, it will be beyond a certain probability level, but not necessarily a one-to-one relationship. This means that not all individuals with a certain described characteristic are arthritic. This leads us to the question, why do we accept a partial relationship rather than a 100% probability in clinical research? A number of factors in clinical research impinge upon statistically significant results that prevent the perfect 100% probability relationships. They are:

- Complex interrelationships among variables where more than one factor contributes to a disability. For example, in arthritis a multifactorial etiology is assumed. However, in clinical research we may be able to identify only some portion of the variance associated with the onset of arthritis.
- Diseases where genetics, age, diet, and numerous other factors influence the course of a disorder. There may be individual factors occurring in the individual, which are very difficult to identify in clinical research during the research study.

- The problem of accurately formulating a diagnosis in chronic disabilities such as arthritis, diabetes, multiple sclerosis, cardiovascular disease, schizophrenia, or ulcerative colitis may affect the results in clinical research. Moreover, the sample may not be a homogeneous group, which could contaminate results.
- The error variance existing in all clinical research, such as measurement of variables, control of experimental conditions, uniformity of subjects, and data collection procedures, that could affect results.

In short, all statistical analysis using hypothesis testing is based on probability. When inferential statistics are applied in a clinical research study, the investigator bases results and conclusions on the probability that any differences between the experimental and control groups are either due to chance or are statistically significantly different.

7.6.2 Procedure for Statistically Testing a Hypothesis

Step 1. State the hypothesis. A null hypothesis is stated unless the researcher is replicating a previous study or has research evidence to support a directional hypothesis.

Null hypothesis is $\bar{x}_1 = \bar{x}_2$ or $r = 0$. Stated in clinical research study: There is no statistically significant difference between means or no significantly statistical relationship between variables.

Directional hypothesis is $\bar{x}_1 > \bar{x}_2$ or r is statistically significant. This is the reverse of the null hypothesis.

Step 2. Select a level of significance. The researcher usually selects the .05 level of significance in the social sciences. This means that the researcher accepts an error level of 5%. The researcher can also state that at a $p < .05$, there is a 95% confidence level that results are not due to chance.

Step 3. Obtain the critical value from the appropriate table for statistical tests based on whether it is one-tailed or two-tailed test, level of statistical significance, and degrees of freedom.

Step 4. Apply inferential statistics and select a procedure or parametric or nonparametric statistical test based on the assumptions underlying the test such as randomness, normal distribution of data, and homogeneity of variance.

Step 5. Calculate the observed value of statistics such as t-observed, F-observed, chi-square or correlation coefficient through a mathematical formula.

Step 6. Accept or reject the research hypothesis (null or directional).

7.6.3 Potential Sources of Research Errors Affecting Statistical Significance

One very important aspect of clinical research is to reduce the possible errors in an experiment that could impact upon the results. These errors include:

- *Hawthorne effect*—attention given to subjects may increase positive outcome and camouflage the true effects of the independent variable or treatment method. When a Hawthorne effect is present, the subject's improvement is due to the attention they receive from the researcher rather than the direct result of the treatment intervention.

- *Placebo effect*—the suggestion that a subject is being given a treatment, such as medication or a procedure, may produce positive expectations within the subject that the treatment will be effective. The subject in a way wills himself or herself to improvement. The placebo produces in the subject a desire for improvement. There is some evidence that a psychophysiological effect occurs from the placebo effect.
- *Honeymoon effect*—a short-term effect of a new treatment procedure that the subject is optimistic will impact upon a disease. The initial enthusiasm disguises the true effects of the treatment procedure.
- *Researcher bias*—the researcher carrying out a clinical treatment program affects the results by the investigator's enthusiasm and desire for the treatment to be effective. The researcher's knowledge of the study may affect its outcome.
- *Test administrator bias*—the individual testing the outcome of treatment method is aware of which subjects are in the experimental or in the control group.
- *Sampling errors*—Lack of a representative sample—the researcher's results are based on a sample from a population that is not representative. The results will be skewed or biased to the research sample selected.
- *Systematic variance*—the researcher fails to control for extraneous variables that could possibly affect the results such as age, gender, intelligence, education, socioeconomic status, or degree of disability.
- *Error variance*—the researcher overlooks or minimizes the effects of anxiety, lack of motivation, inattention, distractive environments, and other unexpected problems in the test environment.

Type I and Type II Errors

All of these factors and other sources of error in an experiment can potentially affect the results of research. The errors in testing a hypothesis are identified as either a Type I or Type II error. These errors result from the researcher accepting or rejecting a hypothesis based on the statistical results. The probability of an error in hypothesis testing is typically accepted at the .05 or .01 level. The researcher has confidence that the results are not due to chance in 95 or 99% of the time. However it is possible that the results are false in five out of a hundred tries or one out of a hundred tries purely on the basis of chance errors. Table 7–9 summarizes the relationship between decision errors and hypothesis testing. The concept in medicine of a false positive or false negative is analogous to describing a Type I or Type II error. A false positive in medicine occurs when a disease is falsely detected, whereas a false negative exists when a disease is overlooked or not detected. Errors in clinical medicine can occur because of human error or in mistaken judgments in interpreting results, the unreliability of the test equipment or procedure, or unexplained or temporary variables in the patient's condition that can lead to a false diagnosis. Often, clinicians will use more than one test as well as repeat tests in order to confirm or validate a diagnosis. Researchers, on the other hand, try to reduce Type I and Type II errors by replicating experiments with representative samples from different geographical areas.

In summary, a Type I error is when a researcher rejects a null hypothesis when it should be accepted. A Type II error is when a null hypothesis is accepted when it should be rejected.

Table 7-9 *Testing the Null Hypothesis, Decision Errors, and Clinical Analogy in Medicine*

Null hypothesis Ho predicts that there is no statistically significant differences between means ($\bar{x}_1 = \bar{x}_2$) or no statistically significant relationship between variables (r = 0).

Decision by Researcher	True Situation	Analogy in Medicine
1. Reject Null Hypothesis: • $\mu_1 \neq \mu_2 \neq \mu_3 \neq \mu_4 \cdots$ • $r \neq 0$	**Type I Error (α):** Researcher rejects the null hypothesis when it should be accepted. In reality, there is no statistically significant difference between means or relationships between variables • $\mu_1 = \mu_2$ • $r = 0$ Researcher should accept the null hypothesis	**False Positive:** Clinician falsely detects the presence of disease or condition when in reality no disease exists. For example, falsely diagnosing breast cancer through mammography screening when in reality breast cancer is not present.
2. Reject Null Hypothesis: • $\mu_1 \neq \mu_2 \neq \mu_3 \neq \mu_4 \cdots$ • $r \neq 0$	**No Error:** Researcher rejects null hypothesis and concludes that there is a statistically significant difference between the means or that r is greater than zero.	**Correct Diagnosis:** Clinician correctly detects presence of disease and concludes a correct positive diagnosis of a pathological condition.
3. Accept Null Hypothesis: • $\mu_1 = \mu_2 = \mu_3 = \mu_4 \cdots$ • $r = 0$	**Type II Error (β):** Researcher accepts null hypothesis when it should be rejected. In reality, there is a statistically significant difference between means or a statistically significant relationship between variables. • $\mu_1 \neq \mu_2$ • $r \neq 0$ Researcher should reject null hypothesis.	**False Negative:** Clinician falsely concludes that based on test results no disease is present when in reality a disease exists.
4. Accept Null Hypothesis: • $\mu_1 = \mu_2 = \mu_3 = \mu_4 \cdots$ • $r = 0$	**No Error:** Researcher accepts null hypothesis.	**Correct Diagnosis:** Clinician correctly concludes that no disease is present.

7.6.4 Exploratory Data Analysis

John Tukey (1977) states that "It is important to understand what you CAN do before you learn to measure how WELL you seem to have done it" (p. v). In clinical research the question that is usually raised is: How effective is a treatment procedure? For example, are Orton–Gillingham reading techniques more effective than traditional basal reading methods in raising reading levels in children with dyslexia? The researcher has to determine at what level of reading achievement significance would be accepted. If the researcher is using a reading achievement test such as the Woodcock Reading Mastery Test—Revised (WRMT–R; Woodcock, 1987), then a definition of significance should be decided upon in advance. Guidelines for the degree of differences between the mean at posttest after intervention should be established. For example, one standard deviation above the mean will show significance. If group one had a mean of 100 and group two had a mean of 85 and one standard deviation equals 15, significance has been demonstrated before a *t* test or ANOVA has been applied to the data. This exploratory data analysis is a method of "eyeballing the data" before applying a statistical test to the results. Exploratory data analysis involves:

1. Calculating group means and standard deviations to determine if the results are clinically significant.
2. Screening results by collapsing data in nominal categories and performing a chi-square test.
3. Describing results in scatter diagrams showing the relationship between variables.
4. Using stem and leaf displays and box plots to tally the frequency count within designated categories.

References: For a more detailed account of exploratory data analysis see C. C. Hoaglin, F. Mosteller, and J. N. Tukey, (1991). *Fundamentals of Exploratory Analysis of Variance*. NY: John Wiley and Sons; and J. W. Tukey, (1977). *Exploratory Data Analysis*. Reading, MA.: Addison-Wesley Publishing Company.

7.6.5 The Concept of Statistical Power and Effect Size

Statistical power is the ability of a statistical test to accurately reject the null hypothesis and to detect a difference between groups when one exists. Statistical power is related to the occurrence of a Type II error when the researcher finds that there is no statistically significant difference between the groups when in reality there is a significant difference. It is affected by the size of the sample, the probability level of significance such as .05 or .01, and the magnitude of the relationship between the variables measured. When large samples are used in a clinical study, any statistical analysis will be powerful. For example, a sample of 100 subjects in a clinical study will be more powerful than a sample of 25 subjects. The researcher will have more confidence in rejecting the null hypothesis with a larger number of subjects than with small size samples. However, statistical significance at a .05 level with large numbers of subjects may or may not demonstrate clinical significance. The power of a test, indicating the ability to reject the null hypothesis, also increases when the researcher is willing to accept a higher probability of error such as .05 (has more power) than the .01 level. What this means is that the researcher is willing to accept more error in interpreting the statistical results. Some researchers recommend a power level of .80 (Ottenbacher & Barrett, 1990). However, for a clinical researcher the major question still remains, Is this treatment method effective? Statistical power should not be manipulated to camouflage clinical results. Clinical research study results should be analyzed to determine if the treatment method is promising, if it is effective with specific patients, and if it can be refined to improve its effectiveness. Statistical confidence should not be compromised to justify the use of treatment methods when they have not demonstrated effectiveness.

Effect Size

In clinical research, the effect size is presented by researchers to demonstrate the difference between treatment methods and their impact on improvement. For example, if a researcher is comparing the effectiveness of two types of hand exercise programs to increase grip strength, the researcher should apply an independent t test to evaluate statistical significance. In addition, the researcher is also interested in looking at the clinical impact of the two treatment techniques. Effect size is an important concept that reflects both the variance between the groups as well as the variance within the groups. The formula for effect size (ES) is:

$$ES = (\bar{x}_1 - \bar{x}_2) / s$$

where s is the pooled standard deviation of both groups.

The effect size is zero when the null hypothesis is true (Cohen, 1977). The effect size also serves as an index of the degree of departure from the null hypothesis. For example, a relatively large effect size can be interpreted to mean that the study has high statistical power in accurately rejecting the null hypothesis. Most researchers have defined small, medium, and large effect sizes. Small effect sizes are about .2, medium effect sizes are about .5, and large effect sizes are about .8.

7.7 Model II: One-Sample Problems (One-Sample t Test)

One-sample t tests are applied to research studies in which the investigator is testing whether a sample mean is equal to, less than, or greater than a given value. An example from environmental science is the sampling of air or water to determine if the air or water is polluted. Scientists concerned with the quality of air and water use one-sample t tests to compare samples with parameter values. These parameter values are health standards that have been predetermined by scientific evidence to be at acceptable health levels. At which point is the air considered to be polluted? What are the accepted levels of bacteria for water consumption? These are problems for one-sample t tests. We can also use one-sample t tests for screening populations. For example, is a group sample above or below normal values in height, weight, cholesterol level, blood pressure, heart rate, and hearing acuity? The procedure for applying a one-sample t test is to compare the sample mean with a parameter value.

Hypothetical Example for Testing for Statistically Significant Differences Between Sample Mean and Parameter Mean Values

Step 1. State the research hypothesis.

a. *Null Hypothesis:* There is no statistically significant difference between the height of adult Japanese-American males and the standard height of all adult American males.

$$\bar{x}_1 = \mu \text{ (mu, parameter mean value)}$$
$$N = 10{,}000$$

b. *Alternative Hypothesis:* There is a statistically significant difference between the height of adult Japanese-American males and the height of all adult American males.

$$\bar{x}_1 \neq \mu \text{ (mu, parameter mean value)}$$

Step 2. Select the level of statistical significance: p. 05
Step 3. Identify the t_{crit} from the t distribution table

a. significance level: p .05
b. two-tailed test of significance
c. $df = N - 1, 10{,}000 - 1 = 9{,}999, t_{crit} = 1.946$

Step 4. Calculate the sample group mean and standard deviation. From a random sample of 10,000 adult Japanese-American males living in the United States, the following data were collected:

$\bar{x} = 64$ in. $sd = 1.8$ in.

Step 5. Identify parameter values. The parameter values[1] for the average adult American males are:

$\bar{x} = 69$ in. $sd = 1.9$ in.

Step 6. Graph normal curve for parameter value. Since the parameter values are a constant, we can use the normal curve to describe the distribution of parameter values. This is shown in Figure 7–29. For a normal distribution with a mean of 69 and a standard deviation of 1.9, we will expect 68% of adult American males to have heights between 67.1 and 70.9 inches.

Step 7. Graph normal curve for sample. This is shown in Figure 7–30.

For the sample distribution with a mean of 64 and a standard deviation of 1.8, we will expect 68% of the adult Japanese-American males to have heights between 62.2 and 65.8 inches.

Step 8. Calculate the t_{obs} using the formula:

---

[1]These are hypothetical values set to explain concepts.

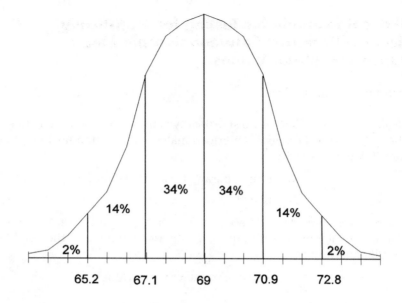

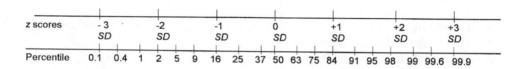

Figure 7–29.   Hypothetical data for typical adult American males depicting a normal distribution in which the mean height is 69 inches and the standard deviation is 1.9. Sixty-eight percent of the adult population should fall between +1 and − 1 standard deviations, or heights of 67.1 and 70.9 inches.

$$t_{obs} = (\bar{x}_1 - \mu) (sd / \sqrt{N})$$

where $\bar{x}$ = sample mean equals 64

sd = sample standard deviation equals 1.8

μ = parameter mean equals 69

N = sample number of subjects = 10,000

$$t_{obs} = (64 - 69) / (1.8 / \sqrt{10,000}) = (-5) / (1.8 / 100)$$

$$t_{obs} = -5 / .018$$

$$t_{obs} = -277.77$$

Step 9. Compare t_{obs} *with* t_{crit}

$t_{obs} = 277.77$ $t_{crit} = 1.946$

$t_{obs} > t_{crit}$

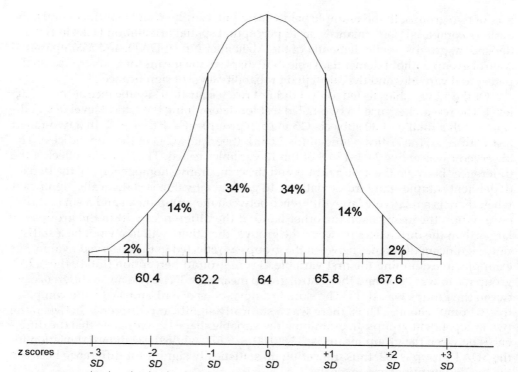

Figure 7–30. Hypothetical data for a sample of 10,000 adult Japanese males depicting a normal distribution in which the mean height is 64 inches and the standard deviation is 1.8. Sixty-eight percent of the adult population should fall between +1 and −1 standard deviations, or heights of 62.2 and 65.8 inches.

Thus the researcher rejects the null hypothesis and concludes that there is a statistically significant difference between the height of adult Japanese-American men as compared to the average heights of all adult American men.

7.8 Model III: Two Independent Groups

7.8.1 Independent *t* Test

The purpose of this statistical model is to test whether there is a statistically significant difference between the means of two independent samples. This is used frequently to test the differences between two clinical techniques applied to an experimental group and a control or comparative group. For example, if a researcher is examining the comparative effectiveness of two treatment techniques in two independent groups, such as Progressive Relaxation Exercise versus Transcutaneous Electrical Nerve Stimulation in reducing pain, then an independent *t* test will be applied to the outcome measure for pain (dependent variable). The *t* test is also applied when the researcher examines whether there is a statistically significant difference in the characteristic abilities of two groups. In the example below from Liu, Gauthier, and Gauthier (1991), the authors compared performances on 12 perceptual spatial orientation tasks in two independent groups: senile dementia of the Alzheimer type (SDAT), and a comparative control group without dementia. Table 7–10 displays the means for both groups on the perceptual variables and the calculated probability level of significance.

Of the 12 variables tested, only 4 did not reach statistical significance at the $p < .05$ level. The researchers used a two-tailed test for determining the critical level of significance with a total n of 30 subjects (15 in each group), at a df of $n - 2$. In a two-tailed test with 28 df, the critical value of t is 2.0484. (See Table C–3 in the appendices). The observed t was above 2.0484 in 8 of the 12 variables tested. The t values reflected the differences between the group means and the comparative homogeneity of the two independent sample standard deviations. In general a t value is statistically significant when there is a relatively large difference between the group mean and a small difference within the groups. On the other hand, if the differences within the groups are larger than the differences between the groups, then there will likely not be a statistically significant difference between the groups as reflected in the observed t value. For example, in examining the first variable, figure-ground perception (total), the SDAT group mean was 26.33 and the control group mean was 36.47. The mean difference between the groups was 10.14. The standard deviations of 6.61 and 4.63 were comparatively homogeneous. Thus, there was a statically significant difference between the two independent groups. In examining the variable shape (visual), note that the differences between the group means is .33 ($10.00 - 9.67$), while the standard deviation for the SDAT group is .82, thus indicating no statistically significant difference between the two independent group means.

Operational Procedure for Testing for Statistically Significant Differences Between Two Independent Samples

Step 1. State the research hypothesis

a. *Null Hypothesis:* There is no statistically significant difference between the mean of group 1 versus the mean of group 2

$$H_0: \mu_1 = \mu_2$$

b. *Directional Hypothesis:* Mean one is significantly statistically different from mean two in a stated direction

$$\mu_1 > \mu_2$$

c. *Alternative Hypothesis:* Mean one does not equal mean two and there is a statistically significant difference between the two means (nondirectional)

$$H_1: \mu_1 \neq \mu_2$$

Step 2. Select the level of statistical significance. In social sciences research, the .05 level of significance is traditionally selected.

Step 3. Decide whether to use a one-tailed or two-tailed test for statistical significance. A two-tailed test is used with a null hypothesis to determine if there are statistically significant differences in either direction of the tail. The model for a two-tailed test are the tails in a normal curve (Figure 7–31).

Table 7–10 Comparison of Performance on Perceptual Spatial Orientation Tasks

Skill	Maximum Score	SDAT Group (n = 15) M (SD)	Control Group (n = 15) M (SD)	p*
Figure–ground perception (total)	48	26.33 (6.61)	36.47 (4.63)	≤.0001
Figure–ground perception (Part 1)	24	16.00 (3.59)	20.53 (1.19)	≤.0002
Figure–ground perception (Part 2)	24	10.33 (4.15)	15.93 (3.90)	≤.001
Shape (visual)	10	9.67 (0.82)	10.00 (0.00)	ns
Shape (tactual)	10	6.13 (2.26)	8.93 (1.34)	≤.0005
Size (visual)	6	6.00 (0.00)	6.00 (0.00)	ns
Size (tactual)	15	14.33 (1.23)	14.87 (0.35)	ns
Position in space (total)	16	11.93 (4.01)	15.33 (0.82)	≤.004
Position in space (Part 1)	8	7.20 (1.42)	7.93 (0.26)	≤.06
Position in space (Part 2)	8	4.73 (2.92)	7.4 (0.74)	≤.002
Spatial relations	15	11.47 (2.67)	14.73 (0.59)	≤.0002
Left–right discrimination	10	9.67 (0.72)	10.00 (0.00)	ns

SDAT = senile dementia of the Alzheimer type; ns = not significant. *Two-tailed t test for independent samples.

Note. From "Spatial Disorientation in Persons with Early Senile Dementia of the Alzheimer Type," by L. Liu, L. Gauthier, & S. Gauthier, 1991, The American Journal of Occupational Therapy, 45, p. 70. Copyright 1991 by American Journal of Occupational Therapy. Reprinted with permission.

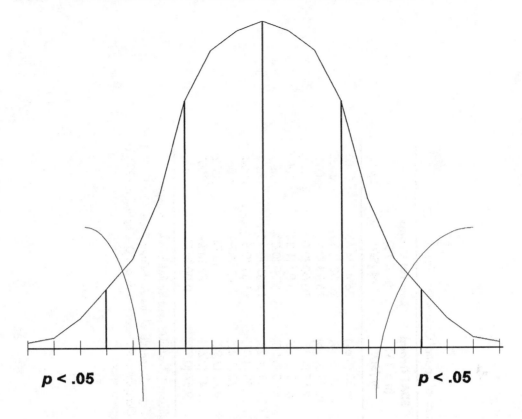

p < .05   **p < .05**

Figure 7–31.   Model for a two-tailed test. A one-tailed test would use only one of the two marked areas.

A one-tailed test is used with a directional hypothesis when the researcher predicts that the experimental group mean will be either statistically greater or lesser than a comparison mean.

Step 4. Look up the critical value (t_{crit}) from the published statistical table. The critical value is determined by:

a.   the degrees of freedom (df)
b.   the level of significance ($p < .05$ or $< .01$)
c.   the direction of the test (one-tailed or two-tailed)
d.   the value of t_{crit} as indicated in the statistical table. (See Appendix C–3.)

Step 5. Calculate the group means and standard deviations.

Step 6. Do an exploratory data analysis to determine if the differences between the two means are clinically significant and that the standard deviations in both groups are approximately equal.

Step 7. Plot a graph. Use the graph mean and raw scores of group 1 and group 2 to visualize whether there seems to be a statistically significant difference between the group means. (See Figure 7–32.)

If there appears to be a difference between the two group means, then go to step 8 and calculate the values.

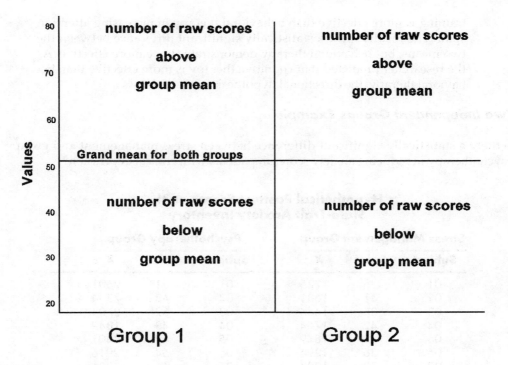

Figure 7–32. Graph to visualize values of scores as a way to estimate possible statistical significance between the group means.

Step 8. Calculate the t_{obs} using the formula.

$$t_{obs} = \frac{\bar{x}_1 - \bar{x}_2}{\sqrt{\{[(n_1 - 1)s_1^2 + (n_2 - 1)s_2^2]/[n_1 + n_2 - 2]\}\{(1/n_1) + (1/n_2)\}}}$$

where $\bar{x}_1$ = mean value of group 1

$\bar{x}_2$ = mean value of group 2

n_1 = total number of cases in group 1

n_2 = total number of cases in group 2

s_1^2 = variance (which is the standard deviation squared) for group 1

s_2^2 = variance for group 2

Step 9. Compare the two values: t_{obs} and t_{crit}.

a. Accept the null hypothesis if t_{obs} is less than t_{crit}.
b. Reject the null hypothesis if t_{obs} is equal to or greater than t_{crit}.
c. Accept the directional hypothesis if t_{obs} is greater than or equal to t_{crit} in the direction that is hypothesized.
d. Reject the directional hypothesis if t_{obs} is less than t_{crit} or if the mean value that is predicted to be greater is less than the mean value of the control or comparative group. For example, a researcher predicts that cognitive

training is more effective than behavioral therapy in increasing attention span. The results show a statistically significant difference between the two means, but behavioral therapy demonstrates to be more effective. As the researcher predicted that cognitive therapy is more effective than behavioral therapy, the directional hypothesis is rejected.

Two Independent Groups Example

Is there a statistically significant difference between stress management and group psychotherapy in reducing anxiety scores in patients with clinical depression?

Hypothetical Posttest Scores on the State-Trait Anxiety Inventory [a]

Stress Management Group			Psychotherapy Group		
Subject	Score	X_1^2	Subject	Score	X_2^2
01	35	1225	01	51	2601
02	41	1681	02	48	2304
03	38	1444	03	52	2704
04	42	1764	04	43	1849
05	43	1849	05	49	2401
06	36	1296	06	54	2916
07	32	1024	07	61	3721
08	40	1600	08	56	3136
09	41	1681	09	54	2916
10	43	1849	10	60	3600
11	42	1764	11	48	2304
12	34	1156	12	46	2116

$\Sigma X_1 = 467$ $\Sigma X_1^2 = 18333$ $\Sigma X_2 = 622$ $\Sigma X_2^2 = 32568$

$\bar{x}_1 = 38.9$ $\bar{x}_2 = 51.8$

Grand Mean $= (\Sigma X_1 + \Sigma X_2) / 24 = (467 + 622) / 24 = 45.37$

[a]Smaller score indicates less anxiety.

Step 1. State the research hypothesis. There is no statistically significant difference between a stress management group and a psychotherapy group in reducing anxiety in a sample of depressed patients. The hypothesis is stated in null form $(\bar{x}_1 = \bar{x}_2)$.

Step 2. Select the level of statistical significance. The p .05 level of statistical significance will be accepted.

Step 3. This is a nondirectional two-tailed test for statistical significance because a null hypothesis was stated.

Step 4. Determine the critical value for t from published statistical tables. (See Table C–3 in the appendices.)

a. $df = n_1 + n_2 - 2 = 22$
b. level of significance $= p$ .05
c. $t_{crit} = 2.0739$

Step 5. Calculate the mean and standard deviations.

Stress Management Group

$\bar{x}_1 = 38.9$
$\bar{x}_1 = \Sigma X_1 \,/\, n = 467 \,/\, 12 = 38.9$
$s_1 = 3.80$

Psychotherapy Group

$\bar{x}_2 = 51.8$
$\bar{x}_1 = \Sigma X_2 \,/\, n = 622 \,/\, 12 = 51.8$
$s_2 = 5.45$

Computational Formula for Standard Deviation.

$$s = \sqrt{[\, n\,\Sigma X^2 - (\Sigma X)^2 \,] \,/\, [\, n\,(n-1) \,]}$$
$$s_1 = \sqrt{\{[\,(12)\,(18333)\,] - (467)^2\} \,/\, [\,12\,(12-1)\,]}$$
$$s_1 = \sqrt{(219996 - 218089) \,/\, [\,12\,(12-1)\,]}$$
$$s_1 = \sqrt{1907 \,/\, 132} = \sqrt{14.44}$$
$$s_1 = 3.80$$
$$s_2 = \sqrt{\{[\,(12)\,(32568)\,] - (622)^2\} \,/\, [\,12\,(12-1)\,]}$$
$$s_2 = \sqrt{(390816 - 386884) \,/\, [\,12\,(12-1)\,]}$$
$$s_2 = \sqrt{3932 \,/\, 132} = \sqrt{29.78}$$
$$s_2 = 5.45$$

Step 6. Exploratory data analysis.

$$\bar{x}_1 - \bar{x}_2 = 38.9 - 51.8 = 12.9$$
$$s_1 = 3.80 \qquad\qquad s_2 = 5.45$$

The mean difference is greater than the standard deviation for group 1 or group 2. Standard deviation difference between the two groups is 1.65. There is a relative homogeneity of variance for the two groups.

Step 7. Exploratory graph analysis. Figure 7–33 shows the graph obtained from the analysis. There appears to be a significant difference between the two groups.

Step 8. Calculate t_{obs}.

$$t_{obs} = \frac{\bar{x}_1 - \bar{x}_2}{\sqrt{\{[\,(n_1-1)\,(s_1^2) + (n_2-1)\,(s_2^2)\,] \,/\, (n_1 + n_2 - 2)\}\,[\,(1\,/\,n_1) + (1\,/\,n_2)\,]}}$$

Group 1

where $\bar{x}_1 = 38.9$
$n_1 = 12$
$s_1^2 = (3.80)^2 = 14.44$

Group 2

$\bar{x}_2 = 51.8$
$n_2 = 12$
$s_2^2 = (5.45)^2 = 29.70$

$$t_{obs} = \frac{38.9 - 51.8}{\sqrt{\{[\,(12-1)\,(14.44) + (12-1)\,(29.70)\,] \,/\, (12 + 12 - 2)\}\,[\,(1\,/\,12) + (1\,/\,12)\,]}}$$

$$t_{obs} = \frac{12.9}{\sqrt{[\,(158.84 + 326.7)\,/\,22\,]\,(.1666)}}$$

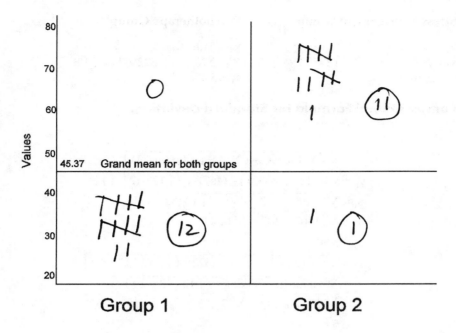

Figure 7–33.   Exploratory graph analysis for hypothetical posttest scores on the State-Trait Anxiety Inventory. The graph shows the difference between scores between two independent groups of patients with clinical depression receiving either stress management training or group psychotherapy. The test performed is an independent *t* test.

$$t_{obs} = 12.9 / \sqrt{(485.54 / 22)(.1666)}$$
$$t_{obs} = 12.9 / \sqrt{3.67}$$
$$t_{obs} = 12.9 / 1.9175$$
$$t_{obs} = 6.72$$

Step 9. Compare t_{obs} and t_{crit}.

$$t_{obs} = 6.72 \qquad\qquad\qquad t_{crit} = 2.0739$$

Examination shows $t_{obs} > t_{crit}$. Reject the null hypothesis. There seems to be a statistically significant difference between the two means, indicating that the stress management group was significantly more effective that the psychotherapy group in the reduction of anxiety in patients with clinical depression.

7.8.2 Mann–Whitney *U* Test

Rationale

The Mann–Whitney, a nonparametric alternative to the independent *t* test, is used to test whether two independent groups have been drawn from the same population. In practice, the Mann–Whitney is used with ordinal scale data.

1. The null hypothesis states that the two independent groups have the same population distribution.
2. An alternative, directional hypothesis is that there is a significant difference between the group means (when the distributions are approximately the same.)

Assumptions

1. Random selection of each group.
2. Two mutually independent groups are compared.
3. The measurement scale is at least ordinal.
4. n for each group is less than 20.

Computation

1. Rank order every raw score combining the two groups (e.g., lowest score in both groups is assigned the rank of 1).
2. When two or more raw scores are the same, average the ranks.
3. Add the ranks for one group, obtaining T_A value.

Formula for Mann–Whitney U Test

$$U_{obs} = [\, n_A n_B \,] + [\, (n_A)(n_A + 1)\,/\,2\,] - [\, T_A \,]$$

where n_A = number of subjects in 1st group
n_B = number of subjects in 2nd group
$T_A = \Sigma_n$ of ranks of first group.

Example

Language intelligibility scores were compared between an experimental and control group after a six-month treatment period. There was no significant difference between the groups on the pretest (two-tailed test, p .05).

The following data were collected:

Experimental Group A			Control Group B		
Subject	Score	Rank	Subject	Score	Rank
101	33	12	201	35	13
102	30	10	202	32	11
103	25	8	203	27	9
104	24	6.5	204	24	6.5
105	22	5	205	21	4
106	19	3	206	18	2
			207	16	1
T_A = 44.5			T_B = 46.5		
n_A = 6			n_B = 7		

$$U_{obs} = [\,(6)\,(7)\,]+[\,6\,(\,6+1\,)\,/\,2\,]-[\,44.5\,]$$
$$U_{obs} = 42+21-44.5$$
$$U_{obs} = 63-44.5$$
$$U_{obs} = 18.5$$

U_{crit}: obtain from table for Mann–Whitney U test (See Appendix C–7.)

$$n_A\,/\,n_B = 6\,/\,7 = U_{crit} = 6\,/\,36$$

If U_{obs} is between 6 and 36, do not reject null hypothesis.

Conclusion

Null hypothesis is not rejected since U_{obs} = 18.5, which is between 6 and 36. Thus the researcher concludes that there is no statistically significant difference in the experimental and control groups in language intelligibility posttest scores.

7.9 Model IV: Paired Data Sample

7.9.1 Correlated *t* Test

The correlated *t* test is applied to data when a researcher compares a group's performance or characteristic on two measures. For example, a researcher compares the difference between pretest and posttest scores of an observed variable. Another example is to compare the difference of two variables in one group, such as intelligence and perceptual motor test scores. The difference between the correlated *t* test and the independent *t* test is that the correlated *t* test is applied with one independent group and two variables, whereas the independent *t* test is applied to scores for two independent groups.

An example of a correlated *t* test was found in a study by McFall, Deitz, and Crowe (1993) entitled "Test-retest reliability of the test of visual perceptual skills with children with learning disabilities." In that study, the authors compared the difference in the score on the same test between 1 to 2 week's time period. The table below describes the means, mean differences, and t_{obs}.

Correlated *t* Tests Between Test and Retest Scores

Subtests	Pretest Mean	Retest Mean	Mean Difference	*t* Value
Visual Discrimination	11.9	13.01	1.1	−1.89
Visual Memory	9.4	10.5	1.1	−2.41*
Spatial Relations	10.4	11.1	.7	−1.76
Form Consistency	8.7	9.4	.7	−1.76
Sequential Memory	8.4	8.4	0.0	1.76
Figure Ground	9.2	9.3	.1	−.11
Visual Closure	9.5	11.4	.9	−3.17**

Note. n = 30; Critical value for t = 2.0452; $df = N - 1 = 30 - 1 = 29$; two tailed test; *p < 05.

There was a statistically significant difference between test and retest means on the variables of visual memory (t_{obs} = 2.41) and visual closure (t_{obs} = 3.17). These *t* values were above the t_{crit} value of 2.0452. The t_{obs} in the other tests were all below 2.045. The negative sign is disregarded in a nondirectional test.

On the basis of a significant statistical difference on these two subtests, the researcher will reject the null hypothesis. The null hypothesis is accepted for the other subtests.

Operational Procedure for Testing for Statistical Significance in a Paired Data Sample

Step 1. State the research hypothesis.

a.   *Null Hypothesis: H_0: $\mu_1 = \mu_2$*
b.   *Alternative Hypothesis: $\mu_1 \neq \mu_2$*
c.   *Directional Hypothesis: H_1: $\mu_1 > \mu_2$*

Step 2. Select the level of statistical significance.

p .05 or .01 level of significance

Step 3. Decide whether to apply a one-tailed or two-tailed test for statistical significance.
Step 4. Look up the critical value for t_{crit} from statistical table.

a.   determine the degrees of freedom: $df = N - 1$
b.   level of significance: p .05 or .01
c.   one-tailed or two-tailed test
d. t_{crit} derived from table of values (See Appendix C–3).

Step 5. Calculate the group means and standard deviations for each variable.
Step 6. Do an exploratory data analysis by determining if mean differences are greater than standard deviations for each variable.
Step 7. Plot a graph (See Independent t Test).
Step 8. Calculate t_{obs} using the formula:

$$t_{obs} = \frac{\Sigma D_1}{\sqrt{[N \Sigma D_1^2 - (\Sigma D_1)^2]/N-1}}$$

where ΣD_1 = Sum of differences between each subject's score on measured variable

ΣD_1^2 = Sum of the squared differences on each score

N = Total number of subjects.

Step 9. Accept the null hypothesis if $t_{obs} < t_{crit}$
Step 10. Reject the null hypothesis if $t_{obs} \geq t_{crit}$

Paired Data Sample

Hypothetical example of correlated t test.

Is there a statistically significant difference between performance IQ scores in adults with traumatic brain injury after undergoing an intensive cognitive retraining program?

Performance IQ Scores

Subject	Baseline (Pretest)	X_1^2	After Treatment (Posttest)	X_2^2
01	97	9409	113	12769
02	106	11236	113	12769
03	106	11236	101	10201
04	95	9025	119	14161
05	102	10404	111	12321
06	111	12321	121	14641
07	115	13225	121	14641
08	104	10816	106	11236
09	90	8100	110	12100
10	96	9216	126	15876

$$\Sigma X_1 = 1022 \quad \Sigma X_1^2 = 104988 \qquad \Sigma X_2 = 1141 \quad \Sigma X_2^2 = 130715$$

Step 1. State the research hypothesis. There is no statistically significant difference between pre- and posttest IQ performance scores in adults with traumatic brain injury who have undergone an extensive cognitive retraining program. This is a null hypothesis ($H_0 : \mu_1 = \mu_2$).

Step 2. The level of statistical significance is p .05.

Step 3. Decide whether to use a one-tailed or two-tailed test. This problem requires a two-tailed test because the hypothesis is stated in null form and the researcher is examining statistical significance without direction.

Step 4. Look up t_{crit} (See Appendix C–3).

a. $df = N - 1 = 9$
b. $p .05$
c. two-tailed test
d. $t_{crit} = 2.2622$

Step 5. Calculate the group means and standard deviations for the baseline and retest conditions.

Group 1

$\bar{x}_1 = \Sigma X / N = 1022 / 10 = 102.2$
$s_1 = 7.74$

Group 2

$\bar{x}_2 = 1141 / 10 = 114.1$
$s_2 = 7.65$

Standard Deviation Computational Formula

$s = \sqrt{[\, N \Sigma X^2 - (\Sigma X)^2 \,] / N (N-1)}$
$s_1 = \sqrt{\{[\, (10)(104988) \,] - (1022)^2\} / (10)(10-1)}$
$s_1 = \sqrt{(1049880 - 1044484) / 90}$
$s_1 = \sqrt{5396 / 90}$
$s_1 = \sqrt{59.95} = 7.74$
$s_2 = \sqrt{\{[\, (10)(130715) \,] - (1141)^2\} / 10(10-1)}$

$$s_2 = \sqrt{(1307150 - 1301881) / 90}$$
$$s_2 = \sqrt{5269 / 90}$$
$$s_2 = \sqrt{58.54} = 7.65$$

Step 6. Exploratory Data Analysis.

$$\bar{x}_1 - \bar{x}_2 = 102.2 - 114.1 = 11.9$$
$$s_1 = 7.74 \qquad\qquad\qquad s_2 = 7.65$$

The mean difference between pre- and posttest scores is greater than the standard deviations for pretest and posttest scores. The difference between the standard deviations is relatively small, indicating a homogeneity of variance for the two groups of scores.

Step 7. Exploratory Graph. This is displayed in Figure 7–34.

For the exploratory data analysis there appears to be a significant difference between the pretest and posttest scores.

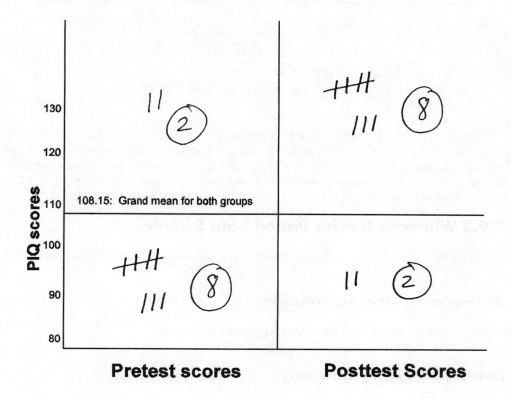

Figure 7–34.   Exploratory graph analysis using hypothetical data. The graph shows differences between pre- and posttest performance IQ scores for a group of adults with traumatic brain damage after cognitive retraining. The statistical test being performed is a correlated *t* test.

Step 8. Calculate t_{obs}.

$$t_{obs} = \frac{\Sigma D_1}{\sqrt{[N\Sigma D^2 - (\Sigma D_1)^2]/(N-1)}}$$

Subject	Baseline Test	Retest	D_1	D^2
01	97	113	−16	256
02	106	113	−07	49
03	106	101	+05	25
04	95	119	−24	576
05	102	111	−09	81
06	111	122	−11	121
07	115	121	−06	36
08	104	106	−02	4
09	90	110	−20	400
10	96	126	−30	900
	1022	1142	$\Sigma D_1 = -119$	$(\Sigma D_1)^2 = 14161$
			$\Sigma D^2 = 2450$	

$$t_{obs} = (-119)/\sqrt{\{[(10)(2450)]-14161/9\}}$$
$$t_{obs} = (-119)/\sqrt{[(24500-14161)/9]}$$
$$t_{obs} = (-119)/\sqrt{10339/9}$$
$$t_{obs} = (-119)/\sqrt{1154.33} = (-119)/33.98$$
$$t_{obs} = -3.5$$

Step 9. $t_{obs} = -3.5$. Using Table C–3 in the appendices, we find that $t_{crit} = 2.2622$. The researcher rejects the null hypothesis and concludes that there appears to be a significant difference between the pre- and posttest scores and that cognitive rehabilitation appeared to be effective in raising Performance IQ scores in this sample of individuals with traumatic brain injury[2].

7.9.2 Wilcoxon Test for Paired Data Samples

The Wilcoxon signed rank test is a nonparametric alternative to the t test for correlated samples.

Assumptions in Applying Wilcoxon

1. Random selection or random assignment of subjects.
2. Measurement scale is at least ordinal.

Example of Applying Wilcoxon

An investigator is interested in comparing the pre- and posttest scores for a group of nine subjects. The null hypothesis is stated, with p .05. The data for this example are as follows:

---

[2]Note that the negative sign in –3.5 does not affect the value. Both positive and negative values are interpreted equally when compared to the t_{crit} value for the table.

Subject	Pretest Raw Score	Posttest Raw Score	Difference	Rank Difference
01	10	12	−2	(−) 4
02	12	13	−3	(−) 7
03	8	6	2	4
04	6	10	−4	(−) 8
05	14	12	2	4
06	7	6	1	1
07	10	12	−2	(−) 4
08	14	16	−2	(−) 4
09	12	18	−6	(−) 9

Stepwise Procedure for Wilcoxon Signed-Rank Test (Example)

Step 1. Calculate the difference between the pre- and posttest raw scores, subtracting the posttest raw scores from the pretest raw scores.

Step 2. Rank order the differences between raw scores from smallest to largest, ignoring the negative or positive signs. Notice that in tied ranks, such as with 2 as a difference, the midpoint of the rank is 4 (2, 3, 4, 5, 6).

Step 3. Sum the positive rank differences:

$$\begin{array}{r} 4 \\ 4 \\ \underline{1} \\ 9 \end{array}$$

Step 4. Sum the negative rank differences:

$$\begin{array}{r} -4 \\ -7 \\ -8 \\ -4 \\ -4 \\ \underline{-9} \\ -36 \end{array}$$

Step 5. Determine T value. T is the absolute value of the smaller sum of the rank differences.

$T = 9$

Step 6. Compare the T_{obs} with T_{crit} from the table for critical values to T. (See Appendix C–8).

T_{crit} for $N = 9$, p .05, two-tailed test. $T_{crit} = 5$

Step 7. If the T_{obs} is equal to or less than T_{crit}, then reject the null hypothesis and conclude that there is a statistically significant difference between the pre- and posttest scores. Because

$T_{obs} = 9$ is greater than $T_{crit} = 5$, we accept the null hypothesis and conclude that there are no statistically significant differences between the pre- and posttest scores.

References: R. Runyon, (1977). *Nonparametric Statistics*. Reading, MA: Addison-Wesley Publishing Company, pp. 107–110, 181.

7.10 Model V: *k*-Independent Samples

7.10.1 Analysis of Variance

ANOVA is a widely used statistical test equivalent to the independent *t* test when testing for significant differences between two means. ANOVA is applied to statistical data when two or more independent group means are being compared. The statistic for the ANOVA is *F*. (*k* Refers to the number of independent groups or conditions in the study.)

$$F = \frac{\text{Variance between groups}}{\text{Variance within groups}}$$

The concept of the ANOVA is that if there are large differences between the group means as compared to relatively small differences within the variances or scores within the group, then a statistically significant result is evident. ANOVA answers the question: Is there a statistically significant difference between the independent groups being tested? For example, does $\mu_1 = \mu_2 = \mu_3 = \mu_k$? ANOVA is always tested by a null hypothesis. When there is a statistically significant result the researcher then carries out a post hoc analysis such as the Scheffé, Duncan Multiple Range, Neuman–Keuls, and Tukey's procedures. These post hoc tests are similar to *t* tests, applied to the data after attaining a significant *F*.

One-Way ANOVA

A one-way ANOVA simply analyzes the group means for statistically significant differences. The hypothetical table of results that follows is a typical example of a one-way ANOVA for comparing the effectiveness of three handwriting programs among 19 children with handwriting problems.

ANOVA Summary Table for Comparing Two Treatment Groups

Source of Variance	df	SS	MS	F
Between treatment groups	2	14	8	4*
Within treatment groups	16	32	2	
Total	18			

*$p < .05$, F_{crit} 3.63

> where SS = sums of squares
> MS = mean squares
> p = number of treatment groups
> N = total number of subjects in all groups

F is a derivative value equivalent to F_{obs} that is compared to the F_{crit} derived from a statistical table of values. For example, the F_{crit} for 2 df (treatment groups $-$ 1) and 16 df [number of subjects (19) $-$ number of groups (3)] with 2/16, p .05 is 3.63. Degrees of freedom (df) is derived from between treatment groups $(p - 1)$ and within treatment groups $(N - p)$.

The result in this hypothetical example shows that there is a statistically significant difference between the three treatment methods for handwriting disorders. F_{obs} 4.00 is $> F_{crit}$ 3.63. Thus, the researcher will reject the null hypothesis.

Example of Two-Factor Anova From the Literature

A one-way ANOVA analyzes the group means for statistically significant differences. The two-factor ANOVA looks at the variables from a two-dimensional perspective. It analyzes interactive effects, such as treatment method and therapist personality or treatment method and patient diagnosis. Palmer (1989) studied two methods of bed transfer following back surgery and examined pain experienced by patients preoperative (day 1) and postoperative (day 2). Results are shown in the following table.

Summary Table of Anova on Pain Rating Scores by Transfer Method and Time

Source of Variance	df	F	p value
Time (pre-post operative)	4	17.196	.000*
Method (2 transfer methods)	1	2.435	.120
Time X Method	4	0.911	.458

*p < .05 significant

The results show that there was a statistically significant difference between pain ratings during pre- and post-operation time periods. There were no statistically significant differences in the two methods of bed transfer nor in the interactional effects of time and method.

Stepwise Procedures for One-Way Anova (Hypothetical Example)

Step 1. State the research hypothesis. The hypothesis is always stated in the null form when using ANOVA. For example, there is no statistically significant difference between electrical stimulation (ES), acupuncture (A), and proprioceptive neuromuscular facilitation (PNF) in improving upper extremity function in patients with chronic hemiplegia.

$$H_0 = \mu_1 = \mu_2 = \mu_3$$

Step 2. Select the level of statistical significance.

p .05

Step 3. Identify F_{crit} from table. (See Table C–4 in the appendices.)

a. df for the numerator = 2 (three treatment groups − 1)
df for the denominator = 15 (number of subjects minus the number of groups: 18 − 3 = 15)
$df = 2 / 15$
b. p .05
c. $F_{crit} = 3.68$

Step 4. Calculate means and standard deviations[3]

ES Group			A Group			PNF Group		
Subject	Score	$X_1{}^2$	Subject	Score	$X_2{}^2$	Subject	Score	$X_3{}^2$
01	23	529	01	13	169	01	33	1089
02	31	961	02	19	361	02	42	1764
03	16	256	03	19	361	03	30	900
04	27	729	04	25	625	04	38	1444
05	32	1024	05	18	324	05	44	1936
06	18	324				06	41	1681
07	38	1444						
$\Sigma X_1 = 185$		$\Sigma X_1{}^2 = 5267$	$\Sigma X_2 = 94$	$\Sigma X_2{}^2 = 1840$		$\Sigma X_3 = 228$	$\Sigma X_3{}^2 = 8814$	
$\bar{x}_1 = 26.4$			$\bar{x}_2 = 18.8$			$\bar{x}_3 = 38.0$		

$$s = \sqrt{[\,N\,\Sigma X^2 - (\Sigma X)^2\,] / N\,(N-1)}$$
$$s_1 = \sqrt{[\,7\,(5267) - (185)^2\,] / 7\,(6)} = \sqrt{2644 / 42} = \sqrt{62.95} = 7.93$$
$$s_2 = \sqrt{[\,5\,(1840) - (94)^2\,] / 5\,(4)} = \sqrt{364 / 20} = \sqrt{18.2} = 4.26$$
$$s_3 = \sqrt{[\,6\,(8814) - (228)^2\,] / 6\,(5)} = \sqrt{900 / 30} = \sqrt{30.00} = 5.48$$

Step 5. Exploratory Data Analysis.

$\bar{x}_1 = 2.64$ $s_1 = 7.93$
$\bar{x}_2 = 18.8$ $s_2 = 4.26$
$\bar{x}_3 = 38.0$ $s_3 = 5.47$
$\bar{x}_1 - \bar{x}_2 = 7.6$ $s_1 - s_2 = 3.67$
$\bar{x}_1 - \bar{x}_3 = 11.6$ $s_1 - s_3 = 2.46$
$\bar{x}_2 - \bar{x}_3 = 19.2$ $s_2 - s_3 = 1.21$

There appears to be a statistically significant difference between the means and a relatively homogenous variance.
Step 6. Exploratory Graph Analysis. This graph is shown in Figure 7–35

$$\text{Group mean} = (\Sigma \bar{x}_1 + \Sigma \bar{x}_2 + \Sigma \bar{x}_3) / (N_1 + N_2 + N_3)$$
$$= (185 + 94 + 228) / (7 + 5 + 6)$$
$$= 507 / 18 = 28.16$$

There appears to be a statistically significant difference between group 2 and group 3.
Step 7. Calculate F.

---

[3]The Fugl–Meyer Postroke Motor Recovery Test Scores wre used for the example. (Range is 0–50.)

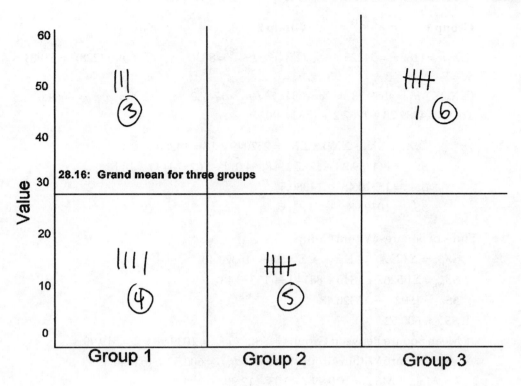

Figure 7–35. Exploratory graph for ANOVA using hypothetical data. The graph shows differences in scores between three different groups.

Summary Table for One-Way Anova

Source of Variance	df	SS	MS	F
Between groups (BG)	2	1039.98	519.99	12.99
Within groups (WG)	15	600.52	40.03	
Total	17			

Formulas for ANOVA

a. $$F = \frac{MS \text{ Between Groups}}{MS \text{ Within Groups}}$$

b. df Between Groups (df_{bg}) = Number of groups minus 1 = (3 − 1) = 2
df Within Groups (df_{wg}) = Total number of subjects in all groups minus the number of groups = 18 − 3 = 15

c. Mean Square Between Groups = SS_{bg} / df_{bg}
Mean Square Within Groups = SS_{wg} / df_{wg}

d. Sum of Squares Between Groups:

$$SS_{bg} = \Sigma \left[(\Sigma X_1)^2 / n_1 \right] + \left[(\Sigma X_2)^2 / n_2 \right] + \left[(\Sigma X_3)^2 / n_3 \right] - \left[(\Sigma X_1 + \Sigma X_2 + \Sigma X_3)^2 / \Sigma N \right]$$

Group 1	Group 2	Group 3
$(\Sigma X_1)^2 = (185)^2 = 34225$	$(\Sigma X_2)^2 = (94)^2 = 8836$	$(\Sigma X_3)^2 = (228)^2 = 51984$
$n_1 = 7$	$n_2 = 5$	$n_3 = 6$
$(\Sigma X_1)^2 / n_1 = 4889.28$	$(\Sigma X_2)^2 / n_2 = 1767.2$	$(\Sigma X_3)^2 / n_3 = 8664.0$

Total = (4889.28 + 1767.2 + 15320.48)

$$(\Sigma X_1 + \Sigma X_2 + \Sigma X_3) / \Sigma N) = 257049 / 18 = 14280.5$$
$$SS_{bg} = [\,(4889.28 + 1767.2 + 8664.0)\,] - [\,(\,257049\,) / 18\,]$$
$$SS_{bg} = 15320.48 - 14280.5$$
$$SS_{bg} = 1039.98$$

e.   Sums of Squares Within Groups

$$SS_{wg} = \Sigma\,(\,\Sigma X_1^2 + \Sigma X_2^2 + \Sigma X_3^2\,) - 15320.48$$
$$SS_{wg} = \Sigma\,(\,5267 + 1840 + 8814\,) - 15320.48$$
$$SS_{wg} = 15921 - 15320.48$$
$$SS_{wg} = 600.52$$

Mean Square Between Groups = $SS_{bg} / df_{bg} = 1039.98 / 2 = 519.99$

Mean Square Within Groups = $SS_{bg} / df_{wg} = 600.52 / 15 = 40.03$

$F = MS_{bg} / MS_{wg} = 519.99 / 40.03 = 12.99$

Step 8. Compare F_{obs} with F_{crit}.

$$F_{obs} = 12.99 \qquad\qquad F_{crit} = 3.68$$

Thus we reject the null hypothesis and conclude that there is a statistically significant difference between the three groups. This confirms our exploratory data analysis.

Step 9. Conduct a post hoc test. If there is a significant F, meaning that the mean values are statistically significant, then the researcher carries out a post hoc analysis. This analysis is parallel to doing independent t tests and determine which pairs of means have statistically significant differences.

There are a number of post hoc tests that are available to the researcher, such as:

- Tukey's Honestly Significant Differences (HSD)
- Neuman–Keuls
- Duncan Multiple Range
- Scheffé

Example of a Post Hoc Analysis.   In the previous example, it was found that F_{obs} is statistically significant when $\bar{x}_1 = 26.4$, $\bar{x}_2 = 18.8$, and $\bar{x}_3 = 38.0$. H_0: Null hypothesis is rejected and we conclude that all the means are not the same. We can now compare each pair of means, such as:

$\bar{x}_1$ compared to $\bar{x}_2$ $\qquad\qquad$ $\bar{x}_1$ compared to $\bar{x}_3$ $\qquad\qquad$ $\bar{x}_2$ compared to $\bar{x}_2$

A significant F means that at least one pair of means are significantly different, that is, the highest and lowest mean. Therefore, $\bar{x}_2$ compared to $\bar{x}_3$ has a statistically significant difference. We do not know whether there is a statistically significant difference between $\bar{x}_1$ and $\bar{x}_2$, and $\bar{x}_1$ and $\bar{x}_3$. A post hoc analysis tests for statistical significant difference in these two situations.

In this example the Tukey (HSD), a widely used post hoc analysis, was selected. The formula for the Tukey is (Gravette & Wellnau, 1985):

$$HSD = q \, (MS_{wg} \, / n \,)$$

where q = a derived table value (See Table C–9 in the appendices: The Student Range Statistic)

MS_{wg} = the value calculated for mean squares within groups and is taken from the ANOVA table. In the above example this value is 40.03.

n = the average of the number of cases in each group. In the above example $n_1 = 7$, $n_2 = 5$, $n_3 = 6$. The average is 6.

k = number of groups (k) = 3

df for MS_{wg} = 15

p .05

$q = 3.67$

$HSD = q \, \sqrt{(\, MS_{wg} \, / n \,)} = 3.67 \, \sqrt{(\, 40.03 \, / \, 6 \,)} = 9.479$

Therefore the mean difference between any two group scores must be at least 9.48 to be statistically significant.

1. $\bar{x}_1 - \bar{x}_2 = 26.4 - 18.8 = 7.6$. Therefore the null hypothesis is accepted and $\bar{x}_1 = \bar{x}_2$.
2. $\bar{x}_1 - \bar{x}_3 = 26.4 - 38.0 = 11.6$. Therefore the null hypothesis is rejected and $\bar{x}_1 \neq \bar{x}_3$.
3. $\bar{x}_2 - \bar{x}_3 = 18.8 - 38.0 = 19.2$. Therefore the null hypothesis is rejected and $\bar{x}_2 \neq \bar{x}_3$.

In conclusion, a post hoc analysis test determines the pairs of means that have statistically significant differences.

Reference: F. J. Gravette, and L. R. Wellnau, (1985). *Statistics for the Behavioral Sciences*. St. Paul: West Publishing Company, pp. 424–425.

7.10.2 Kruskal–Wallis Test for k Sample

The Kruskal–Wallis test is a nonparametric alternative to the one-way ANOVA when comparing three or more independent groups.

Assumptions

1. Random selection or random assignment of subjects to each independent group.

2. Ordinal scale measurement.
3. Each group should have at least five subjects.

Example of Applying Kruskal–Wallis

Step 1. The investigator hypothesizes that there is no statistically significant difference between the three groups.

Group 1	Raw Score	Group 2	Raw Score	Group 3	Raw Score
Subj 101	10	Subj 201	14	Subj 301	12
102	8	202	12	302	14
103	6	203	10	303	7
104	10	204	8	304	6
105	12	205	9	305	10
106	14				

Step 2. Rank order every raw score, combining all groups (in this example, three groups) with the lowest score assigned a rank of 1. In this example, subject 303's raw score of 4 is assigned the rank of 1.

Subject	Raw Score	Rank	
101	10	8.5	
102	8	4.5	
103	6	2.5	
104	10	8.5	
105	12	12	
106	14	15	$\Sigma_{ranks} = 51$
201	14	15	
202	12	12	
203	10	8.5	
201	8	4.5	
205	9	6	$\Sigma_{ranks} = 46$
301	12	12	
302	14	15	
303	4	1	
304	6	2.5	
305	10	8.5	$\Sigma_{ranks} = 39$

Note. n = 16

Step 3. Sum the ranks for each group.

Group 1	Group 2	Group 3
8.5	15	12
4.5	12	8.5
2.5	8.5	12
8.5	8.5	1
12	4.5	2.5
15	6	8.5
$\Sigma = 51$	$\Sigma = 46.0$	$\Sigma = 39.0$
$n_1 = 6$	$n_2 = 5$	$n_3 = 5$

Step 4. Calculate the formula for Kruskal–Wallis (H_{obs})

$$H_{obs} = 12 / [\, N\,(N+1)\,]\,[\,\Sigma\,(T_1^2 / n_1) + (T_2^2 / n_2) + (T_3^2 / n_3)\,] - [\,3\,(N+1)\,]$$

where $N = n_1 + n_2 + n_3 = 16$

$T_1^2 = (\Sigma_{ranks})^2 = 51^2 = 2601$

$T_2^2 = 46^2 = 2116$

$T_3^2 = 39^2 = 1521$

$H_{obs} = 12 / [\,16\,(17)\,]\,[\,\Sigma\,(2601 / 6) + (2116 / 5) + (1521 / 5)\,] - [\,3\,(17)\,]$

$H_{obs} = [\,12 / 272\,]\,[\,433.5 + 423.2 + 304.2\,] - [\,51\,]$

$H_{obs} = [\,.044\,]\,[\,1160.9\,] - [\,51\,] = 51.08 - 51$

$H_{obs} = .08$

Step 5. Calculate H_{crit} for p .05, df = number of groups (k) − 1 = 2.

$H_{crit} = 5.99$ (Use Chi-Square table, Appendix C–10, to test for statistical significance)

Step 6. Compare H_{obs} (.08) with H_{crit} (5.991). If H_{obs} is equal to or more than H_{crit}, reject the null hypothesis. In this example the null hypothesis is smaller and we conclude that there is no statistically significant difference between the three groups tested.

7. 11 Model VI: Correlation (Pearson and Spearman Correlation Coefficients)

What is correlation? What is the difference between an associational relationship and causality? How do we graph the relationship between variables? What is a correlational matrix? What is a regression line? What is the difference between the Pearson correlation coefficient and the Spearman rank order correlation coefficient? All of these questions relate to the correlational model in statistics.

Definition of Correlation

Correlation is the reciprocal relationship between two variables. It is a general concept that assumes that variables can be measured and correlated. The index of the degree of relationship between two variables is the correlation coefficient. This index can range from zero, which indicates no relationship, to $+1.00$ or -1.00, which indicates a perfect correlation between two variables. For example, a correlation coefficient of .30 indicates a low correlation, whereas .90 is a high correlation. The symbol for correlation is r. A correlational relationship indicates an association between variables; it does not indicate a causal relationship.

Example of a Correlation in the Literature

In Table 7–11 the investigator examined the relationship between stress and leisure satisfaction among therapeutic recreation personnel. The table is a correlational matrix that measures the degree of associations between five variables. Each variable is correlated with each other. The Personal Strain Questionnaire component of the Occupational Stress Inventory, as developed by Osipow and Spokane (1987), and the Leisure Satisfaction Scale was administered to 159 individuals who were members of the National Therapeutic Recreation Society. Data were gathered through a mail questionnaire.

Fifteen correlation coefficients (r) were completed to construct the correlational matrix table. The researchers used the p .05 for level of statistical significance. Although statistical significance may be reached at $r = .21$ for 83 df ($N - 2$), (p .05 and a two-tailed test), it is important to note that with correlations, statistical significance is not as important as establishing a clinical level of correlation. For example, in establishing an acceptable reliability for a test, many researchers will accept Pearson correlation coefficients of $r = .80$ or above as acceptable. In the example in Table 7–11, for example, $r = .60$ is considered by some researchers to be low to moderate in clinical significance. In understanding the correlational results, it is important to note that the square of r is the proportion of variance in one variable that is associated with another variable. If $r = .60$, the proportion of variance accounted for is only .36, which means that .64 is that portion of the variance that is not accounted for. Correlation is a measure of predicting the value of one variable Y (unknown) if another variable X is known. If there is a high correlation between the two variables, (e.g., $r = .90$), then the researcher has a high degree of confidence in predicting "if X, then Y." The degree of confidence in the relationship is more important in clinical research than the statistical r value.

Table 7–11   *Correlation Coefficients Between Ratings on Personal Strain Questionnaire and Leisure Satisfaction Scale*

	Vocational	Psychological	Interpersonal	Physical	Total
Psychological	.65*	—			
Interpersonal	.46*	.57*	—		
Physical	.44*	.61*	.43*	—	
PSQ Total	.75*	.87*	.75*	.81*	—
Leisure Satis.	−.21	−.30*	−.24*	−.39*	−.37*

* = significant at .05; $N = 85$.

Note. From "The Relationship Between Stress and Leisure Satisfaction Among Therapeutic Recreation Personnel" in P. H. Cunningham and T. Bartuska, 1989, *Therapeutic Recreation Journal, 23*(3), p. 69. Copyright 1989, *Therapeutic Recreation Journal.* Reprinted with permission.

In the example illustrated in Table 7–11 there are comparatively high correlations between the Personal Strain Questionnaire (PSQ) Total and the subscales of the PSQ. Comparatively low to moderate correlations exist between the Leisure Satisfaction Scale and the subscales of the PSQ. In other words, the clinician could not predict with confidence that persons with higher levels of leisure satisfaction would experience less stress than persons who have low satisfaction with their leisure. On the basis of these results, the researchers should conclude that there is not a strong relationship between stress and leisure satisfaction even through there is a significant statistical relationship at the p .05 level.

Stepwise Procedure for Correlation

Step 1. State the research hypothesis: For example, there is no statistical significant relationship between variable X and variable Y. (Null hypothesis, r = .00 or below predetermined level of correlation.)

Step 2. Determine the degree of relationship that will be acceptable for significance.

a. In establishing test–retest reliability, a correlation coefficient of r = .80 or above is considered acceptable (Anastasi, 1988).
b. In clinical research, a correlation coefficient of below r =.60 is moderate to low.

Step 3. Collect data and arrange raw scores into table. For example:

Subjects	Variable X Raw Score	Rank	Variable Y Raw Score	Rank	d (difference in ranks between X and Y)	d² (difference squared)
1	31	7	45	5	2	4
2	22	5	58	8	-3	9
3	19	4	57	7	-3	9
4	16	3	48	6	-3	9
5	78	8.5	61	9	-0.5	0.25
6	3	1	36	4	-3	9
7	93	10	18	3	7	49
8	78	8.5	88	10	-1.5	2.25
9	23	6	9	1	5	25
10	15	2	12	2	0	0
	ΣX = 378		ΣY = 432		Σd=0[a]	Σd^2 = 116.5

Note. d = difference in ranks between *X* and *Y*; *d²* = difference squared.
[a]Note that in computing the differences (*d*), the sum of the rank differences should equal zero, when taking into conderation the negative and positive signs.

Step 4. Rank order each raw score, with lowest score being assigned rank of 1. Note: for tied ranks, take the midpoint of the rank. For example, a raw score of 78 occupies ranks 8 and 9 and becomes rank of 8.5.

Step 5. Do exploratory data analysis. Note in Figure 7–36 that each point in the scatter diagram is a coordinate value. It appears from the scatter diagram that there is a low moderate correlation between the two variables.

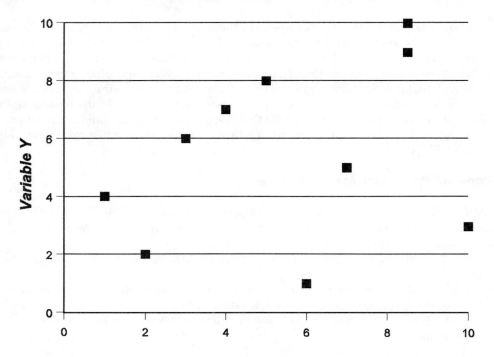

Figure 7–36.   Exploratory data on a scattergram using the ranks of the scores. Notice that each point is a coordinate value. There appears to be a low to moderate correlation between the two variables.

Step 6. Calculate Spearman rank correlation coefficient and estimate degree of relationship between the two variables (X and Y). The formula for Spearman r_s is:

$$r_s = 1.00 - [\,(6)\,(\Sigma d^2\,)\,/\,N^3 - N\,]$$
$$r_s = 1.00 - [\,(6)\,(116.5)\,/\,1,000 - 10\,]$$
$$r_s = 1.00 - [\,699\,/\,990\,]$$
$$r_s = 1.00 - .71$$
$$r_s = .29$$

The exploratory data analysis indicates that there is a low correlation between the X and Y variables.

Step 7. Calculate the Pearson r correlation coefficient. The Spearman (rank order) is a good screening test for the Pearson (product–moment), which is a more accurate test because the Pearson r computes raw scores whereas the Spearman r_s computes ranks, which are transformed scores. The reader shall note that the Pearson r, which is a parametric test, should be applied to interval or ratio scale data. The Spearman r_s is a nonparametric statistical test that can be used with ordinal scale data. As the reader will note interval scale data can be transformed to ranks (ordinal scale data).

The formula for the Pearson r product–moment correlation is:

$$r = [N\Sigma XY - (\Sigma X)(\Sigma Y)] / \sqrt{[N\Sigma X^2 - (\Sigma X)^2][N\Sigma Y^2 - (\Sigma Y)^2]}$$

Calculation for Pearson r Product–Moment Correlation.

Subject	X	X²	Y	Y²	XY
01	31	961	45	2025	1395
02	22	484	58	3364	1276
03	19	361	57	3249	1083
04	16	256	48	2304	768
05	78	6084	61	3721	4758
06	3	9	36	1296	108
07	93	8649	18	324	1674
08	78	6084	88	7744	6864
09	23	529	9	81	207
10	15	225	12	144	180
	378	23642	432	24252	18313
	$\Sigma X = 378$	$\Sigma X^2 = 23{,}642$	$\Sigma Y = 432$	$\Sigma Y^2 = 24{,}252$	$\Sigma XY = 18{,}313$

$N = 10$ $\Sigma X^2 = 23{,}642$

$\Sigma XY = 18{,}313$ $\Sigma Y^2 = 24{,}252$

$\Sigma X = 378$ $(\Sigma X)^2 = 142{,}884$

$\Sigma Y = 432$ $(\Sigma Y)^2 = 186{,}624$

$r = [(10)(18{,}313)] - [(378)(432)] / \sqrt{[(10)(23{,}642) - 142{,}884][(10)(24{,}252) - 186{,}624]}$

$r = (183{,}130 - 163{,}296) / \sqrt{(236{,}420 - 142{,}884)(242{,}520 - 186{,}624)}$

$r = (19{,}834) / \sqrt{(93{,}536)(55{,}896)}$

$r = 19{,}834 / 72{,}307$

$r = .274$

The Pearson r of .274 is very similar to the Spearman r_s of .29. In both computations the correlation is low and will not be clinically significant as only a small portion of the variance is accounted for.

Step 8. Calculation of Regression Line. A regression line describes the relationship between variable X and variable Y. The formula for the regression line is

$$Y = bX + a$$

where Y is a predicted variable from the known X value and the b is the slope of the line and a is the Y intercept. The regression line that is calculated assumes that if a perfect correlation 1.00 exists between two variables, then one could predict the Y value if the X value is known. For example, if we derive the formula for a specific regression line to be:

$$Y = .30X + 1.50$$

$$\text{and } X = .500$$

$$Y = .30(5.00) + 1.50$$

$$Y = 1.5 + 1.5$$
$$Y = 3.00$$

So if $X = 5.00$, then $Y = 3.00$ in this example. The calculation of a regression line is useful when there is a high correlation between two variables. On the other hand, a low correlation of $r = .29$ would not warrant constructing a regression line.

The computational formula for the slope is:

$$b = [N(\Sigma XY) - (\Sigma X)(\Sigma Y)] / [N\Sigma X^2 - (\Sigma X)^2]$$

The formula for the Y intercept is

$$a = Y - bX$$

Step 9. Identify the critical values for the Spearman rank order correlation coefficient.

a.   Determine number of subjects (N)
b.   Significance level, such as p .05, p .01
c.   Directional or nondirectional hypothesis

For example, with $N = 10$, p .05, nondirectional test, $r_{s(crit)} = .648$. (See Table C–6 in the appendices.) In the example above $r_{s(obs)} = .29$. In this result, the researcher will accept the null hypothesis and conclude that there is no statistically significant relationship between the two variables.

Step 10. Identify the critical values for the Pearson product–moment correlation.

a. $df = N - 2$
b.   Significance level
c.   directional or nondirectional test.

In the example as shown, $df = 8$, p .05, nondirectional test, $r_{crit} = .6319$. (See Table C–5 in the appendices.) Since $r_{obs} = .27$, the null hypothesis is accepted and the researcher concludes that there is no statistically significant relationship between the two variables.

The reader should note that as the N increases, the $r_{crit} = $ decreases. For example, for 100 df, p .05 < level of significance, $r_{crit} = .1966$, while for 20 df, $r_{crit} = .4227$.

7.12 Model VII: Observed Frequencies (Chi-Square)

When researchers work with nominal scale data, they frequently are concerned with differences in the number of cases falling into discrete categories such as improved/not improved, or active/disengaged. The major purpose of this statistical model is to test whether their are statistically significant differences between the observed and the expected frequencies of two independent groups. For example, this model could be applied if a researcher is interested in determining whether there is a gender difference in the distribution of individuals with multiple sclerosis in a population where there are 51% females and 49% males. Is there a statistically significance difference between the number of males as compared to females who have a diagnosis of multiple sclerosis? In this hypothetical example the researcher will compare the observed differences between the number of males and females diagnosed with multiple sclerosis with the expected prevalence, that is, 51% for females and 49% for males.

Example of Chi-Square

In an example from the literature, the investigators examined the factors influencing the successful outcome of tracking individuals with severe psychiatric illnesses in the community as compared to in the hospital. In Table 7–12 the investigators compared the patients treated at home with patients admitted to a hospital in relation to where they were assessed during a psychotic episode.

Formula for Chi-Square.

$$\chi^2_{obs} = \Sigma (O - E)^2 / E$$
$$\chi^2_{obs} = [(51 - 42)^2 / 42] + [(3 - 11)^2 / 11] + [(11 - 10)^2 / 10] + [(0 - 2)^2 / 2]$$
$$+ [(13 - 22)^2 / 22] + [(13 - 6)^2 / 6] + [(5 - 5)^2 / 5] + [(3 - 1)^2 / 1]$$
$$\chi^2_{obs} = 1.92 + 5.81 + .09 + 2 + 3.68 + 8.16 + 0 + 4$$
$$\chi^2_{obs} = 25.66$$
$$\chi^2_{crit} = 7.815 \ (3 \ df, p < .05). \text{ (See Table C–10 in the appendices.)}$$

Conclusion.   The researchers rejected the null hypothesis and concluded that there is a statistically significant difference where patients are assessed if they are treated at home or admitted to a hospital. From the results, the researchers concluded that if patients are assessed at home, they will have a significantly less probability of being admitted to a hospital for a psychiatric illness. The results of the study reinforced their hypothesis that home treatment is a feasible alternative to hospital treatment for many individuals with psychiatric illness. The application of chi-square is an appropriate statistical test when comparing nominal categories of data. It is a simple but powerful statistic that can be applied to outcome studies of clinical populations.

Table 7–12   *Location of Assessment During a Psychiatric Episode*

Location of Assessment	Patients Treated at Home		Patients Admitted to Hospital		Total Patients
	Observed	Expected	Observed	Expected	
Home	51	42	13	22	64
Hospital	3	11	13	6	16
Outpatient Clinic	11	10	5	5	16
Police Station	0	2	3	1	3
	65	65	34	34	99

Note. From "Home Treatment for Acute Psychiatric Illness," by C. Dean and E. M Gadd, 1990, *British Medical Journal, 301,* p. 1023. Copyright 1990, *British Medical Journal.* Reprinted with permission.

Operational Procedure of Observed vs. Expected Frequencies (Chi-Square)

Step 1. State the research hypothesis. The null hypothesis is: There is no statistically significant difference between the observed versus expected frequencies in normal groups ($\chi^2_{obs} < \chi^2_{crit}$). The alternative hypothesis is: There is a statistically significant difference between the observed versus expected frequencies in nominal groups ($\chi^2_{obs} \geq \chi^2_{crit}$).

Step 2. Select the level of statistical significance. This is usually *p*. 05.

Step 3. Determine the degrees of freedom (df) for the contingency table.

$$df = (r - 1)(c - 1)$$

r = number of rows in the table

c = number of columns in the table

For example, in a 2 × 2 contingency table, the degrees of freedom is 1. In a 3 × 6 contingency table, *df* = 10.

Step 4. Identify χ^2_{crit} (chi-square critical) from the statistical table of values. The critical value is determined by:

a.   level of significance
b.   *df*

For example, χ^2_{crit} = 18.307 for *p* .05, nondirectional test, with *df* = 10. (See Table C–10 in the appendices.)

Step 5. Identify the discrete nominal categories being compared. For example, diagnostic groups, gender, and health-care settings.

Step 6. Determine the number of columns and rows in the chi-square contingency table. Chi-square contingency tables are based on the number of columns and rows being compared. Contingency tables range from two rows and columns (2 × 2 contingency table) to larger number of rows and columns, such as (2 × 3), (3 × 5), (6 × 8).

Step 7. Tabulate the observed number of frequencies within each discrete category or group.

	Nonsmokers		Smokers		
	Observed	Expected	Observed	Expected	
Lung Cancer	500	1,000	1,500	1,000	2,000
No Lung Cancer	4,500	4,000	3,500	4,000	8,000
	5,000		5,000		10,000

The researcher counts the number of individuals with lung cancer who were smokers or nonsmokers in a population.

Step 8. Calculate the expected frequencies based on the probability of chance. The expected frequencies in a cell are computed by multiplying the total frequencies of a row that contains the cell by the total frequencies of the column that contains the cell and dividing this product by the total number of cases in the population. In the example above, the expected frequencies for nonsmokers with lung cancer is equal to:

(2000) (5000) / 10,000 = 1,000.

Step 9. Calculate chi-square (χ^2_{obs}). The formula for chi-square is:

$$\Sigma = (O - E)^2 / O$$

where Σ = grand sum of all the cells

O = observed frequency in each cell

E = expected frequency in each cell

Step 10. Compare the two values: χ^2_{obs} *and* χ^2_{crit}. (See Table C–10 in the appendices for critical score.)

a. Accept the null hypothesis if χ^2_{obs} is less than χ^2_{crit}.
b. Reject the null hypothesis if χ^2_{obs} is equal to or more than χ^2_{crit}.

Observed Frequencies, Chi-Square Example

Research Problem. Is cognitive–behavioral treatment as effective as antidepressant medication in treating individuals with clinical depression?

Step 1. Research hypothesis. Null hypothesis: There is no statistically significant difference between the number of individuals with depression who improve with medication (Med) and those who receive cognitive–behavioral treatment (CBT).

Step 2. Level of significance: p .05

Step 3. Determine the df from contingency table.

$$df = (r - 1)(c - 1)$$
$$df = (2 - 1)(3 - 1) = 2$$

Step 4. Identify χ^2_{crit} *from the statistical table of values.*

a. *p .05*
b. *df = 2*
c. χ^2_{crit} = 5.99 (See Table C–10 in the appendices.)

Step 5. The nominal categories are: (a) those individuals treated with CBT who regressed, (b) those individuals treated with CBT who showed no improvement, (c) those individuals treated with CBT who improved, (d) those treated with meds who showed no improvement and (e) those treated with meds who improved.

Step 6. There are two rows and three columns: (2 × 3 contingency table).

Step 7. Enumerate the observed number of frequencies within each nominal category and place in 2 × 3 contingency table.

	Regressed		No Improvement		Improvement		
Treatment	O	E	O	E	O	E	**Totals**
Cognitive-Behavioral	20	24.70	40	57.64	150	127.64	210
Medication	40	35.29	100	82.35	160	182.35	300
Totals	60		140		310		510

In this example, 210 individuals received CBT and 300 individuals received medication. A total of 510 individuals with depression were included in the study. Out of 310 individuals who improved, 160 received medication while the remaining 150 received CBT. The rest of the group (200 individuals) showed either no improvement (remained the same) or regressed.

Step 8. Calculate the expected frequencies for each nominal category or cell based on the formula. "To complete the expected frequency of any cell, multiply the marginal total for the row that contains the cell by the marginal total for the column that contains the cell, and divide this product by the total number of cases in the table" (McCall, 1986, p. 321).

$$CBT \text{ (Regressed)} = (210)(60) / 510 = 24.70$$

$$CBT \text{ (No improvement)} = (210)(140) / 510 = 57.64$$

$$CBT \text{ (Improved)} = (210)(310) / 510 = 127.64$$

$$Med \text{ (Regressed)} = (300)(60) / 510 = 35.29$$

$$Med \text{ (No improvement)} = (300)(140) / 510 = 82.35$$

$$Med \text{ (Improved)} = (300)(310) / 510 = 182.35$$

Step 9. Calculate chi-square (χ^2_{obs}).

$$\Sigma = (O - E)^2 / E$$

$$\chi^2_{obs} = [(20 - 24.70)^2 / 24.70] + [(40 - 57.64)^2 / 57.64] + [(150 - 127.64)^2 / 127.64] + [(40 - 35.29)^2 / 35.29] + [(100 - 82.35)^2 / 82.35] + [(160 - 182.35)^2 / 182.35]$$

$$\chi^2_{obs} = .89 + 5.39 + 3.91 + .62 + 3.78 + 2.73$$

$$\chi^2_{obs} = 17.32$$

Step 10. Compare χ^2_{obs} with χ^2_{crit}

$$\chi^2_{obs} = 17.32$$

$$\chi^2_{crit} = 5.991$$

Reject the null hypothesis. There is a statistically significant difference between CBT and medications in the treatment of depression. It appears that CBT is more effective than medication in the improvement of depression in this hypothetical example. One hundred fifty of the 210 individuals, or 71%, of the CBT group improved while 160 out of the 300 individuals, or 53%, of the medication group improved.

7.12.1 Kappa

Purpose

The purpose is to determine the degree of agreement between two or more judges independently ranking a variable. It can be used to measure interrater reliability. Kappa can range from +1.00 to −1.00.

Assumptions

1. The units are independent, that is, are completed by independent observations.
2. The categories are nominal scale measurements, are fully mutually exclusive and exhaustive.
3. The judges operate independently.
4. There are no criteria for correctness, choices, clinical judgement, or client attitudes.
5. Judges have equal competence, education, or ability to make ratings.
6. There are no restrictions placed on ranking or rating the variable.

Formula

$$\text{Kappa} = P_o - P_c / 1 - P_c$$

where P_o = the observed proportion of agreement

P_c = the proportion of agreement expected by chance alone.

Example

In a hypothetical observation, two independent observers rate the level of depression indicated by a behavioral scale. One individual is observed by two independent raters during 10 sessions to evaluate the level of depression (i.e., low depression, LD; medium depression, MD; and severe depression, SD). Each category of depression is operationally defined and each rater has been trained previously using a standardized rating scale. They independently observe a patient on a ward applying a behavior rating scale. Is there a high interrater relationship between the two observers, using a standardized rating scale? The data from the observations follow:

Sessions	Observer 1	Observer 2	Agreement
1	LD	MD	no
2	MD	MD	yes
3	LD	LD	yes
4	MD	MD	yes
5	LD	LD	yes
6	LD	LD	yes
7	MD	MD	yes
8	LD	MD	no
9	MD	MD	yes
10	LD	LD	yes
Totals	**6 LD, 4 MD, 0 SD**	**4 LD, 6 MD, 0 SD**	**Agreements: 8/10 = 80%**

Stepwise Procedure

Step 1. Place data into a 3 × 3 contingency table to display agreements. Use three categories of depression, MD, LD, and SD.

	LD	MD	SD	Marginal totals
LD	4	2	0	6
MD	0	4	0	4
SD	0	0	0	0
Marginal totals	4	6	0	(10)

Notice that there were 4 instances of both observers agreeing on low depression and 4 instances of both observers agreeing on moderate depression. There were no observations of severe depression. The agreements will always be the numbers in the diagonal cells when there are 2 observers and 1 subject. Also note that when adding frequencies in cells that observer one usually is on the Y axis and observer two is on the X axis of the table. In this example the discrepancy between the two raters occurred in the cell containing 2. This is where observer 1 rated subject twice as LD and observer 2 rates the same subject for sessions 1 and 8 as MD.

   Step 2. Calculate for kappa applying the formula.

$$\text{Kappa} = P_O - P_C / 1 - P_C$$

P_o is obtained by adding all the frequencies in the cells that both observers agree.

Observer 2

Observer 1	11	12	13
	21	22	23
	31	32	33

Each cell is numbered to represent the rating of each observer. For example, cells 11, 22, and 33 represent agreements of observers 1 and 2. On the other hand, cell 21 represents discrepancy between observers 1 and 2.

   P_o = the frequency of agreement over the total number of observations (N). The formula is

$$P_o = (n_{11} + n_{22} + n_{33} + n_{ii} \cdots)$$

where n_{ii} = and other cells

$n_{11} = 4$
$n_{22} = 4$
$n_{33} = 0$
$P_o = 8/10 = .80$

The marginal total is the sum of each row or column.
   P_c = marginal totals of observer times marginal totals of observer 2, divided by the total number of observation periods of sessions squared.

$$P_c = \{[(6)(4)] + [(4)(6)] + [(0)(0)]\} / 10^2$$
$$P_c = [(24) + (24) + (0)] / 100$$

$P_c = 48 / 100 = .48$

kappa $= (.80 - .48) / (1 - .48)$

kappa $= .32 / .52 = .61$

A kappa of .70 is considered to indicate an acceptable level of agreement (Sattler, 1988). The results indicate a slightly lower interrater agreement than what statisticians consider acceptable interrater reliability. Note that the percentage of agreement, that is, 80%, is uncorrected for chance. From a pragmatic perspective, kappa should always be interpreted in terms of its value to the clinician. In this example, the clinical researcher would interpret a kappa of .61 as acceptable.

References: For further information see J.Cohen, (1960). "A Coefficient of Agreement for Nominal Scales," *Educational and Psychological Measurement*, 20, 37–46; and J. M. Sattler, (1988). *Assessment of Children* (3rd ed.). San Diego: Sattler Publishing Co.

7.13 Statistical Software Packages

Although the authors have used hand calculations to solve the examples presented in this book, in actuality, many statistical problems can be solved through one of a number of statistical packages available for computers. Three widely used computer programs designed for the health and social sciences include the following:

Statistical Package for the Social Sciences (SPSS)

This program is a data analysis package for research scientists and is widely used within the social science fields as well as other disciplines. SPSS includes the capabilities to perform basic analyses (e.g., frequencies, correlations) and more advanced analyses (e.g., regression, ANOVA, general linear models, contingency tables, factor and discriminant analysis, nonparametric statistics, and time series). It can be used in DOS, Windows, and MAC environments. More information about SPSS can be obtained through the company at 1–800–543–2185.

SAS System

This statistical package is an integrated system of data access, management, analysis, and presentation, which is not limited to a particular computer system. The software is available for mainframes as well as PCs. Basic and advanced statistics are available, and the analysis can be integrated into a presentation for any type of reporting needs. Training and support are available. Further information regarding SAS can be obtained through the World Wide Web at http://www.sas.com/soft.

SYSTAT

This statistical package is a menu-driven data analysis tool that enables data to be analyzed in basic statistics (e.g., descriptive, *t* test, correlation) and more advanced statistics (e.g., ANOVA, multiple regression, and factor analysis). As with most packages, graphics are available. The package is available for DOS environments and Windows environments.

CHAPTER
8

Selecting a Test Instrument

For all such areas of research—and for many others—the precise measurement of individual differences made possible by well-constructed tests is an essential prerequisite.—A. Anastasi, (1988). *Psychological Testing* (p. 4).

• •

8.1 Key Concepts in Testing
8.2 Early History of Test Development
8.3 Outline of Overall Evaluative Process of Testing
8.4 Characteristics of a Good Test in Clinical Research
8.5 Assumptions in Clinical Evaluation
8.6 Major Purposes of Testing in Clinical Research
8.7 Conceptual Model for Selecting a Test Instrument for Clinical Research
8.8 Bibliographic Sources
8.9 Test Instruments
    8.9.1 Individual Intelligence Tests
    8.9.2 Achievement Tests
    8.9.3 Group Intelligence and Achievement Tests
    8.9.4 Tests for Special Populations
    8.9.5 Child Development
    8.9.6 Visual and Auditory Processing, Motor, and Language Tests
    8.9.7 Behavioral Checklists
    8.9.8 Prevocational Tests
    8.9.9 Vocational Interest Tests
    8.9.10 Outcome Measures and Functional Assessment
    8.9.11 Functional Evaluation of Physical Capacity, Work Aptitude, and Independent Living
    8.9.12 Objective Personality Tests
    8.9.13 Neuropsychological Batteries
8.10 Reviewing and Evaluating Tests
8.11 Criterion-Referenced Tests and Normative-Referenced Tests
8.12 Test Publishers
8.13 Ethical Considerations in Testing

Operational Learning Objectives

By the end of this chapter, the reader should be able to

1. define key concepts in testing
2. discuss the early history in the development of testing
3. identify the major purposes of testing
4. know where to look for bibliographies of tests in books and in test catalogues

315

5. know how to select a test for a specific function and target population
6. know how to evaluate reliability and validity of tests
7. know how to incorporate test into a research proposal
8. determine the skills necessary in:
    a. administering tests
    b. scoring tests
    c. interpreting results of tests
9. develop an objective attitude in selecting a test instrument and evaluating its effectiveness
10. identify the potential sources of error in testing

8.1 Key Concepts in Testing

In order to understand testing and evaluation, one should be able to define the key concepts. How is a test defined? How does the evaluator determine what is normal behavior and what is atypical behavior? Why are tests used? What are potential sources of error in testing? What is the difference between norm-referenced and criterion-referenced tests? These key concepts, listed in Table 8–1, are elaborated upon within this chapter.

8.2 Early History of Test Development

Tests have been used for generations to make employment and educational decisions. For example, in the twelfth century, the Chinese used civil service examinations to make hiring decisions. The ancient Greeks administered physical and intellectual tests as part of the educational process. In Europe, from the time of the Middle Ages, universities gave tests as part of the process of awarding professional degrees and bestowing hon-

Table 8–1   *Key Concepts in Tests and Measurements*

- A *test* is essentially an objective and standardized measure of a sample of behavior (Anastasi, 1988).
- A *measurement scale* is a system of assigning scores to a trait or characteristic.
- A *major purpose* of a test is to predict future performance based on a current sample of behaviors.
- An *extremely important quality* of a test is to accurately detect change in an individual's behavior.
- The *value* of a test depends on its purposes, ability to predict outcome, and the degree of consistency and precision in defining a variable.
- The *degree of accuracy* of a test is based on its ability to be consistent (reliability) and to test what it claims to measure (validity).
- The *sources of error in measurement* are derived, for example, from the unreliability of the instrument, bias of the test administrator, unreliability of the client, and undesirable test environment.
- *Distributions of data* from heterogeneous populations tend to be normally distributed while data from homogeneous populations tend to be skewed.
- A *norm-referenced test* is a standardized sampling of behavior that uses data from a heterogeneous group of individuals in interpreting results.
- A *criterion-referenced test* is a standardized sampling of behavior that bases performance on accepted standards of competency.

ors. In the United States, procedures for testing applicants to the United States Civil Service were introduced in 1883. However, not until the nineteenth century, when an interest in providing humane treatment to individuals with mental retardation and mental illness arose, were tests developed that could identify and distinguish between mental retardation and emotional disturbance (Anastasi, 1988; Sattler, 1988). (See Table 8–2 for a summary of major events in test development.)

Traditionally, test theorists have taken the viewpoint that the majority of a population will perform equally on many functions and that there is a normally distributed continuum of abilities. Thus, researchers involved in early test development sought to demonstrate what was normal in an effort to identify those individuals who differed significantly from the normal population. Sir Francis Galton (1822–1911), advocating the importance of individual differences, postulated that differences in physical characteristics such as vision, hearing, reaction time, and physical strength could be used to determine mental capabilities. He tried to validate his beliefs through the use of statistical methods developed by Karl Pearson (1957–1936). Although he was unsuccessful in showing that mental abilities were related to physical characteristics, our use of a normative sample is a direct result of his hypothesis (Swanson & Watson, 1989). James McKeen Cattell (1860–1944), an assistant to Galton, supported Galton's views that "mental

Table 8–2   *History of the Test Movement*

Theorist	Occupation	Contribution to Testing
Esquirol	Physician	Classified individuals with mental retardation into various levels of retardation; believed that language provided the best measure of intelligence.
Sir Francis Galton	Biologist	Theorized that physical traits (visual and hearing acuity, muscular strength) and reaction speed could serve as a measure of gauging intellectual abilities.
Paul Broca	Surgeon	Proposed a relationship between the volume of the brain and intelligence.
James McKeen Cattell	Psychologist	Developed norms in sensory, motor, and simple perceptual processes for comparing individuals, helping to create the concept of mental measurement.
Emil Kraepelin	Psychiatrist	Developed assessment of daily living skills based on perception, memory, attention, and motor functioning. Interested in the clinical examinations of psychiatric patients: tests of critical functions were designed to measure practice effects in memory and susceptibility to fatigue and to distraction.
Alfred Binet	Psychologist	Along with Simon, developed a test that identified children who could not benefit from formal education. This instrument consisted of short tests measuring perception, judgment, comprehension, and reasoning.
H. H. Goddard	Educator	Introduced Binet's scale in America, adding categories of intellectual ability and identifying "morons" and "idiots."
Lewis M. Terman	Psychologist	Popularized and revised Binet's scale by including tasks to identify superior adult intelligence and by assigning age equivalents to items.
Robert M. Yerkes	Psychologist	Instrumental in developing the Army Alpha, a verbal test, and the Army Beta, a visual test, for group testing. He also espoused the idea of point-scales rather than age-scales.

(continued)

Table 8–2 *(continued)*

Theorist	Occupation	Contribution to Testing
Charles E. Spearman	Psychologist	Proposed that intelligence was composed of a primary factor (g) and specific factors (s).
Louis L. Thurstone	Psychologist	Proposed that intelligence was composed of several different factors, which he called primary mental abilities, all of which could be considered equally important.
David Wechsler	Psychologist	Developed the Wechsler-Bellevue, the precursor to the Wechsler Scales. This test had a verbal scale and a performance scale.
Raymond B. Cattell	Psychologist	Along with John Horn, proposed that intelligence was composed of fluid (nonverbal, novel, relatively culture-free) and crystallized reasoning (acquired skills strongly dependent upon culture).
J. P. Guilford	Psychologist	Attempted to link theory to test development by proposing a three-dimensional Structure of Intellect with 120 factors that led to a test that measured each factor.
Jagannath Das	Psychologist	Used an information-processing model to describe cognitive functioning. Information is obtained through two distinct methods: simultaneously and sequentially.
Howard Gardner	Psychologist	Proposed that there are several autonomous intellectual competencies or multiple intelligences, which are manifested differently in different individuals.

tests" measuring sensory and physical abilities differentiated individuals. Although he found no relationship between these abilities and school achievement, he contributed to the understanding of tests and measurement by demonstrating that mental ability could be examined empirically (Sattler, 1988).

Eduardo Séquin (1812–1880) also believed that individuals could be differentiated by sensory and motor-control abilities. While Galton had believed that the differences were inherent and unchangeable, Séquin believed that training in these areas could result in improvement in intellectual potential. Currently his materials, such as the form board (a task in which individuals place wooden or plastic shapes into puzzle frames) are used as a part of a test battery for young children (Swanson & Watson, 1989).

One of the first attempts to classify individuals with mental retardation was made by Jean Esquirol (1772–1840). He recognized that individuals with mental retardation had diverse abilities and concluded that language development was the most important characteristic for distinguishing between degrees of intellectual capacity. His appreciation for the importance of language in the development of intellectual capacity influenced the development of intelligence tests (Anastasi, 1988).

While researchers in the United States tried to measure intellectual development through performance on sensory and motor tasks, clinicians in Germany turned toward more complex and abstract tasks as a means of measuring aptitude. Emil Kraepelin (1855–1926), recognizing the importance of measuring skills needed for daily living, developed a battery that measured such skills as perception, memory, motor functioning, and attention. H. Ebbinghaus (1850–1909), requested by teachers in Germany to develop an aptitude test, produced a timed completion task consisting of reading passages from which words had been left out. This test was a forerunner of group intelligence tests. He also produced tests that assessed arithmetic and memory skills. Carl Wernicke (1849–1905), noted for his work on aphasia and brain localization, investigated individual differences in verbal conceptual thinking and generalization.

Influence of Binet on IQ Testing

In 1905, Alfred Binet, a French psychologist, and a colleague, Theodore Simon, were commissioned by the French government to develop a test that would identify those children who could not benefit from formal education. The content of Binet's test came from educational research and through a deductive analysis of the factors that underlie academic achievement. The Binet–Simon test was developed pragmatically, without a theory of intelligence to guide its contents. However, the influence of individuals such as Esquirol and Séquin was apparent in that Binet included items measuring sensory perception, motor control, and language. In addition, the Binet–Simon intelligence test

> had several unique characteristics: (1) questions were arranged in a hierarchy of difficulty, (2) levels were established for different ages (establishment of mental age), (3) a quantitative scoring system was applied, and (4) specific instructions for administration were built into the test. (Swanson & Watson, 1989, p. 9)

The initial test consisted of 30 items related to following simple directions, defining words, constructing sentences, and answering judgmental questions of a psychological nature.

Binet's test was translated into English by H. H. Goddard (1866–1957) in 1910 and Lewis Terman (1977–1956) in 1916 for use in the United States (Sattler, 1988; Swanson & Watson, 1989; Terman & Merrill, 1972). Whereas Binet had perceived his instrument as a way to identify those students who needed to be instructed through alternative methods, Goddard in the early nineteen century, linked intelligence test scores to occupation and social status (Gould, 1981). Terman extended Binet's test by adding additional items suitable for testing adults and by adding the concept of "mental quotient" to that of mental age. Terman's revision became known as the Stanford–Binet, so named because he was a professor at Stanford University in California.

Alternative Tests to the Binet

Binet's test and revisions by Terman were developed on the premise that one's ability to successfully complete a particular task was related to developmental level. Thus, in a heterogenous set of items arranged in a developmental sequence, age scores could be assigned based on the ability of a majority of children at a given age level to do a particular task. Mental ability was determined by obtaining a ratio between the obtained age score and one's chronological age. Tests that use this format to find mental abilities are said to have an age-scale.

Discontent with age scores lead individuals such as Robert M. Yerkes (1876–1956) and David Wechsler (1896–1981) to develop tests with a radically different scoring format. Rather than using age-score, similar items were put together and points were assigned to each item. Then the raw score, determined by the number of points received, was converted into standard scores and an overall score. Scales with this type of scoring are known as a point-scale. The IQ scores derived in this manner are called Deviation IQs. At this time, most tests developed for school-age children, adolescents, and adults use the point-scale, whereas developmental scales, developed for infants, toddlers, and preschoolers, use an age-scale.

Another concern regarding intelligence testing was the emphasis on verbal reasoning seen on the Stanford Binet. Tests such as the Leiter International Performance Scale (LIPS; Leiter, 1948), the Arthur adaptation of the Leiter International Performance Scale (Arthur, 1949), the Kohs Block Design Tests (Kohs, 1923), and the Culture-Fair Intelligence Scale (Cattell, 1950) were developed to counterbalance the highly verbal influence of the Stanford–Binet. The Wechsler–Bellevue, developed in 1939 by Wechsler, consisted of a verbal and a performance scale. This test, based on Wechsler's conception that intelligence was global, included tasks from various sources (e.g., Kohs Block Design Test; Army Alpha and Army Beta). Although the items have changed over time, many of the same types of items are included in the present-day Wechsler scales (Sattler, 1988).

Factor Analytical Theories of Intelligence

With the development of computers and more advanced statistical methods (e.g., factor analysis), the concept of intelligence has changed drastically. While both Binet and Wechsler believed that intelligence was composed of many different abilities, neither one had proposed a theory that identified the components of intelligence. Binet had used items that he believed would assess skills necessary to succeed in an academic setting. Wechsler, on the other hand, had borrowed from a number of available tests, all of which he believed were factors in the construct of intelligence (Sattler, 1988). It fell to theorists like Charles E. Spearman (1863–1936), Edward L. Thorndike (1874–1949), and Louis L. Thurstone (1887–1955) to suggest the components contained in the construct of intelligence. In general, there were three viewpoints regarding the structure of intelligence:

1. Intelligence was composed of a primary factor called *g* made up of complex mental tasks such as reasoning and problem-solving, and specific factors called *s* which required less complex processes such as speed of processing, visual–motor, and rote learning (Spearman, 1927).
2. Intelligence was multifactorial and similar abilities clustered to form more complex skills (Thorndike, 1927).
3. Intelligence comprised primary factors (e.g., verbal, perceptual speed, inductive reasoning, work fluency, and space or visualization) rather than a single unitary factor (Thurstone, 1938).

More recently, others (e.g., Guilford, Sternberg, Gardner) have proposed alternative theories to account for the nature of intelligence. J. P. Guilford (1897–1987), in an effort to link theory to intelligence tests, proposed in *The Nature of Human Intelligence* (1967) that human intellect could be understood by a three-dimensional model, which he called the Structure of Intellect. This structure contained (a) 5 operations, which defined the way we process information (e.g., divergent or convergent); (b) 4 contents, which defined the manner in which the material is presented (e.g., visual or verbal), and (c) 6 products, which defined the outcome of the mental process (e.g., units or classes). By using combinations of one attribute from each dimension, 120 factors of intelligence can be identified (5 operations × 4 contents × 6 products). Theoretically, if one were to assess a student in each of these 120 factors, one would have a better understanding of how the student learns and could provide an appropriate educational program for that student. Unfortunately, Guilford's model has not been widely accepted, nor has it been used in many research studies.

Raymond B. Cattell and John L. Horn (Cattell, 1963; Horn, 1968) agreed with Guilford that intelligence was not a unitary concept, but disagreed in the specific components comprising intelligence. They suggested, instead, that intelligence is made up of two constructs, fluid and crystallized. Tasks considered to be fluid intelligence include unlearned, culture-free, novel experiences in which adaptation or generalization of previously learned tasks is required (e.g., nonverbal analogies, block building, speed of processing, and problem-solving). Crystallized intelligence, on the other hand, is defined as acquired knowledge, such as what is learned in school or in cultural experiences. Examples of tasks measuring crystallized intelligence include vocabulary tests, verbal analogies, rote learning, and rule learning. Two tests that were developed using the concept of crystallized and fluid intelligence are the Stanford–Binet Intelligence Scale— Fourth Edition (SBIS:FE; Thorndike, Hagen, & Sattler, 1985) and the Kaufman Adolescent and Adult Intelligence Test (KAIT; Kaufman & Kaufman, 1993).

Alternative Theories of Intelligence

Although factor analysis theories of intelligence are still the most widely accepted, two additional approaches to intelligence should be mentioned. One approach, information processing, involves the understanding of the ways in which individuals take in and transform the information so that it can be used. While information processing is frequently linked with memory processes, the concept has been extended by individuals such as Das (Das, Kirby, & Jarman, 1975), and Campione and Brown (1978). Das conceptualized intelligence as having two processes: (a) simultaneous, in which information is processed in a spatial, gestalt manner, and (b) sequential, in which material is sequenced in temporal order. Campione and Brown theorized that intelligence consisted of structures that enabled learning (e.g., memory and efficiency) and an executive system that controlled and managed the components involved in problem-solving (e.g., knowledge, metacognition, and use of learning strategies). The latter theory has led special educators to emphasize the use of strategies in the learning process as a means of improving problem-solving and learning. Continued research is needed to identify ways to teach learning strategies so that learners can benefit from the process.

A second approach to intelligence other than factor analysis is that proposed by Howard Gardner. Gardner (1983), in *Frames of Mind: The Theory of Multiple Intelligences*, proposed that there are several autonomous competencies, each of which can be thought of as separate intelligences. Although he has only identified six of these separate intelligences (linguistic, musical, logical-mathematical, spatial, bodily-kinesthetic, and personal), he suggests that there may be others. Gardner's theory has taken hold in many educational circles, and curriculums have been developed to encourage development of each of these.

Group Aptitude and Achievement Tests

Although the early IQ tests were administered individually, the advent of the First World War resulted in a need for group aptitude (mental ability) testing. In 1917, Yerkes, an American psychologist and professor at Yale, was appointed by the American Psychological Association to develop group mental tests that could effectively evaluate military recruits. Working with Goddard and Terman, Yerkes developed the Army Alpha, a verbal test, and the Army Beta, a perceptual test, to be administered to recruits who failed the Army Alpha. Although the army made little use of these tests, the major result of these tests was the obtaining of normative data on 1.75 million men and the recognition that levels of "intelligence" could now be obtained through group testing. What transpired after that was the massive development and the multiplication of group testing for all groups in society. Students and job applicants were routinely administered tests to determine aptitude and achievement. Two factors led to this phenomenon of mass testing: (a) individuals could be tested simultaneously with less time and personnel needed to administer the tests; and (b) simplified instructions enabled individuals without professional training in testing to administer the tests. Thus many professionals working with groups (e.g., teachers, therapists, counselors, personnel directors) are able to administer group tests (Anastasi, 1988; Gould, 1981).

Although group testing developed because of the need to determine intellectual ability, issues regarding academic achievement soon became a concern of the nation. Group written examinations were first introduced in the Boston schools in 1845 as a substitute for individual oral examinations. The Stanford Achievement Test, developed in 1923, was the first achievement test to be standardized by using statistical principles of measurement. The practice of mass educational testing continues today at the national level, where students enrolled in public schools are administered a group achievement test during the spring semester. Entrance into postsecondary schools is partially based on the results of the American College Test (ACT) and the Scholastic Aptitude Test (SAT) tests. Entrance into a profession is routinely accompanied by a test (e.g., Graduate Record Exam [GRE], Graduate Management Admissions Test [GMAT], Law School Admissions Test [LSAT]), developed specifically to evaluate proficiency and knowledge of the profession.

8.3 Outline of Overall Evaluative Process of Testing

The steps in the overall evaluative process of testing are listed in Table 8–3 and are elaborated upon in the following section.

The first step in the process of testing is to determine what is to be measured and to operationally define the variable. The researcher must be precise and state clearly what is to be discovered. For example, a clinical researcher is interested in evaluating reading progress. Reading, however, consists of a number of different areas, such as the ability to read a list of words by sight, factual and inferential comprehension, and structural and phonetic analysis. Although it is possible to evaluate total growth in reading, an understanding of the reason for the progress necessitates an understanding of changes in each of the various components of reading.

Once the researcher has identified the function to be measured, he or she selects an instrument to measure that function. Often a published instrument is available. In a way, published instruments may be better because of the known psychometric properties. However, it may be that there is no instrument and the researcher has to develop one. This is frequently true when designing an interview or survey questionnaire. (See methodological research in Chapter 3.)

Table 8–3   *Steps in the Evaluation Process*

1. Identify the function to be measured.
2. Identify a published instrument to measure condition, or develop a new standardized procedure for evaluation of function.
3. Identify the skill level necessary to use a test instrument.
4. Identify the possible factors in the environment, tester, subject, or test instrument that can potentially distort the test results.
5. Identify the target population for which the test is intended and for which norms have been established.
6. Strictly follow the directions and procedures for administering and scoring the test, or modifying the test procedure to enable the client with disabilities to perform at a maximum level.
7. Interpret the results based on
   a. norm-referenced data based on the general population
   b. criterion-referenced data for client performance or competence

If the clinical researcher chooses to use a published instrument, then it will be necessary to determine what qualifications are needed to administer the test. Qualification levels are set by the APA Standards for Educational and Psychological Testing, and most test publishers adhere to this policy. Level A requires no special qualification, Level B requires at least a BA in psychology, counseling, or closely related field and relevant training, and Level C requires a graduate degree in psychological education or closely related field and training, *or* membership in a professional association that requires training and experience in the ethical and competent use of testing (e.g., APA, NASP), or license or certification from an agency that requires training in testing.

The fourth step in the process involves identifying the possible factors in the environment, tester, subject, or test instrument that can potentially distort the test results. These factors are outlined in Figure 8–1. The researcher will want to eliminate as many of these factors as possible.

Once the researcher has identified the variable to be measured, the tests to be used, and the potential error factors that need to be eliminated or reduced, the researcher needs to identify the target population for which the test is intended and for which norms have been established. Sometimes this will seem unclear. For example, a clinical researcher may want to examine the psychological effect and impact or behavior that a child with disabilities has on a parent. The target population may, at first, appear to be the parent. However, the question being asked is how the child with disabilities impacts upon the parent. Although a questionnaire will be given to the parents, items on the instrument will relate to the child with disabilities. Therefore, the target population is in reality the child.

Whether the clinical researcher is administering a standardized test or one which he or she developed, it is important to administer the instrument in the same way every time. An alteration in the test directions or administration will confound the results and make them unreliable. When the directions or procedures are altered or modified, this must be stated in the final report. Keep in mind that the alteration or modification of administering a test will make the norms invalid.

Test Instruments	Administration	Client	Environment
• low reliability • low validity • lack of normative data • cultural bias	• improper training • not following directions precisely • incorrect scoring • incorrect interpretation of data • lack of rapport • imprecise use of stop watch and test materials • developmentally inappropriate test	• lack of motivation • fatigue • language differences or deficits • motor disability • high anxiety • lack of concentration • poor sustained attention • acute psychotic symptoms • poor understanding of test directions	• noisy • poor lighting • interruptions • poor seating • too cold or too hot • poor air quality

Figure 8–1.   Potential sources of error in test administration. Errors come from four main areas: the instrument itself, the administration of the test, the client or subject, and the environment.

The final step is to interpret the results based on either the typical performance as determined by the norms from a general population or a standard that has been set prior to the administration of the test. For example, a researcher wants to see the effect of a particular reading program that emphasizes phonetic analysis. The researcher has a choice of measurements: (a) a standardized test that measures phonetic analysis and compares the results of the group with the expected performance based on the general population, or, (b) an inventory of phonetic elements before and after the study to determine changes.

8.4 Characteristics of a Good Test in Clinical Research

The accuracy and precision in evaluating a client's performance or improvement in a clinical research study depends upon the quality of the test instrument. What are the characteristics of a good test instrument? What are some essential questions in evaluating the purposes and "goodness" of a test?

- What is the population for whom the test is targeted (e.g., children with learning difficulties, individuals with schizophrenia, persons with muscular dystrophy)?
- What are the specific purposes of the test (e.g., planning treatment goals, determining prognosis, establishing baseline data, or documenting progress)?
- What are the areas of function identified in the test (e.g., social development, prevocational, personality, leisure interests, perceptual–motor abilities, ADL skills, academic achievement, cognitive level)?
- What are the methods used to evaluate a client? Primary sources for evaluating a client include:
  - *medical records:* demographics, previous treatment, and outcomes
  - *educational records:* educational attainment, achievement scores
  - *clinical observation of performance:* therapists and teacher observations
  - *interviews:* formal or unstructured individual interviews
  - *objective tests:* objectively scored paper and pencil tests, performance scales, and verbal tests
  - *survey questionnaires:* group tests, forced choice or open ended
  - *self-reports:* evaluation of treatment effectiveness through client's perspective
  - *reports from peers, teacher/therapist, or family:* informal reports or observations
  - *biomechanical or physiological measurement of human factors:* machine monitoring, test procedures
- Is there a standardized procedure or manual of instructions in administering the test and interpreting results? Are there tables of normative data?
- Are there special skills or certification that are necessary to administer, score, and interpret results of the test?
- Is the scale of measurement used in collecting data identifiable (i.e., continuous, such as interval or ratio; or discrete, such as nominal or ordinal)?
- Are error factors controlled that can potentially interfere with obtaining reliable test results?
- Are research data reported (such as those derived from previous studies, including reliability, validity, and normative scores?

8.5 Assumptions in Clinical Evaluation

What are some of the assumptions in clinical evaluation that guide a clinician in assessment? The major assumptions are outlined below.

- Evaluation is an essential factor in the treatment process. It is used to determine the client's abilities, interests, potentials, and work traits.
- Evaluation is used to establish baseline data so as to compare with outcome results.
- Evaluation is based on reliable and valid instrumentation. The degree of accuracy in measurement depends on the degree of reliability (consistency) and validity (accuracy).
- Error is always present to a degree in evaluation, owing to anomalies in the examiner's presentation of test materials, degree of anxiety of fatigue, client's motivation, less than perfect reliability of test, and a less than ideal testing environment. Test scores obtained are a sample of the client's performance and represent an approximation of abilities within a given time frame.
- The reliability of the test score is increased by eliminating potential error factors that could danger or distort the test results.
- Evaluation can provide data for documentation and the basis for establishing clinical efficacy and quality assurance. Evaluation is an excellent method for objectively determining client progress.

8.6 Major Purposes of Testing in Clinical Research

The major purposes of testing are as follows:

- Establish baseline data (experimental research—pretest)
- Evaluate outcome or effectiveness of treatment procedure (experimental research—posttest)
- Assess the degree of relationship between two variables (correlational research)
- Evaluate quality of health care or education progress for accreditation (evaluative research)
- Assess developmental landmarks (developmental research)
- Assess individual values, interests, or attitudes (survey research)
- Evaluate differences between groups (correlational, experimental research)
- Evaluate functional assessment (screening target population)

8.7 Conceptual Model for Selecting a Test Instrument for Clinical Research

The decision to select a test from a published source or to construct a new test in order to measure a defined variable is a frequent dilemma. The measuring instrument is an essential part of a research study and represents the operational definition of a variable. Figure 8–2 shows this process.

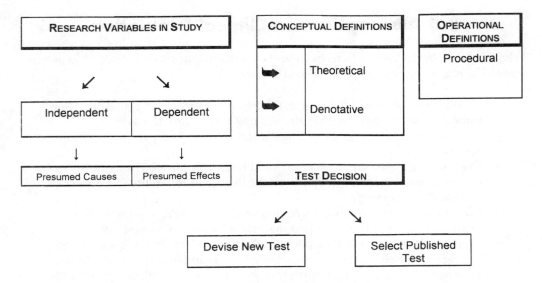

Figure 8–2. Critical steps in determining the test instrument to use.

The conceptual definition of a variable should lead the investigator to a specific test that is the most appropriate one in operationally defining a variable. In clinical research it is crucial that the investigator select a measuring instrument that has a high reliability and is a valid measurement of outcome. Measuring improvement in such areas as personality, physical capacity, cognitive functions, independent living skills, vocational skills, and perceptual-motor abilities depend directly on the adequacy and sensitivity of the instrument to measure changes. A crude measuring device that does not have the capacity to record subtle changes in an individual's functioning or behavior is either of limited or of no value to the researcher.

When deciding on the instrument to use for the outcome measure, the researcher must ask the following questions:

- What is the target population?
  Examples include:
  - normal children, adolescents, adults, elderly
  - intellectual deficit
  - psychiatric diagnosis
  - physically challenged (specify diagnosis)
  - social, economic variables
  - demographic variables
- What are the specific areas of function to be measured?
  Examples of these areas include:
  - manual dexterity
  - intellectual aptitude
  - vocational interests
  - academic achievement
  - personality
  - job readiness
  - attitudes toward work

- work experiences
- work tolerance
- social skills
- self-care
- communication
- mobility and transportation
- Where will the client be assessed?
Some places for assessment include:
  - home
  - sheltered workshop
  - clinical environment
  - school
  - office
  - hospital
- What are the methods for evaluating function?
Some methods include:

  - observation of performance
  - paper and pencil test
  - interview
  - self-report
  - direct measure of function through standardized test instrument
  - evaluation by teacher, therapist, or parent
  - work samples
- Is the test reliable and valid?

  - Are there standardized directions for administration?
  - Are norm scores available for comparison purposes?
  - How many subjects were used in collecting norm values?
  - How was reliability of the test established (e.g., test–retest, split half, equivalent forms)?
  - How was the validity of the test established (e.g., concurrent, construct, predictive)?
- Are the test results easily interpreted?
- What is the scale of measurement (i.e., ordinal, nominal, interval, or ratio)?

8.8 Bibliographic Sources

Another consideration for testing involves asking the question, Where can I find the most appropriate test instrument? Examples of and names of tests instruments can be found in a number of sources, including:

- Books on psychological testing, such as the following:
Anastasi, A. (1988). *Psychological Testing* (6th ed.). New York: Macmillian.

  Power, P. (1991). *A Guide to Vocational Assessment* (2nd ed.). Austin, TX: PRO–ED.

  Sattler, J. M. (1988). *Assessment of Children* (3rd ed.). San Diego: Sattler Publishing.

  Lezak, M. (1984). *Neuropsychological Assessment* (2nd ed.). New York: Oxford University Press.

Hemphill, B. J. (Ed.). (1988). *Mental Health Assessment in Occupational Therapy: An Integrative Approach to the Evaluative Process*. Thorofare, NJ: Slack.

Cronbach, L. J. (1984). *Essentials of Psychological Testing* (4th ed.). New York: Harper and Row.

Mental Measurements Yearbook, Mental Measurements Supplement, or Tests in Print, published by The University of Nebraska Press. In 1989 the MMY began an alternate-year publication schedule with the *Supplement to the Mental Measurements Yearbook* or *MMY-S*.

Cole, B., Finch, E., Gowland, C., & Mayo, N. (1994). *Physical Rehabilitation Outcome Measures*. Toronto, ON: Canadian Physiotherapy Association.
This text includes 60 outcome measures that are currently used by physiotherapists in Canada. Each test is described and reliability and validity data are presented. The tests are organized into four categories: adult motor and vocational activity measures, back and/or pain measures, cardiopulmonary measures, and developmental measures.

- Catalogs of tests, such as the following (a more complete list is found in section 8. 12): Psychological Corporation, PRO–ED, and Western Psychological Services (WPS)
- Vocational rehabilitation centers
- Specialists in work assessment

8.9 Test Instruments

Testing materials and instruments can be found for almost every functional area that one might want to assess. Table 8–4 lists some categories of tests. The following paragraphs and sections describe a few tests in each of the functional areas. We have tried to select tests that are commonly used or are important for specific reasons (e.g., they have normative data for populations of individuals with special needs; they are used more frequently by allied therapists, school psychologists, or teachers; they have high validity or reliability). We recognize that not all tests are listed. For a more complete list, the reader should refer to one of the books on assessment and testing listed in above or to a publisher's catalog (listed at the end of the chapter in Section 8.12). As a caution, however, tests are developed or revised yearly, and even the most up-to-date book may not have a description of the test. In case of doubt, it is wise to contact the publisher directly.

8.9.1 Individual Intelligence Tests

Because special training is required for administering and interpreting individual intelligence tests, it is possible that the clinical researcher will not be administering these tests. Group tests of intelligence, however, such as the Slosson Intelligence Test—Revised (SIT–R; Nicholson & Hibpshman, 1990), Lorge–Thorndike (Lorge & Thorndike, 1966), and the Otis–Lennon Tests of Mental Ability (OLSAT; Otis & Lennon, 1989), are routinely used in public schools and require no special skills in administering and scoring. Regardless of whether the clinical researcher administers the test or obtains the IQ score from available records, the score is useful when doing clinical research. For example, the IQ score may be used to screen candidates for a research project in order to insure that all subjects have average intelligence. Frequently the IQ score is used as a covariate, as its use in this procedure may result in equalization of subjects. For this reason, a review of the most widely used tests of intelligence is appropriate for a book on research. In cau-

Table 8–4   *Categories of Testing*

Achievement Tests (Individual and Group)
Adjustment to Disability Questionnaires
Behavioral Checklists
Child Development Tests
Functional Assessment
Health Questionnaires
Intelligence Scales (Individual and Group)
Language Tests
Motor Instruments
Neuropsychological Testing
Outcome Measures
Perceptual Process Instruments
Personality Tests (Objective and Projective)
Physical Capacity Tests
Prevocational Tests
Vocational Tests
Vocational Rehabilitation Evaluation Systems and Vocational Capacity Assessments

tion, the investigator should be aware of the fact that intelligence tests yield global scores of intelligence and may be strongly affected by academic learning and social class.

Some of the more frequently used individually administered tests of intelligence are summarized in Table 8–5. A few of these tests are described below. Group IQ tests, often used within the school setting, are described later in this chapter in section 8.9.3.

Kaufman Assessment Battery for Children (K-ABC; Kaufman & Kaufman, 1983a, 1983b) is an individually administered test of intelligence and achievement for ages 2 years 6 months to 12 years 6 months based on Das' (Das, Kirby, & Jarman, 1975 Das & Molloy, 1975;) theory of sequential and simultaneous processing. An achievement battery is separate from the tests of intelligence. The sequential tasks include memory for words, numbers, and hand movements, and the simultaneous tasks include visual closure, memory for faces, nonverbal analogies, and block designs. A nonverbal score, especially useful for children with language delays or differences, can be computed. The standardization sample included representative proportions of Caucasians, Blacks, Hispanics, Native Americans, Asians, and children with exceptional needs. Separate percentile ranks are available for different socioeconomic levels.

Slosson Intelligence Test—Revised (SIT–R; Nicholson & Hibpshman, 1990). This individually administered screening test of crystallized verbal intelligence provides information regarding the need for further in-depth evaluation. Items cover areas in general information, social judgement, arithmetic, similarities and differences, vocabulary, and auditory memory. The test is easy to administer and score and is designed for use by anyone who has completed an introductory course in tests and measurements (e.g., therapists, teachers, counselors). Although reliability and validity are reported to be high, Salvia and Yssledyke (1995) report that "the norm sample for this test is inadequately described [and e]vidence for reliability and validity are inadequate" (p. 355). Caution is suggested in using this test for more than a quick screening instrument.

Stanford-Binet Intelligence Scale—Fourth Edition (SBIS:FE; Thorndike, Hagen & Sattler, 1985) is an individually administered intelligence test based on the theory of fluid/crystallized intelligence (Cattell, 1963; Horn, 1968). Fifteen subtests contain items of vocabulary, verbal reasoning, numerical reasoning, copying of designs using blocks and paper/pencil, numerical reasoning, and memory for visual and verbal material. All sub-

Table 8-5 *Frequently Used Intelligence Tests*

Test	Target Population	Publisher	Scores Obtained	Strengths	Weaknesses
Kaufman Adolescent and Adult Intelligence Test (KAIT; Kaufman & Kaufman, 1993)	age 11 years 0 months through age 85	Riverside	general intelligence based on a crystallized/fluid reasoning theory	• de-emphases speed and fine-motor coordination • an expanded battery includes tests of delayed memory • well-written manual with emphasis on interpretation	• high cultural bias on some subtests • standardization sample limited in western states
Kaufman Assessment Battery for Children (K-ABC; Kaufman & Kaufman, 1983)	2 years 6 months to 12 years 6 months	Riverside	sequential, simultaneous, and mental processing; academic achievement	• high reliability scores, especially for achievement scale • separate academic achievement scales • based on theory of neurological functioning • nonverbal scale available • separate percentiles for SES categories	• inconsistent concurrent and construct validity across ages, although they generally fit theoretical constructs • limited number of subtests within the sequential scale
Slosson Intelligence Test—Revised (SIT–R; Nicholson & Hibpshman, 1990)	norms available for ages 4 to 18	Slosson	crystallized verbal intelligence	• easily administered screening instrument to determine need for further testing • can be used by anyone with a beginning course in testing	• no age range identified by authors • adaptations suggested, but no data on effects of adaptations • reliability and validity data is poorly reported
Stanford–Binet Intelligence Scale—Fourth Edition (SBIS:FE; Thorndike, Hagen, & Sattler, 1985)	age 2 years 0 months through adult	Riverside	general intelligence (*g*) and specific intelligence (*s*)	• adequate validity • measures short-term memory separately	• lengthy administration time for older individuals

Test	Age Range	Publisher	What It Measures	Strengths	Cautions
Stanford–Binet Intelligence Scale—Form LM (SBIS–LM; Terman & Merrill, 1973)	age 2 years 0 months through adult	Riverside (discontinued with completion of SBIS:FE)	general intelligence (g), mental age	• many developmental items at lower level, so useful for children under 5 years	• lengthy administration time for older individuals • gives mental age and total score, without examining skills • highly verbal
Wechsler Adult Intelligence Scale—Revised (WAIS–R; Wechsler, 1981; new revision due in 1996)	age 16 years 0 months through adult	Psych. Corp.	verbal and nonverbal intelligence, with specific skills identified in subtests	• high test-retest reliability • high concurrent validity • verbal or performance scores can be used separately for populations with disabilities	• verbal scale highly correlated with academic achievement
Wechsler Intelligence Scale for Children—Third Edition (WISC–III; Wechsler, 1991)	age 6 years 0 months through 16 years 11 months	Psych. Corp.	verbal and nonverbal intelligence; supplemental indexes measure processing speed and attention	• high test-retest and split-half reliability • high concurrent and construct validity • separate scales can be used independently for populations with disabilities • index scales provide further analysis of abilities	• verbal scale highly dependent upon school experiences
Wechsler Preschool and Primary Intelligence Scale—Revised (WPPSI–R; Wechsler, 1989)	age 3 years 0 months to 7 years 3 months	Psych. Corp.	verbal and nonverbal intelligence	• high internal consistency	• lengthy administration time for younger children

jects are administered the first six subtests. The selection of additional subtests administered are based on the age of the subject individual and the score obtained on the vocabulary subtest. The fifteen subtests yield scores on four scales (*Verbal Reasoning, Visual/Abstract Reasoning, Quantitative, Short-Term Memory*), as well as a Composite or total score. Qualitative scoring allows for comparisons of strengths and weaknesses. Computer scoring is available.

The Wechsler Scales are individually administered intelligence tests that yield verbal and nonverbal IQ scores. Items on the verbal portion include vocabulary, verbal reasoning, short-term auditory memory, practical judgment, and knowledge of general information. The nonverbal scale consists of timed performance items, including block design, puzzle building, visual memory, and a pencil/paper coding task. Each scale has an alternate or optional subtest. Three different editions cover the age span from 3 years through adult. Use of either the Verbal or Performance scale can obtain an estimate of cognitive functioning when used with populations of individuals with special needs.

Wechsler Adult Intelligence Scale—Revised (WAIS–R; Wechsler, 1981), designed for individuals age 16 and above, has all of the features of the Wechsler tests described above. The Verbal scales alone can be used with people with visual or motor handicaps; nonverbal scales can be used with those with language difficulties. Additional norms are available for the elderly. Use of supplemental materials incorporates the WAIS-R into a neuropsychological tool (WAIS-R-NI; Kaplan, Fein, Morris, & Delis, 1991). Computer scoring is available. The test is being newly standardized and is due to be published in 1996.

Wechsler Intelligence Scale for Children—Third Edition (WISC–III; Wechsler, 1991) is designed for children ages 6 year 0 months to 16 years 11 months. It has all of the features described above as well as some additional features. There are ten core subtests and three supplemental subtests (verbal digit span, mazes subtest, and visual processing speed). Factor analysis using all 13 subtests yields 4 indexes: Verbal Comprehension, Perceptual Organization, Processing Speed, and Freedom from Distractibility. Additional studies have been made with various clinical groups (i.e., gifted, mental retardation, learning disabilities, attention deficit-hyperactivity disorder [ADHD], conduct disorders, epilepsy, speech–language delays, and hearing impairments), and suggestions and cautions are mentioned in the manual.

Wechsler Preschool and Primary Scale of Intelligence—Revised (WPPSI–R; Wechsler, 1989) is individually administered and designed for children ages 3 years 0 months to 7 years 3 months. The revised edition contains full-color artwork for subtests of general information, numerical reasoning, and similarities. In addition to a measure of visual–motor integration, there is also a measure of visual recognition and discrimination, allowing the examiner to identify weaknesses. A sample of 1700 children were used in standardizing the test. Age, race, gender, geographic region, parents' education, and parents' occupation were stratified.

8.9.2 Achievement Tests

Achievement tests are designed to measure one's achievement within the school setting. There are two kinds of achievement tests: (a) general achievement tests, which survey the domains of reading, writing, and mathematics; and (b) specific achievement tests, which evaluate more fully each of the skills area (e.g., reading decoding and reading comprehension or math computation and math problem solving). Achievement tests differ in format (multiple choice versus short answer) rather than in the types of scores that can be obtained. Most achievement tests yield grade and age equivalents, standard scores, and percentiles. Some achievement tests also yield normal curve equivalents

(NCEs; required for Title I services), and stanines. Since the passage of PL 94-142 and now the Individuals with Disabilities Educational Act (IDEA) , virtually all newly published achievement tests are based on a mean of 100 and standard deviation of 15, as are most intelligence tests. Thus, evaluators can determine if there is a discrepancy between intellectual aptitude (IQ) and achievement. Frequently used achievement tests are summarized in Table 8–6, and the most frequently used tests are described below.

Kaufman Test of Educational Achievement (K-TEA; Kaufman & Kaufman, 1985) is an individually administered achievement test for grades 1–12. The test consists of a brief form (which takes 20–30 minutes) and a comprehensive form. Responses are made by recall and short- answer format. Norm-referenced scores are available for reading (decoding and comprehension), mathematics (computation and application), and spelling. An error analysis form, available on the comprehensive form, enables the examiner to further analyze performance based on the expected performance for the grade level (e.g., criterion-referenced). Grade norms and normal curve equivalents (NCEs) are available for spring and fall performance. A computer program is available for quick scoring and analysis.

Peabody Individual Achievement Test—Revised (PIAT–R; Markwardt, 1989) is a norm-referenced, individually administered achievement test using a multiple-answer format for reading comprehension, spelling, and mathematics; and short-answer responses for reading recognition and general information. The written expression subtest has two levels: a prewriting task, and a writing task requiring the student to write a short story. The multiple-choice format is helpful for students with language or motor difficulties. Computer program makes scoring easy.

Wechsler Individual Achievement Test (WIAT; Psychological Corporation, 1992) is a newly developed, norm-referenced, individually administered global achievement test. The test is composed of eight subtests: (a) seven subtests measuring the various aspects of learning disability as defined by PL 94-142 (basic reading skill, reading comprehension, mathematics reasoning, mathematics calculation, listening comprehension, oral expression, and written expression), and (b) spelling. The test can be used as a screening test by administering the basic reading skill, mathematics reasoning, and spelling subtests.

Wide Range Achievement Test—3 (WRAT–3; Wilkinson, 1993) is a norm-referenced global achievement test measuring decoding, spelling, and mathematics computation. Two equivalent forms allow for pre- and posttesting. Normative data are available by age. Reading must be individually administered; spelling and mathematics can be administered in a group.

Woodcock–Johnson—Revised, Tests of Achievement (WJ–R; Woodcock & Johnson, 1989) is a norm-referenced test of achievement. The test is divided into two batteries: a standard form that evaluates reading, mathematics, and written language, and a supplemental form that evaluates skill development in word attack, handwriting, proofing, and writing speed. When used with a companion battery, Woodcock–Johnson—Revised, Tests of Cognition (Woodcock & Johnson, 1989), academic–aptitude discrepancies can be identified. Computer scoring is available.

KeyMath—Revised: A Diagnostic Inventory of Essential Mathematics (KeyMath-R; Connolly, 1988) is an individually administered mathematics test that examines basic skills, whole and rational number operations, and applications of concepts. The mathematics standards developed by the National Council of Teachers of Mathematics are reflected in this test, making it easy to identify those areas in which a student is deficient. Two parallel forms allow for pre- and posttesting. Reliability and validity are adequate for the total score, but not for individual subtests or domains. A computer program makes scoring easy.

Woodcock Reading Mastery Test—Revised (WRMT–R; Woodcock, 1987) is a norm-referenced individually administered reading test that measures six areas of reading:

Table 8-6 *Frequently Used Individually Administered Tests of Achievement*

Test	Target Population	Publisher	Scores Obtained	Strengths	Weaknesses
Kaufman Test of Educational Achievement (K-TEA; Kaufman & Kaufman, 1985)	grades 1 through 12	AGS	math, reading, spelling and composite score	• provides qualitative assessment based on expected achievement • brief and comprehensive forms • objective scoring • psychometrically sound, with high reliability and validity	• content for brief form is poorly defined and varies across grades • no test of written or oral language is included
KeyMath—Revised: A Diagnostic Inventory of Essential Mathematics (KeyMath–R; Connolly, 1988)	grades K through 9	AGS	specific math skills, including basic concepts, applications, operations, and total test	• equivalent test forms • behavioral objectives linked to Items • table of specifications developed to guide content	• no reliability data for domains • no evidence of construct validity
Peabody Individual Achievement Test —Revised (PIAT-R; Markwardt, 1989)	grades K through 12	AGS	academic achievement in reading, mathematics, written language, and general information	• multiple-choice format for some subtests is helpful for students with language or motor difficulties • reliability and validity appear adequate	• multiple-choice format allows for guessing • norms do not represent national census data for some grade levels
Wechsler Individual Achievement Test (WAIT; Psych. Corp., 1992)	grade K through 12	Psych. Corp.	general and specific academic skills specifically comprising the areas defined by PL 94-142 for learning disabilities	• excellent psychometric properties • only achievement test to include listening comprehension and oral expression • co-normed with the WISC-III	• may be lengthy in time if all subtests are administered • provides fall and spring norms for grade and age rather than continuous norms

Test	Publisher	Ages	Description	Strengths	Weaknesses
Wide Range Achievement Test—3 (WRAT-3; Wilkinson, 1993)	Jastek	age 5 to 75	general measure of reading, mathematics, and spelling	• adequate reliability and construct validity • screening test that is easily administered and scored • spelling and mathematics subtests can be administered in small groups	• questionable content validity (measures only decoding and computation) • incomplete standardization data
Woodcock Johnson—Revised, Tests of Achievement (WJ-R; Woodcock & Johnson, 1989)	Riverside	ages 2 through 90, grades K through 16.9	comprehensive measures of reading, mathematics, written language, and general information	• two equivalent forms for test-retest • adequate psychometric properties • preschool and postsecondary norm	• "spelling" subtest includes capitalization, punctuation, grammar, and spelling • scoring is difficult without the computer program • scoring of written expression subtest can be cumbersome and subjective
Woodcock Reading Mastery Tests—Revised (WRMT-R; Woodcock, 1987)	AGS	Ages 5 to 75	specific reading skills, including readiness, decoding, sight word, and comprehension	• provides continuous year norms for grade and age • high reliability and validity • two equivalent forms for test-retest	• passage comprehension tested by "fill in the blank," requiring adequate language abilities • scoring is difficult without the computer program

readiness, letter recognition, decoding (sight words and phonetic analysis), and comprehension (word and passage comprehension). Subtests cluster to obtain a total score and scores in readiness, basic reading, and comprehension. The test is used frequently in clinical research as an outcome measure of academic achievement. Computer scoring is available.

8.9.3 Group Intelligence and Achievement Tests

Group intelligence and group achievement tests differ from individualized tests in their format and in the way that they are administered (Salvia & Ysseldyke, 1995). Group tests are generally paper/pencil tests which may be given in one or more sessions. The emphasis in group tests may be on speed (e.g., timed tests) or on accomplishment (e.g., power tests). Group tests are generally scored by machine and usually provide such scores as percentile, NCEs, grade and/or age equivalents, aptitude scores, and achievement levels. In many cases group intelligence tests are used to screen individuals to determine the need for further diagnostic testing in order to determine eligibility or need for special services (Salvia & Ysseldyke, 1995). Some of the more common group tests are discussed below and summarized in Table 8–7.

Iowa Tests of Basic Skills (ITBS; Hoover, Hieronymus, Frisbie, & Dunbar, 1993) are comprehensive, norm-referenced group tests, designed for use in grades K through 9. These tests measure skills in vocabulary, reading, mathematics, writing, listening, science, and social studies. Schools using the tests can have results reported by (a) type of school (public, Catholic, or other private schools); (b) SES level (high or low), and (c) demographic information (local, national, large city, or international). Hand or computerized scoring is available.

Otis–Lennon School Ability Test, Sixth Edition, Form I, (OLSAT; Otis & Lennon, 1989). This is a group-administered test designed to be an objective measure of ability that enables teachers to make appropriate instructional planning. Tasks include pictorial, verbal, figural, and qualitative measures of reasoning, memory, recall, application, and generalization. It can be used in conjunction with a standardized achievement test (i.e., Stanford Achievement Test) for determining academic–aptitude discrepancies. The verbal scores are better predictors of reading ability, and the nonverbal scores are better predictors of math ability. Two forms for pre- and posttesting are available. The test can be machine scored.

Raven's Progressive Matrices Test (RPM; Raven, 1963, 1992, 1993; Raven, Court, & Raven, 1977) include a three-level series of nonverbal tests designed to measure eductive ability for all age levels between 5 and adult. Eductive ability measures one's ability to develop insights, to generalize a concrete relationships, and to make sense of a complex situation. The raw score is converted into a percentile score, which can then be converted into standard scores. Separative normative data is available for various nationalities and ethnic groups (e.g., British, American, Native-American). When used with the *Mill Hill Vocabulary Scales* (also published by Psychological Corporation), an estimate of verbal and nonverbal cognition is obtained.

Stanford Achievement Test Series (Psychological Corporation, 1990, 1992) are a group of three measures which together assess students from kindergarten through community college. Each measure in the series includes a basic battery, which assesses general achievement in reading and mathematics, or a complete battery, which assesses reading, mathematics, science, and social studies. Standardization for these tests were completed concurrent with standardization for the OLSAT. As a result, comparison tables for ability and achievement are available.

Table 8-7 *Frequently Used Group Intelligence and Group Achievement Tests*

Test	Target Population	Publisher	Scores Obtained	Strengths	Weaknesses
Iowa Tests of Basic Skills (ITBS; Hoover, Hieronymus, Frisbie, & Dunbar, 1993)	grades K through 9	Riverside	broad general achievement	• development and standardization are excellent • scores can be personalized to meet school needs	• reliability depends upon the grade level • standard scores computed based on a median score
Otis-Lennon School Abilities Test, Sixth Edition (OLSAT; Otis & Lennon, 1989)	grades K through 12	Psych. Corp.	general verbal and nonverbal intelligence	• moderate to high reliability • spring or fall norms • when used with the SAT, academic-achievement discrepancies can be obtained	• although demographics were considered in the standardization, stratification was not used • limited validity data
Raven's Progressive Matrices (RPM; Raven, 1963, 1992, 1993; Raven, Court, & Raven, 1977	3 levels to cover ages 5 through adult	Psych. Corp.	nonverbal general intelligence	• highly cultural free • provides norms for nationalities and ethnic groups • untimed	• total score consisting of a percentile which can be translated into a standard score
Stanford Achievement Tests (Psychological Corporation, 1990, 1992)	3 levels which cover K through community college	Psych. Corp.	broad academic achievement, including science and social studies	• when administered with the OLSAT, provides academic-achievement discrepancy • special editions for visually impaired and deaf • norm-referenced and criterion-referenced	• timed test • validity depends on the similarity of curriculum with the content of the test • may not be appropriate for students with special needs

The oldest measure, the SAT, is intended for use with first grade through ninth grade. Two special editions of the SAT are available: (a) one in either braille or large print for students who have visual impairments, and (b) a visual test for students who are deaf. Norms for these editions were obtained using the respective populations.

8.9.4 Tests for Special Populations

A limited number of standardized tests have been developed to use with populations with special needs. For example, the Leiter International Performance Scale (LIPS; Leiter, 1948) and the Arthur Adaptation of the LIPS (Arthur, 1949) were originally developed to use with subjects who did not speak English. Subsequently, they have been used with individuals who are deaf or who have language disorders/delays. The Stanford–Binet Intelligence Scale (Terman, 1916; Terman & Merrill, 1937; Terman & Merrill, 1973) was adapted to use with subjects with visual impairments (Hayes, 1942, 1943), while The Pictorial Test of Intelligence (PTI; French, 1964) and the Columbia Mental Maturity Scale (CMMS; Burgemeister, Blum, & Lorge, 1972) were designed to work with students with speech/language deficits or motor problems. Unfortunately, most of these tests have outdated norms and their value in determining an intellectual level is limited. Many are no longer published. Finally, many of the newer intelligence tests (WISC-III, K-ABC) have recommendations for testing populations who are deaf, blind, or motorically impaired. Occasionally, separate norms are presented for individuals from a minority ethnoculture. Whenever possible, it is best to use portions of standardized and reliable tests to obtain information (e.g., the verbal portion of the Wechsler scales for individuals who are blind, the nonverbal portion of the Wechsler scales for individuals who are deaf or who have language differences or delays).

When the severity of disability interferes with obtaining reliable and valid results from a standardized test, the current philosophy is to use tests that measure functional abilities related to independence, communication, and self-help. This type of evaluation is called a *functional analysis of behavior* because the intent of the assessment is to identify the causes or reason for the behavior. When the behavior is maladaptive, the functional analysis of behavior guides treatment and intervention. For example, an individual who displays self-abusive behavior is utilizing maladaptive behavior in order to communicate some need. The use of a functional analysis of behavior may reveal reasons for the behavior and feasible treatment methods. The researcher interested in assessing the value of different interventions on maladaptive behavior, or changes in skill level as a result of intervention, will likely use a functional assessment as a pre- and post-outcome measure.

In general, assessments of this type use many of the developmental tests, prevocational and vocational evaluations, and outcome measures (identified in the next sections) and criterion referenced tests (identified in Section 8.11). Other examples of functional tests include the Developmental Assessment for the Severely Handicapped (DASH; Dykes, 1980), the Learning Accomplishment Profile (LAP; Sanford & Zelman, 1981), the Uniform Performance Assessment System (Haring et al., 1981), and the Behavioral Characteristics Progression Checklist (Santa Cruz County Superintendent of Schools, 1973).

8.9.5 Child Development

The basic assumption underlying all child development scales is that development is vertical, sequential, and hierarchical. Arnold Gesell and his associates in the Children's

Development Laboratories at Yale University during the 1920s and 1930s used observational analysis of children's behavior to develop norms. Gesell provided the earliest data correlating age with task attainment in such areas as perceptual–motor, language, and personal–social. Since Gesell, other developmental researchers have provided data demonstrating that the growth of human abilities are linked to a biological clock that determines when behavior unfolds at certain critical periods along an age continuum. Differences among child development tests are based on the factors identified and the methods used for assessment. These tests also vary in the time involved in administering a test and in the requirements needed to validly interpret results. For example, the Denver Developmental Screening Test takes about 15 minutes to administer by nonprofessional health aides, whereas the Gesell Developmental Scale requires at least two hours to administer by a professionally trained psychometrician. Examples of the most widely used child development scales are described below and are summarized in Table 8–8.

McCarthy Scales of Children's Abilities (MSCA; McCarthy, 1972) is individually administered and assesses cognitive and motor abilities. Features include an additional memory scale. The test is used frequently by developmental psychologists to obtain an estimate of development level. Because it is related highly to school skills, the scores can predict school achievement. Children with learning disabilities or language disorders have difficulties with this test. Future norms are planned.

Bayley Scales of Infant Development—II (BSID–II; Bayley, 1993) is the newly revised norm-referenced test that assesses children's developmental levels. The test may be given to children from birth through 42 months. It assesses functioning in the areas of language, motor, cognitive, and behavior. Standardization was good, reliability is .78 or above. Because the test has been newly rewritten, validity information is limited.

Battelle Developmental Inventory (BDI; Newborg, Stock, & Wnek, 1984) is a norm- referenced inventory that assesses functioning in five domains, each of which are divided into smaller subdomains. The five domains are personal–social, adaptive (e.g., independent functioning, self-help skills), motor, communication, and cognition (e.g., memory, reasoning, judgment). A screening battery is available. Also available are modifications that can be used to adapt the test for students with disabilities.

Denver Developmental Screening Test—II (Frankenburg, Dodds, Archer, Shapiro, & Bresnick, 1990) is a quick screening tool that can be used to identify those children who are developing slower than the majority of children at the same age. The test can be administered by most professionals with little training.

Miller Assessment For Preschoolers (MAP; Miller, 1988) is a norm-referenced test that examines abilities in sensory; motor; cognition; verbal and nonverbal memory, sequencing, and comprehension; and intersensory integration. The scoring parameters, which include the categories of not-at-risk, perhaps-at-risk, and at-risk, allow for nonlabeling of children while still monitoring progress.

Peabody Developmental Motor Scales (PDMS; Folio & Fewell, 1983) is an individually administered, norm-referenced motor test consisting of two scales: Gross Motor and Fine Motor. Norms are available for children between birth and 83 months. Adequate reliability and validity are available. The test is normally administered by motor therapists (occupational and physical therapists), but, with training, other allied therapists and special educators can administer it.

Preschool Language Scale—III (PLS–III; Zimmerman, Steiner, & Pond, 1992) is an individually administered test that examines receptive and expressive language of children birth through age 6 in a play-like setting. Credit is given for spontaneous responses that occur during the evaluation but are not a direct response to a particular question. A Spanish version is available.

Table 8-8 *Frequently Used Tests of Child Development*

Test	Publisher	Age Range	Variables Measured	Strengths	Weaknesses
McCarthy Scales of Children's Abilities (MSCA; McCarthy, 1972)	Psych. Corp.	ages 2½ through 8	general intelligence, verbal, nonverbal, motor, and memory abilities	• highly related to school tasks • tasks are enjoyable • given quickly	• high level of language needed to do well • inadequate standardization • age-scaled
Bayley Scales for Infant Development—II (BSID-II; Psych. Corp. 1993)	Psych. Corp.	birth through 42 months	overall developmental level, motor, and behavioral	• high reliability • well-designed instrument to assess developmental level	• correlations with other tests range from (.42 to .75) • validity evidence is limited
Battelle Developmental Inventory (BDI; Newborg, Stock & Wnek, 1984)	AGS	birth to 8 years old.	general reasoning, in personal social, communication, adaptive, motor, and cognition	• individual language, cognitive, motor, and social functioning scores obtained • interesting for children • screening version available • administration and scoring are quick and easy	• validity data is limited • reliability is on unspecified number of subjects
Miller Assessment For Preschoolers (Miller, 1988)	Psych. Corp.	2 years 0 months through 5 years 8 months	cognition, motor, verbal and nonverbal abilities, and integration of abilities	• interesting for children • can be given quickly • reliability and validity appear adequate • scoring parameters prevent labeling	• screening instrument • difficult test to learn to give
Preschool Language Scale—3 (PLS-III; Zimmerman, Steiner, & Pond, 1992)	Psych. Corp.	birth through age 6	receptive and expressive language skills	• allows for spontaneous responses • can be used as a criterion referenced test • reliability and validity appear adequate • Spanish version available	• takes up to 30 minutes to administer • requires additional objects not included in the kit

8.9.6 Visual and Auditory Processing, Motor, and Language Tests

A basic assumption in learning is the ability to understand or process information that is seen, heard, or felt, and to express oneself in these same modalities. For example, an individual may hear and understand what is said, and, as a result, may respond, either by speaking aloud or by writing. On the other hand, individuals with learning difficulties, brain damage, stroke, or other neurological impairments may have an inability to process information in one or more modalities (i.e., visual, auditory, motor, or tactile). In these cases, therapy or special education may be employed in order to improve the processing deficit. Pre- and posttests may be used to determine changes in processing. The standardized instruments described below and in Table 8–9 are a few of the more frequently used instruments measuring visual or auditory processing, visual–motor integration, fine and gross motor, or language.

Bruinicks-Oseretsky Test of Motor Proficiency (BOMPT; Bruininks, 1978) is an individually administered test of fine and gross motor skills for typical and atypical students. It

Table 8–9 *Tests for Visual and Auditory Processing, Motor, and Language*

Visual Processing	Auditory Processing	Motor Proficiency	Language Tests
	Variables Assessed		
visual discrimination	visual discrimination	fine motor	articulation
figure ground	figure–ground	gross motor	receptive vocabulary
closure	closure		receptive language
sequencing	sequencing		expressive language
spatial orientation	memory		pragmatics
memory			
visual–motor			
	Examples of Tests		
Bender Visual Motor Gestalt Test (Bender, 1938)	Test of Auditory Perceptual Skills (TAPS; Gardner, 1985)	Brunicks–Osteresky Motor Proficiency Test (BOMPT; Bruininks, 1978)	Clinical Evaluation of Language Functions—Revised (CELF–R; Semel, Wiig, & Secord, 1987)
Test of Visual Perception (nonmotor) (TVPS; Gardner, 1982)	Detroit Test of Learning Aptitude—3 (DTLA–3; Hammill, 1991)		Peabody Picture Vocabulary Test—Revised (PPVT–R; Dunn & Dunn, 1981)
Developmental Test of Visual Motor Integration (VMI; Beery, 1989)			Token Test (DiSimoni, 1978)
			Expressive One-Word Picture Vocabulary Test—Revised (EOWPVT–R; Gardner, 1990)

can be used as an outcome measure to evaluate motor training programs. A brief form is available. Age equivalents are available for the complete battery.

Developmental Test of Visual-Motor Integration (VMI; Beery, 1989) can be administered either individually or as a group assessment of visual–motor skills. The paper–pencil test can be given in 10–15 minutes. Clients draw up to 24 shapes beginning with vertical and horizontal lines and ending with overlapping triangles. The test is reported to be culture-free.

Bender Visual Motor Gestalt Test (Bender, 1938) is widely used as a clinical research instrument. It is individually administered and assesses visual motor maturation in children. Qualitative analysis can be used to screen for mental retardation, regression, loss of brain function, organic brain defects, and personality deviations for individuals of all ages. The test consists of 9 cards which the test administrator shows to the client to draw free-hand on a blank sheet of blank paper. The test is not timed.

Detroit Tests of Learning Aptitude—3 (DTLA–3; Hammill; 1991) is an individually administered test originally developed by Baker and Leland in 1934. Other tests in an updated series include preschool (ages 3 years 0 months to 9 years 11 months) and adolescents and adults (age 16 through 79). On the DTLA–3, 11 subtests combine to provide composite scores in verbal and nonverbal processing, attention to stimuli, and visual–motor performance. Computer scoring makes the tests easy to score.

Test of Auditory Perceptual Skills (TAPS; Gardner, 1985) is an individually administered test that measures auditory skills in discrimination, sequential memory, word memory, sentence memory, interpretation of directions, and processing. There are two levels: (a) age 2 years 0 months through 11 years 11 months, and (b) age 12 through 15. It is easy to give and quick to score.

8.9.7 Behavioral Checklists

Behavior rating scales are used by therapists, teachers, and clinicians to obtain information about a client's behavior. Usually the rating scales are paper–pencil instruments filled out by the client's parents or family. Occasionally, rating scales may be completed by a member of the peer group (e.g., another student in the classroom), or as a self-report measuring.

Although rating scales are widely used, there are some disadvantages and cautions to be considered when using them. Because the rating scale is a subjective measurement, response bias is possible. For example, the responder may rate the individual either too harshly or too positively (e.g., Halo effect) than is realistic. Or, the respondent may restrict the scores to the central range of the scale, leaving the impression that the individual being rated has few strengths or weaknesses. Second, results from rating scales obtained from different settings (e.g., individual therapy and large classroom setting) may show very different scores. This is frequently due to the client's varied behavior in different settings. Finally, differences obtained on the scales may occur because of the day on which the rating scale was completed (Martin, Hooper, & Snow, 1986), thereby reflecting the behavioral variability of either the respondent or the client. For these reasons, more than one informant should be used to complete the rating scale. If possible, each informant should complete a couple of rating scales over a short period of time.

Some of the more widely used scales are described below. Other examples can be found in the publishers' catalogs.

Behavior Rating Profile—2 (2nd ed.; BRP–2; Brown & Hammill, 1990) is a comprehensive measurement scale that utilizes individual measures obtained from parents, teachers, the student, and peers to develop a total picture of the target child's behavioral status. Validity and reliability appear high. There are comparisons of profiles for students who are learning disabled, gifted, mentally retarded, emotionally disturbed, or typical. The instrument is available in Spanish.

Devereau Scales of Mental Disorders (Naglieri, LeBuffe, & Pfeiffer, 1994) and *Behavior Rating Scales—School Form* (Naglieri, LeBuffe, & Pfeiffer, 1992) are newly revised rating scales that allow teachers and professionals to evaluate and identify behavior in individuals ages 3 through 18 that might suggest severe emotional disturbance. The former rating scale also identifies individuals who might be at risk for emotional or behavioral disorders. Both forms are valuable for designing treatment and measuring outcome of treatment. Reliability and validity are good. Both instruments can be used easily with the DSM-IV.

Conners Teacher Rating Scales (CTRS; Conners, 1989b) and *Conners Parent Rating Scales* (CPRS; Conners, 1989a) are a companion set of rating scales designed to identify individuals with behavioral difficulties. Five primary factors discriminate between conduct disorders, anxiety disorders, learning problems, psychosomatic concerns, and hyperactivity. Reliability and validity are adequate. The rating scales have also been used successfully with cross-cultural populations.

The Way I Feel About Myself: The Piers–Harris Self-Concept Scale (Piers & Harris, 1984) is a self-report scale designed for children in grades 4 through 8. The subject reads each of the 80 declarative statements and indicates whether the statement item describes him- or herself or not. Although the test was developed for research, validity data appears adequate. Reliability data is not available. Standardization is poor, as all the subjects used for standardization were from a single school district.

8.9.8 Prevocational Tests

In assessing an individual's prevocational ability an evaluator seeks information on basic ability levels required for specific occupations. Most prevocational tests involve some aspect of motor coordination. Such tests as the Bennett, Crawford, Stromberg, and O'Connor (see Table 8–10) require the subject to perform tasks using small tools in an assembly operation. The tests purport to measure skill proficiencies related to industrial work. Other tests have been devised, such as the San Francisco, to evaluate work behavior at a sheltered workshop as indicative of vocational aptitude. Other work sampling tests not included in this survey, such as the Tower (developed at the Institute of Crippled and Disabled in New York) and the Singer System, are more elaborate methods for assessing vocational aptitude in various industrial occupations. There are many self-devised, unpublished, prevocational tests that are used in sheltered workshops, occupational therapy clinics, and special schools. Some of the more common prevocational tests are listed in Table 8–10.

8.9.9 Vocational Interest Tests

Most investigators constructing vocational interest tests assume that

- Vocational interests are stable characteristics.
- Vocational interests can be measured by paper and pencil tests.
- Vocational interests are grouped around clusters of interest.
- Individuals in occupations share common interests and characteristics.
- There is a positive relationship between vocational interests and choice of occupation.
- Job satisfaction is related to vocational interest and aptitude.

Table 8-10 *Prevocational Tests*

Test	Publisher	Age Level	Administration Time	Method of Assessment
Crawford Small Parts Dexterity Test	Psych. Corp.	adolescents through adults	9 to 25 minutes	speed test for fine motor coordination using tweezers and small pins
Stromberg Dexterity Test	Psych. Corp.	adolescents	5 to 10 minutes through adults	speed test for motor coordination
O'Connor Tweezer Dexterity Test	Stoelting Corporation	adult	10 minutes	speed test for fine motor coordinaiton
Stoelting Laboratory	Stoelting Corporation	adult		simulates factory assembly work
Minnesota Rate of Manipulation	Western Psychological	grade 7 to adult	30 to 50 minutes	speed test for motor coordination using blocks and formboard
Purdue Pegboard	Science Research Associates	adult	5 ot 10 minutes	speed test, measuring manual dexterity, using pegs, washers, and collars
San Francisco Vocational Competency Test	Psych. Corp.	adolescents through adults with mental retardation	10 minutes	30 item behavior rating code, measuring vocational competence–Motor skills, cognition, dependability, responsibility, and social–emotive

The Strong Vocational Interest Test (SCII; Strong, Campbell, & Hansen, 1985) and the Kuder Occupational Interest Survey (Kuder, 1960) are the two tests most widely used by clinical psychologists and social researchers. Table 8–11 lists the most widely used tests available for measuring vocational interest.

8.9.10 Outcome Measures and Functional Assessment

There is a rising trend in health care to demonstrate effectiveness and client satisfaction. Outcome measures have been designed to evaluate the overall functional status of clients who have received treatment and rehabilitation services in hospitals, outpatient clinics, rehabilitation centers and home environments. These outcome measures (Keith, 1984) are usually designed for specific populations such as individuals with stroke, brain injury, spinal cord injury, low back pain, psychological diagnoses, and developmental disabilities. The outcome measures evaluate the client's ability to perform functional activities of daily living, the degree of pain intensity, ability to work, to engage in leisure activities, to have restful sleep, to drive, to be mobile in the community, to communicate, to ambulate, to academically achieve, and to perform other activities related to functional abilities. Following is a list of some commonly used outcome measures for rehabilitation. (Also see Applegate, Blass, & Williams, 1990. For assessment of outcome in education, see Sattler, 1988).

- The Levels of Rehabilitation Scale (LORS–II; Carey & Posavac, 1980), designed to obtain functional ratings from individuals who are in hospital-based rehabilitation programs.
- The Katz Index of Independence in ADL (Katz, Ford, Moskowitz, Jackson, & Jaffe, 1963), developed for use with rehabilitation in patients.
- The Functional Assessment Screening Questionnaire (Granger & Wright, 1993), an instrument used with patients who have undergone rehabilitation.
- Global Assessment of Functioning (American Psychiatric Association, 1994), used with individuals with psychosocial diagnoses.
- The Multilevel Assessment Instrument (Lawton, Moss, Fulcomer, & Kleban, 1982), designed for older individuals.
- Unified ADL Evaluation form (Donaldson, Wagner, & Gresham, 1973).
- Functional Life Scale (Sarno, Sarno, & Levita, 1973).
- The Community Integration Questionnaire (Willer, Ottenbacher, & Coad, 1994), used with individuals with traumatic brain injury.
- Barthel Index (Mahoney & Barthel, 1965), designed to evaluate the degree of assistance required by an individual on ten items of self-care and mobility.
- The Health Status Questionnaire (Tarlov, Ware, Greenfield, Nelson, Perrin, & Zubkoff 1989), used to assess the functional status of adults with chronic illnesses.
- The Sickness Impact Profile (Gilson et al., 1975), used to assess a patient's function in such areas as sleep and rest, work, social interactions, leisure, and emotional behavior.
- Functional Independence Measure (Keith, Granger, Hamilton, & Sherwins, 1987), designed as a tool to evaluate the patient's ability to complete activities of daily living.

Table 8-11 *Vocational Interest Tests*

Test	Publisher	Age Level	Administration Time	Method of Assessment
Strong Vocational Interest Test (SCII)	National Computer Systems	College students, adults	1 hour	Forced choice paper and pencil test measuring interest in specific occupations
Kuder Occupational Interest Survey	Science Research Association	High school, adults	1 hour	Forced choice paper and pencil test measuring interest in specific occupations
Geist Picture Interest Inventory	Western Psychological	Junior high school to adult	½ hour	Picture selection test measures occupational interest. Spanish and deaf forms available
Wide Range Interest-Opinion Test	Jastak	Junior high school through adult	1–2 hours	Picture format measuring occupational interests. Specifically designed for who are blind. Computer format is available, to take in two sessions.
Reading-Free Vocational Interest Inventory	Elbern Publishers	Junior high through adult	½ hour	Picture format measuring occupational interests. Specifically designed for individuals who can't read or who are mentally retarded.
Gordon Occupational Checklist	Psych. Corp.	Junior high to high school	½ hour	Subject underlines preferred activities. Scoring identifies major occupational areas of interest.
California Occupational Preference System (COPS)	Educational and Industrial Testing Service	High school to adult, professionals	½ hour	System includes an aptitude test (CAPS), interest inventory (COPS), and values test (COPES), which together result in a profile of occupations keyed to the *Dictionary of Occupational Titles*

8.9.11 Functional Evaluation in Physical Capacity, Work Aptitude, and Independent Living

Tests of functional capacity, vocational aptitude, and independent living assess the degree to which an individual can live and work independently in the community. They assess an individual's ability to perform physical movements as they relate to work, vocational activities, and activities of daily living. These measures are extremely important to rehabilitation research in determining whether an individual can return to work or live in independent housing.

Functional capacity evaluations are comprehensive and systematic approaches that measure the client's overall physical ability such as muscle strength, endurance, joint range of motion, ambulation, sitting, standing, and lifting. *Work samples* are well-defined activities that are similar to actual jobs. They can be used to assess an individual's vocational aptitudes, worker characteristics, and vocational interests. *Independent living measures* test the degree to which an individual can perform the activities of daily living. They include self-care, communication, leisure, shopping, mobility, and related areas. Table 8–12 summarizes information about each of these areas and gives examples of evaluation instruments.

8.9.12 Objective Personality Tests

Measurement of personality variables through paper and pencil tests are widely used in research studies of treatment outcome in psychiatry. The Minnesota Multiphasic Personality Inventory, first published in 1942, is the most extensively used test for diagnosing psychological maladjustment. The researcher using objective personality tests should use caution in interpreting results. The methods of administering the tests and the subject's attitude toward the tests can potentially affect the results. Factors such as noise distractions, unmotivated and uncooperative subjects, and subject faking (sometimes referred to as *malingering*) are some of the problems encountered in personality testing. The ethical consideration in personality testing is another major consideration. The researcher should make efforts to ensure the anonymity and confidentiality of the subject. Most of the tests can only be given by evaluators training in personality assessment. Some of the more common tests are described in the following paragraphs.

- *Minnesota Multiphasic Personality Inventory—2* (MMPI–2; Hathaway & McKinley, 1970) consists of 550 true–false items used for measuring adjustment on 10 psychiatric diagnostic scales. The test takes from 2 to 3 hours and is given to adults.
- *Million Adolescent Personality Inventory* (MAPI; Million, Green, & Meagher, 1982) is a personality test for adolescents ages 13 and up. The test is written in language understood by adolescents, and is based on a model of personality development rather than clinical pathology. The paper and pencil test must be scored by computer through the National Computer Systems is required.
- *Edwards Personal Preference Schedule* (Edwards, 1959) has 225 paired forced choice items used to measure specific personality characteristics in adults. It is available through the Psychological Corporation.
- *Personality Inventory for Children* (PIC; Wirt, Lachar, Klinedinst, & Seat, 1984) is a questionnaire containing true–false items that are completed by an infor-

Table 8–12 *Functional Assessment of Physical Capacity, Work Aptitude, and Independent Living*

	Functional Capacity Evaluation	Work Sample Systems	Independent Living Measures
Purpose	To evaluate a person's functional physical abilities as they relate to work performance (Lechner, Rother, & Straaton, 1991)	It is used to assess an individual's vocational aptitudes, worker characteristics, and vocational interests (Nadolsky, 1974)	To assess activities of daily living skills the client needs to function successfully in the community (Power, 1991)
Sample of Variables Assessed	• range of motion • muscle strength • coordination • manual dexterity • muscular endurance • position tolerance	• vocational potential in various fields • gross and fine manual dexterity • visual and tactile discrimination • work habits	• social skills • self-care • safety and health • communication • transportation • money management • homemaking • leisure activities
Examples of Widely Used Instruments	BTE (1992): Published by the Baltimore Therapeutic Equipment	*McCarron–Dial:* Available from McCarron–Dial, P.O. Box 4628, Dallas, TX 75245	Kohlman Evaluation of Living Skills (KELS; Thomson, 1992)
	KEY (Key, 1988): Available from KEY Functional Assessments, Minneapolis	*MICRO-TOWER:* Available from ICD Rehabilitation and Research Center, 340 East 24th St., New York, NY 10010	The Barthel Index (Granger & Greer, 1976)
	Isernhagen (1988)	*JEVS Work Samples:* Available from Vocational Research Institute 1528 Walnut St. Philadelphia, PA 19102	Independent Living Behavior Checklist (ILBC; West Virginia Research and Training Center, 1 Dunbar Plaza, Suite E, Dunbar WV 25064.)
	Blankenship (1989)	Valpar 3801 East 34th St. Tucson, AZ 85713	The Milwaukee Evaluation of Daily Living Skills (MEDLS; Leonardelli, 1988)

Examples of Widely Used Instruments

Work Capacity Evaluations (Matheson, 1988)

The Physical Work Performance Evaluation (Lechner, Jackson, Roth, & Straaton, 1994)

Smith FCE (Smith, Cunningham, & Weinberg, 1986)

Singer Vocational Evaluation
80 Commerce Drive
Rochester, NY 14623

Talent Assessment Programs (TAP)
P.O. Box 5087
Jacksonville, FL 32207

Hester Evaluation System (HES)
Educational Systems, Inc.
P.O. Box 10741
Chicago, IL 60610

The Katz Index of Independence in ADL (Katz, Ford, Moskowitz, Jackson, Jaffe, 1963)

Vineland Adaptive Behavior Scale (Sparrow, Balla, & Ciocchetti, 1984; AGS)

Kenny Self-Care Evaluation (Schoening & Iverson, 1968)

mant (usually the parent). Scoring results in a profile composed of 12 clinical scales. The inventory is designed for children ages 3 through 16.

*   *Children's Depression Inventory* (CDI; Kovacs, 1992), available through the Psychological Corporation, consists of 27 self-rating items in which the client must choose between one of three sentences that best describes his or her experience in the past two weeks. High scores result in possible depression. The test is designed for ages 7 to 17 and takes about 15 minutes.
*   *California Life Goals Evaluation Schedules* (Hahn, 1969) consists of 150 hypothetical questions that are rated to provide scores in 10 life goals. It is available through Western Psychological Services.
*   *Sixteen Personality Factor Questionnaire* (5th ed.; 16PF; Cattell, Cattell, & Cattell, 1993) is a forced choice test used for measuring 16 independent factors of personality. It is designed for high school, college, and adult subjects and takes about an hour to administer. It is available through Psychological Corporation.
*   *California Psychological Inventory* (CPI; Gough, 1987) is available through The Psychological Corporation and appropriate for age 14 through adult subjects. It consists of 480 true–false items, which are used for measuring 18 personality traits.

8.9.13 Neuropsychological Batteries

Clinical neuropsychology is a relatively new field that attempts to relate behavior to brain functioning. Neuropsychological testing is requested by clinicians, therapists, and educators in special cases. For example, neuropsychological testing is usually requested when a client has sustained a traumatic or acquired brain injury. Neuropsychological testing may also be requested when a more specific understanding of an individual's strengths and weaknesses is desired. Although individual neuropsychological tests can be given, frequently neuropsychologists use a specific battery of tests generated by their particular philosophical stance.

The *Halsted–Reitan Neuropsychological Test Battery* consists of up to 37 individual tests, each of which must be administered to obtain a complete profile of an individual's brain functioning. Diagnosis is dependent upon (a) comparing the client's score with a comparison group, (b) comparing scores between individual tests, and (c) comparing differences between scores performed on the right or left side of the body. Based on the profile of scores, treatment for deficits are suggested.

A. Luria (1980) developed a second approach to neuropsychological testing by developing specific test items that would allow the clinician to identify the way in which a person approached a task. The *Luria–Nebraska Neuropsychological Battery* (LNNB; Golden, Purisch, & Hammeke, 1985) is an outgrowth of Luria's work. Although this battery is not frequently used, it does provide information for the clinician regarding brain–behavior relationships.

Edith Kaplan, using the philosophy and work of Luria, has proposed a third approach to neuropsychological testing. She proposed that an evaluation should result in an understanding of the way in which a person approaches a task, regardless of which tests are used. This method, called the Boston process approach, relies less on specific instruments and more on observation of behavior during the evaluation. All neurological functioning (e.g., cognitive, perceptual, memory, language, organization, and personality) is evaluated in this approach. The Wechsler Adult Intelligence Scale—Revised—

Neuropsychological Instrument (WAIS–R–NI; Kaplan, Fein, Morris, & Delis, 1991), developed by the Psychological Corporation is an example of an instrument using the Boston process approach.

Clinical researchers may not, at first, be involved in neuropsychological testing as part of their research. However, information obtained from these tests, as well as use of pre- and posttest data can be useful as outcome measures in examining the relationship between changes in behavior and interventions.

8.10 Reviewing and Evaluating Tests

For the researcher, the selection of a valid and reliable instrument is critical. The knowledge in assessing the adequacy of a measuring instrument is extremely important in view of the literally thousands of tests that are published by test corporations. Before the clinical researcher chooses a test to use in research, the purpose for the test must be determined. Does the researcher need to screen participants for normal intelligence or average achievement? Is adaptive behavior a concern? If the purpose of the investigation is to evaluate the effect of a treatment on reducing high blood pressure, the researcher will want to make sure that all subjects have clinically significant hypertension.

The next step to determining which test to use is to review tests available in the area for which the test is to be used. The tests need to be reviewed for psychometric properties, including reliability, validity, and measurement scales. If there are special qualifications in administering the test, the researcher must know who is able to administer the test and how long it will take to administer. The following outline and examples of reviews of tests will illustrate the manner in which tests are analyzed (Stein, 1988).

Outline for Reviewing Tests

1. Title
2. Date published, date revised
3. Authors
4. Publisher: Distributor of test, or where test available
5. Target Population: What was the original sample that data were collected from in terms of age, diagnostic group, and geographical location? Is there a specific target population for which the test is appropriate?
6. Variables Assessed: What are the specific areas of function, behavior, or personality that are being assessed? What are the major stated purposes of the test?
7. Measurement Scales: What is the level of measurement in the test?

    A. Qualitative (subjective judgment)

      i. Nominal scale of measurement refers to evaluating variables using independent categories such *as can or cannot perform a specific task.*

      ii. Ordinal scale of measurement refers to evaluating variables using magnitude and ranking such as *completely dependent in task, needs assistance,* or *independent functioning.* Variables can also be rated on a numerical scale from 1 to 5, for example, where 1 indicates *no self-care* and 5 indicates *cares for self independently.*

    B.   Quantitative (objective evaluation)

        i.   Interval scale of measurement refers to scoring variables on a continuous scale with equal distances between score values. Pulse rate, blood pressure, height, and weight are usually measured on interval scales using tests that produce mathematical data.

        ii. Ratio scale of measurement incorporates the concept of an absolute zero.

  8. Administration of Instrument: Who administers the test and when is it administered? How long does it take to administer? Is there special training to administer the test? Are special materials or environments required?

  9. Scoring and Interpretation of Results: Are there overall scores or subtest scores derived from the test results? Are there norms available to interpret raw scores? How are the results used in treatment planning, documentation of progress, and discharge recommendations?

 10. Test Reliability and Validity

 11. Other Comments: Included in this section are miscellaneous comments such as the theoretical orientation or conceptual framework of the test and its appropriateness for the clinical researcher.

 12. References: Includes books, journals, test manuals, and other sources where the test has been published or critically evaluated.

Example of Test Review: Intelligence Test

  1. *Wechsler Intelligence Scale for Children—Third Edition* (WISC–III)

  2. Originally published in 1949, revised in 1974, and newly revised in 1991

  3. David Wechsler

  4. Psychological Corporation

  5. The standardization sample for the *WISC–III* included 2200 English-speaking subjects. Two hundred children, 100 males and 100 females, in each of 11 age groups (age 6 years 0 months through 16 years 11 months) were used. Data collected in 1988 from the Bureau of Census were the basis for the sample, which was stratified according to race, ethnicity, geographic region, and parent education. Data were collected from both private and public schools. Seven percent of the standardization sample contained children classified as learning disabled, speech–language impaired, emotionally disabled, or physically challenged. Five percent of the sample included children from gifted and talented programs.

  6. The test is designed to test intelligence through a number of different subtests. The subtests assess different aspects of intelligence, and the combination of these subtests are believed to measure behavior considered to be a part of intelligence (*WISC–III Manual*, 1991). Individual subtests measure abstract reasoning, memory, perception, or language development. The purposes of the test as noted in the manual include psychoeducational assessment, diagnosis of exceptionality, clinical and neurological assessment, and research.

  7. The level of measurement is both continuous and discrete.

Because there is no absolute zero, the ratio scale is not available. An IQ score of 100 is not twice as high as an IQ score of 50. IQ scores can be grouped into classifications such as borderline (70–80), average intelligence (90–110), and superior (120 and above).

8. The test must be administered by someone trained in the clinical administration and interpretation of standardized tests. In addition, the examiner should have experience with children of various cultures, ages, and educational levels. Training to give this test is available through The Psychological Corporation and in most clinical psychology and school psychology programs. The regular battery of subtests takes between 50 and 70 minutes, and the additional supplementary subtests take an additional 10 to 15 minutes. The test should be administered in one session if at all possible. The test should be administered in a well-lighted, quiet environment.

9. Five verbal subtests combine to obtain the Verbal Scale Score and five nonverbal subtests combine to obtain the Performance Scale Score. The Full Scale Score is obtained by adding the Verbal Scale Score and the Performance Scale Score. These scores, in turn, are converted into the VIQ, PIQ, and FSIQ through normative tables for age levels at 3-month intervals. The supplementary scales (Verbal Comprehension, Perceptual Organization, Perceptual Speed, and Freedom from Distractibility) are converted into index scores. Scores range from 40 to 160. Confidence intervals and percentile scores are available. Mean and median age scores can be obtained and may be useful for qualitative analysis. Results can be used to determine deviation from the normal population (e.g., mental retardation, giftedness), as well as predict expected school achievement. Changes in IQ scores can be indicative of neurological impairment or emotional disturbance. Discrepancies between the obtained IQ score and school achievement suggest the presence of a learning disability, whereas lack of a discrepancy in the presence of a score that is below average may suggest that the individual is a slow learner. Analysis of subtest scores may indicate cognitive strengths and weaknesses.

10. Reliability coefficients for all but two of the subtests (Coding and Symbol Search) were obtained by split-half methods. Average reliability coefficients for all subtests ranged between .69 and .87; for the IQ scales from .91 to .95; and for the index scores from .85 to .94. Test–retest stability using a median retest interval of 23 days showed average coefficients ranging from .87 to .94 for the IQ scores. Interscorer reliability for the subtests requiring more judgment (i.e., Similarities, Comprehension, Vocabulary, and Mazes) ranged between .92 and .98.

Validity was measured by internal validity examined through a review of correlations between subtests. Moderate correlations were noted, with the Verbal Scale subtests ($r = .76$ to .87) correlating more highly with each other than the Performance Scale subtests ($r = .56$ to .80) did. High correlations were noted between VIQ and FSIQ (.92) and the PIQ and FSIQ (.90). In addition, the Verbal IQ correlated more highly with the Full Scale IQ (.92) than the Performance IQ did (.90). The high correlations provide evidence of convergent validity.

Exploratory and confirmatory factor analysis suggest a four-factor construct within the WISC–III. These factors were named as Verbal

Comprehension, Perceptual Organization, Freedom from Distractibility, and Processing Speed. These four factors held for clinical groups such as attention-deficit hyperactivity disorder (ADHD), gifted, and mental retardation.

      Comparison studies using the WISC–III with other intelligence tests revealed adequate convergent and discriminate validity. Correlations between WISC–III and the WISC–R IQ scores (VIQ, PIQ, and FSIQ) ranged from .81 to .90. Similar correlations were seen between the WISC–R and the WAIS–R. Correlations between the WISC–III and the WPPSI–R IQ scores ranged from .73 to .85. Moderate correlations were noted between the WISC–III and the Otis–Lennon School Ability Test Scores (OLSAT; r = .64 to .73). Correlations between tests of perceptual processing (e.g., Halsted–Reitan and Benton Revised Visual Retention Test) were low, as were correlations between the WISC–III and the Wide Range Achievement Test—Revised (WRAT–R; .11 to .41). This would suggest that the WISC–III measures different abilities than those measured by either the neurological scales or the achievement test.

11.   Validity studies suggest that the construct measured by the WISC–III is separate from academic achievement or perceptual functioning. Because it was developed along the same lines as the other Wechsler Intelligence Scales, we may presume that the test measures general intelligence (g) as well as specific factors of g.

12.   Kaufman, A. S. (1994). *Intelligence Testing with the WISC–III*. New York: Wiley.

8.11 Criterion-Referenced Tests and Normative-Referenced Tests

Until recently, most tests were normative-referenced tests, or NRTs. These tests, described previously, were developed to classify individuals into levels of instructional groups. The scores obtained by the normative sample on a norm-referenced test are distributed along a normal curve. Raw scores obtained by individuals taking a norm-referenced test are compared to the normative sample and can be converted into standard scores and percentiles.

      There are several advantages to NRTs. Individuals taking the test are compared to the general population. Thus, the performance of a student or patient can be judged to be typical or atypical. Because NRTs are usually commercially published, psychometric characteristics such as reliability and item analysis are carefully considered in the development. Additionally, standardization of an NRT includes administering the test to large samples of individuals stratified across many socioeconomic groups, ages, ethnic backgrounds, and educational levels. In this way, raw scores obtained from a given individual can be compared to the raw score obtained by most of the population having the same characteristics.

      At the same time, there are disadvantages to an NRT. Because the tests are broad measures of a subject and contain a limited number of items from many areas within that subject, they are often referred to as survey tests. It is not uncommon for an NRT designed to be used in grades 1 through 12 to include only 100 sight words. Because there is no national or state curriculum, the content found on the test may not match the curriculum of a particular school or community. Finally, since the number of items in each area is limited, the test results cannot be used to measure small gains in progress. Likewise, there is limited value for using the results of an NRT in determining an instructional or therapeutic program.

The purpose of NRTs is (a) to compare an individual's achievement or performance with other individuals of the same age, educational level, and socioeconomic status and (b) to obtain information regarding the normal population. When these tests are used with atypical populations, there may be a bias, which results in systematic error. In spite of these disadvantages, NRTs are useful in clinical research.

In testing circles during the last 20 years there has been a growing interest in devising criterion-referenced tests in lieu of norm-referenced tests (Deno, 1985). Criterion-referenced tests (CRTs), first proposed by Glaser (1963), use content or curricular domains to set the standard of performance. They compare the performance of an individual to a specified level of mastery or achievement rather than to a normative population. Because the performance is compared to a criterion, performance on these tests allows the therapist or teacher to suggest specific classroom goals and objectives to use in program planning. Progress can be monitored more effectively and more discretely.

CRTs are based on a comprehensive theory that generates ideas for a specific content domain. In CRTs, items are selected systematically to represent the content domain. For example, if an investigator is interested in determining the reading ability of students, the first task would be to determine the dimensions of the reading concept from the theoretical and experiential perspectives. The investigator would use the theoretical framework to guide the writing of test items, making sure that each aspect of the framework is covered by test items in the CRT. Operational performance standards, obtained by surveying a representational sample of the general population, are used in writing test items. For example, a survey of second graders would reveal that most of them could read 90% of the most commonly used words. The operational performance standard, therefore, might be set at a criterion level of 90% accuracy for reading these words.

One example of criterion-referenced testing occurs when measuring an individual's independent living skills. For instance, in the criteria of dressing completely, we might include the act of putting on all clothes right-side out and frontwards, tying shoes, and fastening all fasteners. The individual's ability to perform this activity is measured by a given standard. Until the individual has mastered the expected standard, competency is not considered to be reached. Social skills and self-help skills are often evaluated by CRTs.

CRTs are sometimes referred to as curriculum based measures (CBMs) or curriculum-based assessments (CBAs). CBAs and CBMs establish a student's instructional needs in relationship to the requirements of the actual curriculum being used. Just as with CRTs, the CBAs and CBMs assess mastery of learning by providing an operational performance criterion as a necessary standard for passing. Although commercial CRTs are available, teachers and allied therapists frequently develop the measurement instrument based on their own criteria.

In summary, a CRT is constructed to obtain measurements that can be interpreted in terms of specific criteria or performance standards. Scores obtained on NRTs, however, are interpreted in terms of comparison to a population. The choice of which test to use depends on the outcome desired. If a researcher is interested in the progress of a particular student over time, a CRT is more appropriate. However, if the researcher is interested in the differences between two groups of subjects, then an NRT may be more appropriate.

A summary of the differences between criterion- and norm-referenced tests is given in Table 8–13. This summary may help in making decisions about which type of test to use.

Table 8–13   *Comparison of Criterion-Referenced Tests and Norm-Referenced Tests*

Criterion-Referenced Tests	Norm-Referenced Tests
• absolute standards of competence or mastery are established based on theory	• relative standards are based on normal standards
• scores are derived from standards of behaviors or competency	• scores are compared to established norms
• scores are interpreted based on what the student can or cannot do and then used diagnostically	• scores are interpreted by percentile ranks, standard scores, and organized along a normal curve
• content or items are comprehensive of domain	• content of items are a sample of domain
• cut-off score for passing is based on minimal standards of competency	• cut-off score for passing is based on pre-established percentile rank
• theoretically all can pass or all can fail	• the number of failures is predicted before test is administered

Applying Criterion-Referenced Concepts to Research

The major content areas for clinical researchers in evaluation include basic living skills, interests, work behavior, and skill attainment. If one uses a criterion-referenced approach to these areas, one should consider the following factors:

- The theory underlying these concepts is identified.
- Research evidence supporting any assumptions of the test are stated.
- The content domain of the test that considers a comprehensive view of skills, interests, and behavior is discussed.
- The specific target population is operationally defined in terms of age, intelligence, education, and degree of disability.
- The test items are generated by selecting representative samples of behavior.
- Performance standards in the test are based on systematically collected data from representative samples of the target population.
- Test items are pilot-tested for clarity and ease of administration.
- Scoring methods are devised that are operationally defined.
- Reliability and validity data are documented.
- A test manual for administering, scoring, and interpreting data is provided.
- The degree of competency in the administration of the test is included in test descriptions.

8.12 Test Publishers

The development of new tests and measuring instruments is a relatively recent event in the allied health professions. The clinical nature of these fields and the service-oriented process of treatment have led to the emphasis in the past on developing new treatment techniques rather than measuring outcome variables. However, as the need for accountability and validation for treatment continue on federal and state governmental levels (e.g., through laws such as IDEA), the use of tests and measuring instruments to justify therapeutic and educational intervention has become more important. Literally hundreds of tests have been developed for use by allied therapists, clinicians, and special educators in the past 10 years.

For the researcher, the selection of a valid and reliable instrument is critical. The knowledge in assessing the adequacy of a measuring instrument is extremely important in view of the literally thousands of tests published by test corporations. In addition to publishing their own tests, most test corporations distribute the most widely used tests. Thus, in general, a researcher is not limited to one corporation to obtain a specific test.

The following list includes test publishers that are frequently used by therapists, school psychologists, and special educators:

- American Occupational Therapy Association (AOTA)
  P.O. Box 31220
  Bethesda, MD 20824–1220
  1–800–729–2682 (members)
  301–652–2682 (nonmembers)

- American Guidance Service, Inc.
  401 Woodland Road
  P.O. Box 99
  Circle Pines, MN 55014–1796
  1–800–328–2560

- California Test Bureau/McGraw-Hill
  10 Ryan Ranch Road
  Monterey, CA 93940–5703
  408–393–0700

- CPPC (Clinical Psychology Publishing Co.)
  4 Conant Square
  Brandon, Vermont 05733
  1–800–433–8234
  FAX: 802–247–6853

- Consulting Psychologists Press, Inc.
  303 East Bay Shore Road
  Palo Alto, CA 94306
  415–691–9143

- Curriculum Associates, Inc.
  P.O. Box 2001
  N. Billerica, MA 01862–0901
  1–800–225–0248
  FAX: 508–667–5706

- Educational Testing Service
  Rosedale Road
  Princeton, NJ 08541
  609–921–9000

- Educational and Industrial Testing Service (EdITS)
  P.O. Box 7234
  San Diego, CA 92107
  619–222–1666

- Flaghouse Rehabilitation
  150 N. Macquesten Parkway
  Mt. Vernon, NY 10550
  1–800–793–7900
  FAX: 1–800–793–7922

- Hawthorne Educational Services
  800 Gray Oak Drive
  Columbia, MO 65201
  1–800–542–1673

- ICD Rehabilitation and Research Center
  340 East 24th St.
  New York, NY 10010
  212–995–9154

- Institute for Personality and Ability Testing (IPAT)
  P.O. Box 1188
  Champaign, IL 61820–0188
  1–800–225–4728

- Lafayette Instrument
  P.O. Box 5729
  Lafayette, IN 47903
  1–800–428–7545
  FAX: 317–423–4111

- McCarron–Dial
  Box 45628
  Dallas TX, 75245
  214–247–5945

- MHS
  908 Niagara Falls Blvd.
  North Tonawanda, NY
  14120–2060
  1–800–456–3003
  FAX: 416–424–1736

- PAR (Psychological Assessment
  Resources, Inc.)
  P.O. Box 998
  Odessa, FL 33556
  1–800–331–8378
  FAX: 1–800–727–9329

- PRO–ED
  8700 Shoal Creek Boulevard
  Austin, TX 78757–6897
  512–451–3246
  FAX: 1–800–FXPROED orders
  only

- Psychological and Educational
  Tests and Remedial Activities
  1477 Rollins Road
  Burlingame, CA 94010–2316
  1–800–523–5775
  FAX: 1–800–447–0907

- Psychometric Affiliates
  Box 807
  Murfreesboro, TN 37133
  615–890–6296

- Riverside Corporation
  A Houghton Mifflin Company
  8420 Bryn Mawr Avenue
  Chicago, IL 60631
  1–800–323–9540
  FAX: 312–693–0325

- Science Research Associates
  P.O. Box 543
  Blacklick, OH 43004–0543
  1–800–843–8855

- Slosson Educational
  Publications
  P.O. Box 280
  East Aurora, NY 14052–0280
  1–800–828–4800
  FAX: 1–800–655–3840

- Stoelting Corporation
  620 Wheat Lane
  Wood Dale, IL 60191–1109
  708–860–9700

- Stout Vocational Rehabilitation
  Institute
  School of Education and Human
  Services
  University of Wisconsin–Stout
  Menomonie, WI 54751
  715–232–1122

- The Psychological Corporation
  Harcourt Brace, Inc.
  Order Service Center
  P.O. Box 839954
  San Antonio, Texas 78204-3954
  1–800–228–0752
  FAX: 1–800–232–1223
  TDD: 1–800–723–1318

- Trace Center Publications and
  Media
  University of
  Wisconsin–Madison
  S–151 Waisman Center
  1500 Highland Ave
  Madison, WI 53705–2280
  608–263–2237

- Valpar International
  Corporation
  P.O. Box 5767
  Tucson, AZ 85703–5767
  1–800–528–7070
  FAX: 602–293–9755

- Vocational Research Institute
  1528 Walnut St.
  Philadelphia, PA, 19102
  215–875–7387

- Western Psychological Services
  12031 Wilshire Boulevard
  Los Angeles, CA 90025
  1–800–648–8857

8.13 Ethical Considerations in Testing

"Competence in test use is a combination of knowledge of psychometric principles, knowledge of the problem situation in which the testing is to be done, technical skill and some wisdom" (Davis, 1974, p. 6). This quote is from the Standards for Educational and Psychological Tests published by the American Psychological Association. In order to protect psychological tests from abuse, standards fall into three areas: guidelines for devising a new psychological test, qualifications for administering tests, and the guidelines for interpreting results. The following guidelines should be adhered to in using tests:

1. The researcher publishing a new test should provide reliability, validity, normative data, scoring procedure, and qualifications for using the test in an accompanying manual.
2. A standardized test procedure should be carefully followed by the tester.
3. Results should be reported that can be compared to specified populations.
4. The researcher using psychological tests should obtain informed consent for the subject and ensure the subject's confidentiality.

Qualification levels are set by the APA Standards for Educational and Psychological Testing. Level A requires no special qualification, Level B requires at least a BA in psychology, counseling, or closely related field and relevant training; Level C requires a graduate degree in psychological education or closely related field and training, or membership in a professional association that requires training and experience in the ethical and competent use of testing (e.g., APA, NASP), *or* licence or certification from an agency that requires training in testing. Almost all publishing companies adhere to this policy. These levels are listed here for the reader's information.

CHAPTER
9

Scientific Writing and Thesis Preparation

Vigorous writing is concise. A sentence should contain no unnecessary words, a paragraph no unnecessary sentences, for the same reason that a drawing should have no unnecessary lines and a machine no unnecessary parts. This requires not that the writer make all his sentences short, or that he avoid all detail and treat his subjects only in outline, but that every word tell.—W. Strunk Jr. and E. B. White, *The Elements of Style* (p. 23)

Operational Learning Objectives

By the end of this chapter, the reader will be able to

1.   state ways to prepare for writing a research paper
2.   name the important divisions of a research paper
3.   identify and correct sexist and racist language in the research paper
4.   use *People First* language
5.   recognize reasons for revising the original draft
6.   write a bibliography using APA format
7.   proof for errors in language mechanics and style
8.   critically evaluate one's own writing
9.   identify the major parts of the final format
10. design a research proposal

9.1 Preparation for Writing

It is as important to prepare yourself for writing as it is to complete the review of literature and collect the data for the research project. Prior to writing the research paper, a number of important processes that facilitate writing should be taken into consideration.

While one hindrance to the completion of the writing task is the failure to actually sit down and write, another hindrance is allowing frequent interruptions during the actual writing period. The first task in the preparation for writing is to get oneself into a proper frame of mind. This includes taking care of as many "settling activities" that might lead to interruptions. This can be likened to an animal preparing to go to sleep: The animal roughs up the bed, circles the bed a number of times, grooms, and finally settles down. Similarly, settling activities for writers include planning a large block of time, getting one's coffee or drink, assembling all the materials needed, finding a quiet, comfortable place (preferably away from a phone), arranging for child care, putting the dog or cat outside, and taking care of any needed personal toiletries. Once one has completed those tasks and is settled, writing is made easier.

Effective writing is a skill that becomes more refined as it is practiced. Clear and simple language is the hallmark of good scientific writing. The most important quality of writing is objective self-criticism. A major block to writing for some individuals is the initial step of organizing their ideas on paper. The desire to write at first as if whatever is put on paper is chipped forever in granite sometimes prevents the flow of ideas.

The place and time in which one writes are important initial considerations also. Some individuals do their best writing during the morning in a quiet, sunny room with a large table where they can spread out reference books, scrap paper, and notes filed in manila folders. Others work better in the late evening. Some individuals are able to work 12–14 hours for several days, followed by several days of complete rest. Some students do their best work in a college library or college cafeteria, despite visual and noise distractions. Some are able to write using paper and pencil, while others compose better on a computer or word processor. Whatever the method and place, it is important that one is sensitive to an environment that facilitates one's most creative writing.

A second consideration in writing is the time schedule. Some writers report that they write in spurts of creative inspiration, while others work daily whether or not they feel inspired. It is important, however, to set aside enough time for writing so that the individual does not feel rushed or under time constraints. Allowing enough time in each setting allows the writer to feel that something can be accomplished. Writing a research paper or article is unlike casual writing, in which an individual can use spare minutes throughout the day to complete the task. Scientific writing takes mental energy and therefore requires concentrated effort.

A third consideration consists of assembling the materials to be used before beginning any writing task. Writing materials (e.g., pens, paper, computer), notecards prepared during the literature review, statistical analyses, and other references should be available and at hand. Just as one would not consider doing therapy without having all the tools and equipment available, one cannot expect to do adequate writing without having the proper tools and materials.

Writing a book, journal article, or thesis requires self-discipline. In a way, the individual should prepare for writing like a boxer trains for a fight. A period of self-toughening and mental rigor prior to writing is important. Some individuals take long walks, ride bicycles for miles, climb mountains, or take part in physical sports in preparation for writing. Others prepare mentally by playing chess, doing crossword puzzles, solving arithmetical problems, reading prolifically in an area, or doing intricate manual work. Sleeping on an idea or letting it brew beneath the surface for a while is also helpful. After the first draft, there will be ample time for revision, which in most cases, will involve excision. For the author or research investigator, the completed document is analogous to giving birth. Writing is a continuous process with much editing and revision. One should be careful not to prematurely abandon the initial efforts.

Previously, in Chapter 4, we talked about choosing a research topic. We stated that while the research topic must be meaningful to the researcher, the implications of the findings should lead to changes in the way in which the disability is viewed. These implications may affect evaluation or treatment of the disability, or result in changes in administrative or educational practices. The purpose of the research paper includes an explanation of why the question was formulated and how the research methodology serves to answer the question. In the final project, that is, the research paper, the writer summarizes the literature, discusses the findings, and makes specific recommendations based on these findings. In this way, the final scientific paper becomes a part of the body of literature, placing the research findings within the context of previous works (Locke, Spirduso, & Silverman, 1987).

A well thought-out research paper requires active contemplation by the writer. The conceptual relationships between previous research and present findings must be considered. The hypothesis or guiding question(s) proposed by the researcher must be concisely and clearly stated and should cover all the points covered in the paper (Slade, Campbell, & Ballou, 1994). The summary and arguments used in the paper to advance one's theory must be compared to viewpoints held by established researchers. On the other hand, a researcher may present findings that are contradictory to accepted beliefs in the scientific community. Under attack, the researcher must be able to defend the validity of the research findings. For example, in spite of common belief that dyslexia is a result of visual–perceptual deficits, such as seeing and writing letters backwards, researchers such as Liberman (1973) and Kamhi and Catts (1989) have espoused the underlying deficit in dyslexia to be language related.

Another essential component for writing a research paper is to understand as fully as possible the literature encompassing the topic being examined. This is accomplished by completing an exhaustive literature review as described in Chapter 5. The researcher will discover quickly, however, that much more literature has been reviewed than will be discussed in the paper. This fact does not minimize the need for an extensive literature review; rather, it emphasizes the need for the researcher to understand and master the relationship of a specific literature within the context of a body of knowledge. For example, a cogent understanding of the methods used to teach students with dyslexia to read requires an examination of landmark studies directly related to the identification and diagnosis of this disability. It is not uncommon to revise the initial hypothesis or guiding question several times, as one's knowledge base increases through reading and reviewing the literature.

Writing and reviewing literature is like an organic process that helps the researcher to modify his or her own thinking while extending his or her own knowledge base. It is a creative process that allows one to be objective and self-critical. This process is sometimes referred to as cognitive dissonance (the state in which there is conflict between one's attitudes and one's behavior, generally resulting in changing one's thinking so that there is equilibrium between the two), reflective decision-making (the process of making decisions by critically examining all sides of the issue), or the Socratic method of learning. All these methods rely on the individual's ability to question and rethink a body of knowledge.

9.2 Outlining the Research Paper

The overall organization of the research study, outlined in Table 9–1, is dictated by tradition. Each of the major sections within the research paper contains specific issues and topics.

I. Introduction to the Research Paper

The first part of the research paper contains a brief introduction to the present study, including the purpose, the research or guiding question(s), and the significance when examined beside findings from landmark studies (Best, 1977). A pivotal part of this portion of the research paper, article, or manuscript is a clear statement of the hypotheses or guiding questions such that they are (a) well understood, (b) lead the reader to anticipate the major sections of the paper, and (c) indicate the direction or argument in which the paper will be written (Winkler & McCuen, 1979). Finally, this part of the research paper should include definitions for any terminology that are uncommon or might not be understood by the reader (Best, 1977).

II. Review of the Literature

The second part of the research paper, which contains the literature review, is, to some extent, a measure of what the student knows about the subject (Best, 1977; Krathwohl, 1988). In some papers, this section and the previous section are written as a single part. In a thesis or dissertation, this section is traditionally identified as Chapter 2 or, if written with the introduction, as Chapter 1.

Table 9–1   *Major Parts of a Research Paper*

I.	Introduction to the Research Paper
	A. Statement of the Research Problem or Guiding Question
	B. Significance of the Research Problem
	C. Purposes of the Study
	D. Specific Definitions or Terms
II.	Review of the Literature
	A. Major Studies
	B. Critical Analysis of Key Studies
III.	Methodology
	A. Research Design
	1. Subjects (Number, Demographic Data)
	2. Procedures (Tests, Collection of Data)
	3. Statistical Analyses
IV.	Results
	A. Presentation and Analysis of Data
	B. Relevant Tables and Figures
V.	Discussion, Summary, Conclusions, and Implications of the Findings
	A. Limitations of the Study
	B. Significance of Study Related to Prior Research
	C. Future Research
VI.	Reference List and Appendices
VII.	Abstract (Placed after the Title Page)

The purpose of this section is to introduce further the reason for the study by reviewing previous research in the same area and by building a background for the study. Although it is not necessary to cite or review every article or book in the subject, as the researcher must presume that the reader has some knowledge in this area, the major studies must be discussed (American Psychological Association, 1994). For example, a student is interested in finding out more about the relationship between cerebral damage and spasticity. In a preliminary literature review, the student will have read or identified a number of articles on the etiology and prognosis of motor dysfunction as well as some clinical descriptions of cerebral damage. A more in-depth review will yield studies regarding the relationship between specific types of cerebral damage as it relates to motor dysfunction. A final review will examine those articles related to cerebral damage and spasticity. Although all of these articles may be important, only the articles related directly to the research question will be discussed at length.

One way to outline this portion of the research paper is to organize the articles reviewed (described in Chapter 5). If note cards were used, organization becomes a logical task of putting the note cards in the order in which they will be discussed. The selection of appropriate articles will be based on the findings as well as on the relationship of the article to the research question being examined. Some note cards will be put aside, as the articles will not be linked directly to the research question. Others will be mentioned only briefly, as a means of building a background underlying the rationale behind the research question. Some of the articles will be especially important in building a strong argument for the research design. A critical analysis of these articles will be an integral part of the literature review. Research literature and theory need to be reviewed and discussed objectively, citing both positive and negative research findings that relate to the present research question. In this way, one can avoid researcher bias, as shown in the following example from literature on treating dyslexia.

A student is interested in the relationship between reading ability and the use of tinted glasses for students with dyslexia. A review of literature identifies studies concerning improvement of reading with tinted glasses: (a) those in which there was no improvement (e.g., Saint-John & White, 1988; Winter, 1987); (b) those in which there was improvement (e.g., Adler & Attwood, 1987; O'Conner, Sofo, Kendall, & Olsen, 1990); and (c) those in which mixed success was noted (e.g., Blaskey, Scheiman, Parisi, Ciner, Gallaway, & Selznick, 1990). Each of these articles should be critically analyzed and critiqued, with special attention given to the methodology used in the studies and the relationship of the findings to the present research question. The student should present studies in which favorable and unfavorable results were found. In doing this, the student demonstrates objectivity in reviewing the literature and avoids research bias.

Once the note cards have been placed in a logical order, a formal outline should be written. There are many ways to write an outline. Some people prefer to use phrases or single words, while others prefer to use sentences for each level. Occasionally, a student may find it easier to jot down a paragraph describing and expanding on the topic. This paragraph becomes the outer edifice of the particular section. Regardless of the method that one chooses when organizing the topics, the outline facilitates the organization of the literature review.

An effective way to organize the outline and make it functional is to use parallel or grammatical structure. For example:

a. planning a therapy session
b. obtaining materials
c. positioning the student

is easier to comprehend than:

    a. plan the therapy session
    b. obtaining materials
    c. to position the student.

Use of parallel or grammatical structures in an outline is effective in clarifying one's writing. (Refer to the Section 9.6 [Format of a Paper] for further discussion regarding parallel structures.)

III. Methodology

The third section of the research paper includes a discussion of the methodology used in the study. This portion of the research paper should be written in a concise and succinct manner, with enough information available so that others can replicate the study.

Traditionally, there are three subdivisions in the methodology section: (a) subjects, (b) the apparatus or tests, and (c) the procedures used for data collection and analysis. Demographic information, such as the number of subjects, ages, gender, and ethnicity, is critical. Other additional demographic information that may be essential for the study might include educational level, socioeconomic level, handedness, disabilities, prior testing, and previous need for therapies or special education. If a control group is used, the demographics of the control group must be contrasted with the experimental group. The manner in which subjects were chosen (e.g., stratified random sample, voluntary response to a newspaper ad) is also described in this section.

A description of the tests or apparatus includes the names of the tests or surveys used, any laboratory equipment needed, and any specific directions or adaptations to the test or procedure which might not be found in a test manual. For example, if only part of an intelligence test is used, one must name the subtests chosen and justify the modification. When a standardized test is used, the reliability and validity of the test (or test portions used) must be indicated. If a survey or questionnaire has been developed for the study, a copy is put into the appendix following the major divisions of the paper.

Finally, the researcher describes the methods of data collection and the statistical procedures used to analyze it (Best, 1977). For example, did the researcher collect data alone, in person, or by telephone? Were others trained to collect the data? If a questionnaire was used, was it mailed or left in a public place for people to fill out as desired? Was a second letter sent as a follow-up? How long did data collection occur? Was it collected in one or two sessions? Was it collected by outcome measures (pre- and posttesting)? What type of statistical procedures were used to analyze the data?

IV. Results

The fourth section of the research paper presents the results and statistical findings from the study without attempting to interpret them. Each hypothesis is discussed separately, with statistical interactions and main effects reported. Tables and figures depicting significant relationships between variables often make the text more understandable; however, they should be self-explanatory and add to the information in the text rather than add new information.

V. Summary, Discussion, and Implications of the Findings

In the final section, the writer summarizes the findings and attempts to interpret them in the context of previous studies in the same field. Conclusions regarding acceptance or rejection of hypotheses are stated in this section. Although statements of generalization can be made here, one must be careful not to overgeneralize or overstate the significance of the findings. The writer should be aware of and state the limitations of the study and express any cautions regarding generalization to populations not included in the sample. Implications for further research, present practice, or policy changes are advanced, along with the arguments for these changes. The internal and external validity of the study should be discussed.

According to Best, the discussion section of the research paper is the most difficult part to write. Inexperienced authors tend to over- or undergeneralize, thinking their results less or more important than the data would support (Winkler & McCuen, 1979). The discussion section should be a critical and analytical summary of the findings rather than a superficial overview of the results. Because this part of the research paper is the most frequently read (Best, 1977), it is crucial that the researcher summarize the results and critically review these findings in the context of prior studies. The usefulness of the research paper, regardless of the findings, can be determined by the way in which the discussion section is written (Best, 1977).

VI. Reference List and Appendices

In the last section of the research paper, the writer needs to list all of the cited references. The writer must be careful not to leave out any reference and to include all information in the citation. There is nothing more frustrating than an incomplete citation when one wishes to obtain further information from the original article. (Refer to Section 9.5 [Bibliography] for further information.)

Sometimes a writer wishes to place a bibliography as well as a reference list into the research paper. A bibliography contains any article, book, or chapter that might be helpful in understanding the topic. A reference list, on the other hand, includes journal articles, books, or other sources used in the research and preparation of the paper and cited within the article (American Psychological Association, 1994). Any additional information (e.g., copy of the survey or test protocol, drawing of specific apparatus) can be placed in an appendix, following the list of references.

VII. Abstract

The abstract of a research study, which is written last and placed at the beginning of the study, contains summary statements of each independent unit or section (i.e., the problem, literature review, research design, methodology, results, discussion, and conclusions). The abstract should contain enough information so that the reader will know the purposes of the study, the specific variables or groups investigated, the number of subjects, the measuring instruments used, the results, and the conclusions presented. An abstract of a research study usually is limited to 150 to 500 words. When preparing an abstract, it is useful to extract key sentences from each part of the study, then integrate the sentences through transitional phrases. Abstracts are extremely important to investigators reviewing literature; it is therefore vital to present as complete a summary of the total study as possible within the number of words permitted. Abstracts are not merely a summary or discussion of the results as perceived by some investigators. An abstract should be a complete statement representative of the total study. Whenever possible, key words or phrases should be identified by the author and placed below the abstract. These key words are used in data retrieval systems (see Chapter 5).

9.3 Writing the First Draft

The first draft is started after completing the outline. As stated above, the outline is important to aid one in organizing the literature review. The writer must be aware that the outline is not set in stone. After the first draft has been written, the organization may need to be revised. Nonetheless, having an outline allows the writer to have a sense of the direction in which the paper is going.

Perhaps the hardest part of writing is putting one's initial thoughts on paper. One should write these initial thoughts with the expectation of revising them later. There will be plenty of time for revision after the first draft has been written. It is expected that the first draft will need to be revised a number of times.

A difficult skill for the inexperienced writer is the ability to use notes effectively. There is a tendency to quote extensively rather than paraphrase the author's words. Frequently, this is due to difficulty in understanding what the author meant. If this is the case, one must do additional reading and studying until the material is completely understood. Although quotes from the original source can be an effective means of relating information, too many quotes make the research paper difficult to read and leave "the impression that students have done [no more than] 'cut and paste' from books and articles they have read" (Winkler & McCuen, 1979, p. 114). It is better to use quotations sparingly, intermixing the quotations with summaries and paraphrases of the original sources. When quoting or paraphrasing, one must document the source. (See section on quotations.)

The literary and scientific styles used for citations are determined often by a particular discipline. The three most commonly used systems are *The Chicago Manual of Style* (University of Chicago Press, 1993), the *Modern Language Association* (MLA; Gibaldi, 1995), the *American Medical Association Manual of Style* (Iverson, 1989), and the *American Psychological Association* (American Psychological Association, [APA], 1994). The latter style is used most frequently in psychology, education, and social and health sciences and will be discussed in this book.

The essential reference book for APA style is the *Publication Manual of the American Psychological Association* (4th edition; 1994), generally available in university or college bookstores. If the university or local technical bookstore does not have one, it can be obtained from the American Psychological Association in Washington, D.C. Because of the extensiveness of the APA style, one will need to refer to this manual frequently. It is wise to get into the habit of referring to the *APA Manual* whenever there is a question about style, language mechanics, or format of the paper. Major highlights of the *APA Manual* will be discussed in the following sections of this chapter; however, because of space limitations, not all topics will be covered in detail.

9.4 Making Revisions

Once the research paper has been written, revisions will be necessary. It is not uncommon to revise the research paper five or six times. Each time the writer reviews the research paper for accuracy and cohesiveness, he or she may discover additional ways for revision or clarity.

The function of revision is to make sure that specific editing requirements have been followed. These editing requirements are summarized in Table 9–2.

9.4.1 Gender or Ethnic Bias

First, the writer will want to make sure that no gender or ethnic bias has been introduced into the paper or into the study. Guidelines have been established by the APA for avoiding sexist and ethnic language in journal articles. Gender bias occurs when the writer uses the term *man* to mean the human race rather than using a less ambiguous term such as *person, people,* or *individual*. Additionally, use of specific gender words (e.g., his, her) or using terms that end in *man* or *men* (e.g., *postman, chairman, policemen*) must be avoided. Stereotyping (e.g., the school psychologist . . . he; mothering) can be avoided by using specific language (e.g., boys enjoyed playing with Legos while girls enjoyed reading), by using parallel language (e.g., *men and women* rather than *men and girls*), or by changing the term to a plural (e.g., *them* instead of *his* or *her*) (American Psychological Association, 1994).

Table 9–2 *Checklist for Proofing One's Article*

1. **Gender and Ethnic Bias**
   - Is the article free of language that might be ambiguous or stereotypical?
2. **People First**
   - Is the manuscript written with the individual emphasized rather than the disability?
   - Have all references to a disability been written in the form *individual with. . .* ?
3. **Grammar**
   - Are there run-on sentences or sentence fragments?
   - Are there split infinitives, dangling modifiers, errors in verb–subject agreement?
   - Is the writing in parallel structure?
   - Are relative pronouns used appropriately?
   - Has a grammatical program been used to check the grammar?
4. **Spelling/Punctuation**
   - Has a speller been used to check spelling?
   - Has the article been reviewed for commas, quotation marks, hyphens, and apostrophes?
5. **Abbreviations**
   - Is the abbreviation placed in parentheses following the full term the first time it is used?
   - Are the Latin abbreviations used correctly and according to APA style?
   - Are abbreviations invented by the author kept to a minimum?
6. **Transitional Words, Phrases, and Sentences**
   - Are there transitional statements or words between ideas?
   - Is there a sense of unity and integration in the paper?
   - Do words such as *however, although,* or *nevertheless* need to be added?
7. **Clarity**
   - Is the language clear and simple?
   - Do any unusual terms need to be explained or defined?
   - Would a figure or table help explain the information?
8. **Organization**
   - Do the hypotheses or guiding question(s) drive the content of the research paper?
   - Is there consistency between sections?
   - Are unnecessary repetitions removed?
   - Is the sequence of the research paper logical and coherent?

Ethnic bias occurs when the writer attributes to a specific ethnic group something that has no supporting data (American Psychological Association, 1994). An example of this stereotyping occurs when one writes "In general, all students with learning disabilities tend to be unmotivated in the classroom." APA suggests that an informal test can be completed by substituting another group (e.g., your own) for the group being discussed. If the writer perceives offense in the revised statement, then bias is probably present.

9.4.2 *People First* Language

A *second reason* for revision is to make sure that the writing is in *People First* language. As a result of the Individuals with Disabilities Education Act (1990), all references to disabilities must be written with the individual placed first. Thus, *child with autism* is correct, while the *autistic child* is incorrect. This convention emphasizes the value of the human being and delegates the disability to secondary importance.

The writer must distinguish also between the terms *handicap* and *disability*. A handicap can be thought of as a disadvantage that makes achievement difficult, whereas a disability is something that an individual is unable to do. For example, a student who is deaf cannot hear; the inability to hear is a disability. However, the lack of hearing only becomes a handicap if the student is unwilling to use a hearing aid, learn sign language, or develop some other method of communicating. Individuals with disabilities are not necessarily handicapped.

9.4.3 Mechanics of Writing

Clear writing requires that one use a formal writing style and that one's writing is grammatically correct. A *third reason* to revise the manuscript is to make sure that there are no grammatical errors. Errors such as subject–verb agreement (e.g., *data is* rather than *data are*), punctuation and capitalization, run-on sentences, and sentence phrases are common for inexperienced writers. Run-on sentences and sentence fragments are an indication that either the writer is careless and has not proofread the research paper or that the writer needs help with writing skills. Other common errors include: (a) failing to use parallel structure for grammatical units (e.g., using different parts of speech in a series or in connecting phrases), (b) having dangling modifiers (e.g., sentences in which the modifier is misplaced such as "It is also believed," rather than "Also it is believed"), (c) splitting infinitives, (d) improperly using relative pronouns, (e) using the passive tense rather than the active tense, and (f) placing prepositions at the end of sentences ("...ethical and legal obligations that special educators are faced with" rather than "ethical and legal obligations which special educators face"). If one is unsure about the proper grammatical structure, a basic grammar book is indispensable. Examples of these errors as well as the correct usage are illustrated in Figure 9–1.

Many excellent references are available that help the writer avoid grammatical errors and improve his or her writing. Major references and computers software programs available for checking spelling and grammar are also listed.

- Strunk, W. Jr., & White, E. B. (1979). *The Elements of Style* (3rd ed.). New York: Macmillian.
  A 92-page gold mine of writing ideas, including rules of usage, principles of composition form, and writing style. The epitome of concise, effective writing.
- American Psychological Association (1994). *Publication Manual of the American Psychological Association* (4th ed.). Washington, DC: Author.

Type	Rules	Incorrect Example	Correct Usage
DANGLING OR MISPLACED MODIFIER OR PARTICIPLE	Modifiers and participles should be put as close as possible to the word they are to modify in order to prevent ambiguity or missing referents.	. . . would first determine. . . . . . local issues in that particular school that affect job satisfaction	. . . would determine first . . . . . . local issues that affect job satisfaction in that particular school
SPLIT INFINITIVES	Place adverbs that modify the verb after the phase "to . . ." rather than between the "to" and the verb.	Administrators have to also keep in mind	Administrators have to keep in mind also . . .
PARALLEL STRUCTURE	Expressions similar in function or content should be in the same grammatical construction.	(a) identification and clarification of . . . (b) assessment of . . . (c) determine whether . . .	(a) identification and clarification of . . . (b) assessment of . . . (c) determination of . . .
RELATIVE PRONOUNS	Use *that* with a restrictive clause (i.e., is essential to the passage).		The students that participated in the races were all second graders.
	Use *which* with an unrestrictive clause surrounded by commas (adds information, but is not essential to the sentence).		The glasses, which were on top of the container, belonged to the student.
	Use *who* in unrestrictive clauses in reference to people.		The students, who were all second graders, won ribbons at the races. (Note the commas in this sentence.)
VOICE (ACTIVE/PASSIVE)	Use the active voice whenever possible.	The authors' purpose for this article was to examine . . .	The authors examined . . .

Figure 9-1. Common errors of writing style. (Adapted from the *Publication Manual of the American Psychological Association* by the American Psychological Association [1994] and *Form and Style* by C. Slade, W. G. Campbell, and S. V. Ballou. [1994].) *(continued)*

Type	Rules	Incorrect Example	Correct Usage
POSSESSIVES	Place an apostrophe after the noun or pronoun to show possession. **Exception:** do not use an apostrophe after the word it when showing possession.	The subjects scores . . . It's major strengths are . . .	The subject's score was . . . The Wechsler has 12 subtests. Its first score is . . . **But:** It's cold (It is cold)
SERIATION	Place elements in a series in parallel form. (See Table 9-4 for correct punctuation.)	. . . asked to read the directions, fill out the information, and then to turn in the form.	. . . to read the directions, fill out the information, and turn in the form.
	When the series of items is written in one sentence, use letters to separate each item. Use commas to separate the items, unless there are internal commas. Use semicolons to separate items of major categories.	The subjects were administered four tests: WISC-III, a test of intelligence; WJ–R, a test of achievement; Bender, a test of visual perception; and WCST, a test of organization.	The subjects were administered four tests: (a) WISC-III, a test of intelligence; (b) WJ–R, a test of achievement; (c) Bender, a test of visual perception; and (d) WCST, a test of organization.
	When each item in the series is placed into separate sentences or separate paragraphs, use numbers to separate the items.		The subjects were administered 3 tests: 1. The WISC-III to assess intelligence 2. The WJ–R to assess achievement 3. The Bender to assess visual-motor integration.
PRONOUNS	Make sure that the referent for the pronoun is clear.	This was completed. Those were put over there.	This test was completed. Those books were put over there, on the bottom shelf.

Figure 9–1. *(continued)*

Type	Rules	Incorrect Example	Correct Usage
PRONOUNS (con't)	Make sure that the pronoun agrees in number with the noun it replaces and/or modifies the noun	His work was placed in their folder. The group took their packages . . .	His work was placed in his folder. The group took its packages . . .
SUBJECT-VERB AGREEMENT	Verbs must agree with the subject, regardless of intervening phrases and/or use of pronouns.	Data is; phenomena is The articles that were taken from a single journal was . . .	Data are; phenomena are The articles that were taken from a single journal were . . .
MISPLACED PREPOSITIONS	Prepositions should not be placed at the end of the sentences.	. . . the next area the clinicians were questioned in . . .	. . . the next area in which the clinicians were questioned.

Figure 9–1. *(continued)*

An exhaustive guide to organizing a journal article for publication. Includes content areas such as headings, quotations, references, tables, figures and graphs, and other matters of style that can keep a writer up all night.

- Turabian, K. L. (1987). *A Manual for Writers of Term Papers, Theses, and Dissertations* (6th ed.). Chicago: University of Chicago Press.
  If the APA style manual is confusing on a question of style Turabian is the final word. These three little books: Strunk and White, *APA Manual*, and Turabian give the student a complete guide to writing a scholarly paper that no professor can fault.

- Slade, C., Campbell, W. G., & Ballou, S. V. (1994). *Form and Style*. Boston: Houghton Mifflin.
  A well-written, up-to-date, and clear guide for writing research papers. Focuses on the processes of writing as well as gives detailed coverage of *The Chicago Manual*, Modern Language Association, and American Psychological Association styles. Helpful for the inexperienced writer, as there are many examples in the text.

- *Roget's Thesaurus* (1994). Miami, FL: Paradise Press.
  An invaluable guide to the writer for selecting the most appropriate word. It is helpful in locating a specific word and in varying language.

- Thomas, C. L. (Ed.). (1993). *Taber's Cyclopedic Medical Dictionary* (17th ed.). Philadelphia: F. A. Davis.
  An essential guide for those researchers needing medical terms defined and clarified.

- *Merriam–Webster's Collegiate Dictionary* (10th ed.). (1993). Springfield, MA: Merriam–Webster.

- Weiss–Lambrou, R. (1989). *The Health Professional's Guide to Writing for Publication*. Springfield, IL: Charles C. Thomas.

- Church, G., & Bender, M. (1989). *Teaching with Computers! A Curriculum for Special Educators*. Boston: Little, Brown.
  This handy book describes software that is intended to help the writer with grammar and spelling.

A *fourth reason* for revision is to check for spelling and punctuation errors. It is critical to check one's spelling with a speller (available with most word processing programs) to insure that there are no errors. One must be careful, however, to read the article and proof for errors, rather than rely on the computerized speller to find all the errors. It cannot find errors when the words are spelled correctly, but misused. For example, if the words *to* and *too* are used incorrectly, the speller will not identify the error.

Punctuation errors must be located and corrected. Figure 9–2, adapted from the *APA Manual* (1994) and Slade, Campbell, and Ballou (1994), summarizes common punctuation rules. Reading the paper aloud is one method to revise the paper and locate errors in punctuation and grammar.

In scientific articles it is common practice to abbreviate terms used repeatedly. For example, proprioceptive facilitation can be abbreviated (PF), neurodevelopmental therapy (NDT), learning disability (LD), perceptual–motor training (PMT), and quality food index (QFI). Abbreviations invented by the writer should be kept to a minimum and used only for terms that are long and frequently repeated. Tables of statistical data containing abbreviations should contain a footnote defining the abbreviations.

	Type	Rule	Example
COMMA	**Seriation**	Use a comma after each word in a series of three or more items.	. . . equipment, apparatus, and tools. . .
	Parenthetical expression	Use a comma before and after a phrase that adds information, but is not essential.	Collaboration can be an informal process, where two individuals meet to discuss a problem, or. . .
	Independent clause	Use a comma to separate independent clauses, but do not use to separate the two parts of a compound predicate.	Five of the subjects were Black, and seven of the subjects were Anglo. (But notice: Six students were in seventh grade and were taking history.)
	Essential or restrictive clauses	Do not use a comma when the modifying phrase is used to identify, limit, or define a word and is essential to the meaning.	The subjects that were used for the control group included seven occupational therapists.
	Dependent clauses	Use a comma rather than a semicolon to separate a dependent and independent phrase.	Although the students with mental handicaps were separated from the general education students, all the subjects were placed into a single group for evaluation.
SEMICOLON	**Independent clauses**	Use a semicolon when the independent clauses are not separated by a coordinating conjunction or when the clauses are separated by a conjunctive adverb.	The apparatus was put on the shelves; the writing materials were put into the desk. The client was interviewed . . .; however, . . .
	Seriation	Use a semicolon when there is a comma contained in any part of the seriation.	. . .: (a) red box, which contained 3 balls; (b) blue box, which contained 2 balls; and (c) yellow box, which contained 6 balls.
COLON	**References**	Use a colon after the place of publication and before the publisher	Boston, NY: Allyn and Bacon.

Figure 9-2. Common errors of punctuation. (Adapted from the *Publication Manual of the American Psychological Association* by the American Psychological Association [1994] and *Form and Style* by C. Slade, W. G. Campbell, and S. V. Ballou [1994].) *(continued)*

Type	Rule	Example
COLON (con't)		
Phrases	Use a colon before a phrase or example of explanatory material with an introductory phrase. If the example is a complete sentence, start it with a capital letter.	The recorded scores were in the following order: 37, 49, 24, 70. The material was made up of the following parts: two blue boxes, each of which contained 4 toys.
QUOTATION MARKS		
Direct quotation	Put quotation marks around any direct quote of 40 words or fewer. If the direct quote is more than 40 words, offset it in a paragraph, and indent on both right and left margins. Cite the reference with the author, date, and page, or just the page in parentheses following the quote.	Locke, Spirduso, and Silverman (1987) caution that "[t]he problem in writing a proposal is essentially the same as in writing the final report" (p. 19). "The problem in writing a proposal is essentially the same as in writing the final report" (Locke, Spirduso, & Silverman, 1987, p. 19).
Titles	Put quotation marks around any title of a chapter or article cited in the text. Do not put around any title in the reference list.	John's review discussed Chapter 2, "The Scientific Method."
Terms	Use quotation marks when introducing a word or phrase used as slang, irony, or invented term. Do not use quotation marks when the word or phrase is used a second time. Do not use with commonly used foreign terms.	Ninja coined the term "normalization". . . But: per se vis a vis
PARENTHESES		
Parenthetical information	Use parentheses to set off material that is independent of the rest of the information. Put punctuation marks inside the parentheses if the material is a sentence and outside the parentheses if the material is a phrase.	The subjects (15 boys and 2 girls) were . . .
References	Enclose citations with parentheses.	(Jones & Smith, 1994); Jones and Smith (1994)

Figure 9–2. *(continued)*

Type		Rule	Example
PARENTHESES (con't)	Abbreviations	Abbreviations should be put in parentheses the first time the full term is used. Thereafter, the abbreviation can be used instead of the full term.	Least restrictive environment (LEA). . . . . . LEA
	Seriation	Enclose the letters used in seriation in parentheses.	(a) . . . , (b) . . . , and (c) . . . .
BRACKETS	Parenthetical material	Enclose parenthetical material that is within parentheses in brackets, unless the use of commas will not confuse the reader.	(The other team [wearing red uniforms]. . .) (Jones and Smith, 1990, denied this allegation.)
	References	Enclose material inserted into a quotation with brackets.	". . . [the students in the study] were asked to come . . ."

Figure 9-2. *(continued)*

Latin abbreviations are useful for shortening sentences. The following are the most commonly used abbreviations in scientific articles:

- ca. (circa): about a certain time, e.g., ca. BC 130
- e.g. (exempli gratia): for example
- et al. (et alii): and others
- et seq (et sequens): and the following
- ibid (ibidem): in the same place
- i.e. (id est): that is to say
- viz. (videlicet): namely, used to introduce lists.

Be sure to refer to the *APA Manual* for the proper way to use abbreviations. For example, the abbreviations i.e. and e.g. must be used within parentheses.

9.4.4 Transitional Words, Phrases, Sentences

A *fifth reason* for revision is to make sure that transitional statements are present so that the flow of ideas is smooth. Writing a well-organized, integrated manuscript requires the use of words and phrases that connect ideas and summarize a section of a paper. In reviewing scientific literature, it is important to integrate the studies under topical areas and to develop a logical sequence. Writing should be coherent. The use of transitional words such as *however, although*, or *nevertheless*, can be used to make the transition smoother and the paper unified. In addition, sentences can be used to permit the smooth transition from one idea to another. The reader should have no difficulty following the train of thought or the arguments used to build a case. Additionally, reading the research paper as a whole will uncover any inconsistencies or repetitions between sections (Slade, Campbell, & Ballou, 1994). Often, having someone unacquainted with the topic read the research paper serves to ensure clarity, understanding, and consistency.

9.4.5 Clarity of Thought

The scientific writer should try to communicate ideas simply and rigorously. Some of the most profound ideas can be expressed in clear, direct language. It is not a sign of intellectual prowess to present ideas so that they are difficult to understand. Therefore, a *sixth reason* for revision is to insure that the paper is written clearly. Scientific writing is particularly prone to abstruseness and ambiguity, especially in clinical areas where language is used loosely, without precise operational definitions. One method of insuring clarity is to include an conceptual or operational definition for unusual terms, or terms specific to a certain discipline. Even if the writer chooses not to create a glossary, uncommon terms must be operationally defined. Use of well thought-out charts, tables, or figures can facilitate the clarity of the research paper. It is not unusual for readers to look at charts, tables, or figures before reading the text, especially when these visual aids provide an overall summary of the principle finding.

9.4.6 Organization

Finally, the author should examine whether the background information is represented accurately, whether ideas unrelated to the topic have been introduced, and whether the hypothesis or guiding statement(s) have directed the writing (Slade, Campbell, & Ballou, 1994). Each statement of results should be supported by data. Differences or contradictions in findings compared to previous studies need to be discussed and, when possible, explained. Finally, the whole research paper should be reviewed for sequence of ideas. Eventually, even though additional changes are possible, the writer must accept the paper as it is.

> the secret of good writing is to strip every sentence to its cleanest components. Every word that serves no function, every long word that could be a short word, every adverb which carries the same meaning that is already in the verb, every passive construction that leaves the reader unsure of who is doing what—these are the thousand and one adulterants that weaken the strength of a sentence. (Zinsser, 1980, pp. 7–8)

9.5 Quotations, Referenced Material, and Bibliographic Citations

Whenever one uses material written by another person, whether the material is directly quoted or only paraphrased, one must make reference to the original author(s). Failure to do so is plagiarism. Some authors (Winkler & McCuen, 1979) have suggested that plagiarism is common in everyday language. Commonly, one might use in speech an example stated in a lecture by a professor and fail to give that professor the credit. In another case one may use a proverb such as "A stitch in time saves nine" and fail to give Benjamin Franklin the credit. While these examples are not routinely considered to be plagiarism, and therefore are generally acceptable in everyday speech, plagiarism is not accepted in a research or scholarly paper.

Plagiarism occurs when a researcher deliberately takes another person's ideas and incorporates them into his or her own writing without giving any credit to the original author. Examples of plagiarism include the following: (a) taking another's research ideas and submitting them as one's own, (b) paraphrasing an article without giving credit to the author, or (c) directly copying part of an article without citing the authors. Any copyright material used without giving credit to the original author is considered plagiarism (Winkler & McCuen, 1979).

If the material used is a direct quote from another author or authors, the writer must cite the author(s), year of publication, and page number of the quotation in the text. There must be no change in spelling, phrasing, capitalization, or punctuation from the original. The exception to this rule is when the first word of a quotation needs to be capitalized or placed in lower case in order to make the statement grammatically correct. When it is necessary to make changes (e.g., when a pronoun must be clarified or a word added to make the content more understandable), the change must be put in square brackets ([ ]). When a word is misspelled or the grammar is incorrect in the original, [*sic*] follows the misspelling or grammatical error to show that the quotation is reproduced exactly. For example, "The article was written by an england [*sic*] author."

A quote can be introduced as part of a grammatical sentence, or it may stand alone as a sentence. When material is omitted from the quotation, then an ellipsis (. . .) replaces the material which is left out. When the quote is more than 40 words, it should stand alone as a separate paragraph. In this case, the quoted material is punctuated, and the reference for the quoted material is placed after the paragraph, in parenthesis and with no punctuation. Examine the following:

> Slang, hackneyed or flippant phrases, and folksy style should be avoided. Since objectivity is the primary goal, there should be no element of exhortation or persuasion. The re-

search report should describe and explain, rather than try to convince or move to action. In this respect, the research report differs from the essay or the feature article. (Best, 1977, p. 317)

When the material has fewer than 40 words, it is placed within the paragraph. The reference is placed in parentheses at the end of the quote. For example: According to Best (1977), "The research report should be presented in a style that is creative, clear, and concise" (p. 317).

When the writer wishes to paraphrase another author's material, then the writer must cite the author(s) and date of publication. Examine the following two examples:

1. Best (1977) suggests that when writing a research article, one must be careful to write concisely and clearly.
2. When writing a research article, one must be careful to write concisely and clearly (Best, 1977; Winkler & McCuen, 1979).

Notice that no page numbers are used in either reference and that the author's name is put within parentheses at the end of the sentence if it has not been used as part of the sentence structure. Additional information regarding common citations of authors in the text is summarized in Figure 9–3.

Whether the writer has quoted the source directly or paraphrased the material, a complete reference must be placed into the references at the end of the research paper. Figure 9–4 summarizes the different styles for common reference citations and Table 9–3 shows some examples of these citations. Further information regarding the appropriate style for dissertations, secondary sources, movies, or films can be found in the *APA Manual*. Regardless of the type of publication, all citations must include enough information so that the reader can locate the original source.

9.6 Format of a Paper

The format of the research paper is dictated by the style of writing used. For journal publications using the APA style, the size of the margins, line spacing, and size of print are specified. Individual professors and non-APA style journals may have different requirements. In a thesis or dissertation, additional sections are required. A typical organization of the sequence for a thesis or dissertation is listed below.

1. Title Page (see Figure 9–5)
2. Approval page indicating names and titles of thesis readers (required for a thesis or dissertation only)
3. Acknowledgments, including individuals who aided in the study and any grant support accepted
4. Table of Contents, including chapter and section headings, appendix, and bibliography
5. List of Statistical Tables
6. List of Illustrations, Photographs, and Figures
7. Abstract
8. The Content of the Text

	FIRST CITATION	ADDITIONAL CITATIONS IN THE TEXT
ONE AUTHOR	Last name, year, page (when applicable) Smith (1994) . . . (p. 94); (Smith, 1994, p. 94)	Last name, year, page, (when applicable) Smith (1994) or (Smith, 1994)
TWO AUTHORS	Last names, "and" or "&", year: Smith and Jones (1994); (Smith & Jones, 1994).	Last names and "and" or "&", year: Smith and Jones (1994); (Smith & Jones, 1994).
THREE TO SIX AUTHORS	Last names, separated by a comma, "and" or "&", year Smith, Jones, Johnson, and James (1994); (Smith, Jones, Johnson, & James, 1994)	Last name of first author, et al., year. Smith et al., (1994); (Smith et al., 1994
SIX OR MORE AUTHORS	Last name of first author, et al., year. Smith et al., (1994); (Smith et al., 1994)	Last name of first author, et al., year Smith et al., (1994)
TWO OR MORE CITATIONS	(James, Smith, & Johnson, 1994; Markley & Bennett, 1994)	(James et al., 1994; Markley & Bennett, 1994)

Figure 9-3. Citations within the body of the text. A citation is for direct quotes and paraphrases of someone else's writing. (Adapted from the *Publication Manual of the American Psychological Association* by the American Psychological Association [1994] and *Form and Style* by C. Slade, W. G. Campbell, and S. V. Ballou [1994].)

	Book	Journal	Chapter from a Book
Author(s)	Last name(s), initials, ... & last name, initials. No punctuation at the end. **Jones, M. J., & Smith J. C.**	Last name(s), initials, . . . & last name, initials. No punctuation at the end. **Jones, M. J., Johnson, P. G., & Smith, J. C.**	last name(s), initials, & last name, initials. No punctuation at the end. **Johnson, M. J., & James, P. G.**
Year	Place the year in parentheses, and put period after the parentheses: **(1994).**	Place year in parentheses and put period after the parentheses. For weekly issues, put the month, date, and year in parentheses: **(1977, October 15).**	Place year in parentheses, put period after the parentheses: **(1994).**
Title of Book, Article, Chapter	Capitalize first word of the book and first word after a colon. End with a period unless there is an edition number. Underline the title of book or put it in italics. **Evaluation of classroom progress.**	Capitalize first word of the journal article and first word after a colon. End with a period. Do not underline the article title or put it in quotations: **Evaluation of classroom procedures.**	Capitalize first word of the chapter from a book and first word after a colon. End the chapter title with a period: **Evaluation of classroom procedures.**
Title of Journal		Capitalize important words in the journal title and underline it. Put a comma after the title: **Journal of Aging,**	
Editor	Place the terms (Ed.). or (Eds.). after author(s). Place a period at the end: **James, J. B., & Jones, J. J. (Eds.).**		Place the words term (Ed.) or (Eds.). after the author(s). Place a period at the end: **In J. C. Jones & M. C. Smith (Eds.), Evaluation procedures pp. 779–89.**

Figure 9-4. Common bibliographic references. These references are listed at the end of the research paper. Additional information regarding the appropriate style for dissertations, secondary sources, movies or films can be found in the *APA Manual*. (Adapted from the *Publication Manual of the American Psychological Association* [1994] and C. Slade, W. G. Campbell, & W. V. Ballou [1994].) *(continued)*

	BOOK	JOURNAL	CHAPTER FROM A BOOK
EDITION	Put the edition number of the book in parentheses following title of the book. Place period at the end: **(2nd ed.).**		
VOLUME		Underline the volume number, place a comma after the number: _17,_	
ISSUE		Only include the issue number if each issue begins with page 1; place the issue number in parentheses after the volume number: _17_ (2),	
PAGE		Place the page number after the volume (or issue) number. Put a period after the page number. Don't use p. or pp.: **79–95.**	Place the page numbers of the chapter inside parentheses after title of the book. Put a period after the parentheses. Use p. or pp.: (pp. 355–390).
PLACE OF PUBLICATION	City, State: Publisher. Boston, MA: Allyn & Bacon.		City, State: Publisher. Boston, MA: Allyn & Bacon.

Figure 9–4. (continued)

Table 9-3 *Examples of Bibliographic Reference*

- ***Book***
  Locke, L. F., Spirduso, W. W., & Silverman, S. J. (1987). *Proposals that work* (2nd ed.). Newbury Park: Sage.
- ***Journal Article***
  Smith, J. C., & Jones, J. M. (1993). Reconstructing the facial features. *Journal of Paleontology, 17,* 339–431.
- ***Chapter***
  Rutter, M., Chadwick, O., & Shaffer, D. (1983). Head injury. In M. Rutter (Ed.), *Developmental Neuropsychiatry* (pp. 83–111). New York: Guilford.

Note. Additional information regarding the appropriate style for dissertations, secondary sources, movies or films can be found in the *APA Manual.* Adapted from the *Publication Manual of the American Psychological Association* (1994) and Slade, Campbell, & Ballou (1994).

Boston University

College of Allied Health Professions

The Effect of Biofeedback
on the
Hyperactivity of a 10-Year-Old Male

by
Barbara Stein, B. S.

Submitted in partial fulfilment
of the
requirements for the degree of

Master of Science

September 1995

Figure 9-5. Example of a title page for a research paper, thesis, or dissertation.

   a. Introduction
   b. Review of the Literature
   c. Methodology
   d. Results
   e. Discussion, including clinical implications of findings and limitations of study
   f. Conclusions and further research
9. Bibliography and References
10. Appendix
11. Vita, listing professional education, work history, and previous publications.

A running title, consisting of three or four words, is placed flush right on the title page. APA style dictates the position of page numbers (usually below the running title), the use of roman and arabic numbers, the type of paper, and the levels of heading. The text should be double-spaced, with quotations that have been indented either single or double space.

9.6.1 Outline of a Research Proposal

1. Title of Study
2. Investigator
3. Date
4. The Research Problem
   a. statement of problem in question form
   b. justification and need for the study
   c. implications of anticipated results in relation to clinical treatment, professional, education, or administrative problems
5. The Literature Review
   a. outline of major areas to be reviewed
   b. plan for search of related literature
   c. annotated bibliographical notation organized under major areas reviewed
6. Research Design
   a. research model, (e.g., experimental, correlational, or methodological)
   b. operational definitions of variables
   c. statement of hypotheses or guiding questions
   d. identification of presumed independent or dependent variables
   e. theoretical explanation underlying study
7. Methodology
   a. procedure for selecting sample and screening criteria for subject inclusion
   b. setting for study and procedure for collecting data
   c. tests, questionnaires, or instruments applied to study
   d. methodological studies to include evaluation of
      • reliability
      • validity
   e. tentative time schedule for study:
      • time period for literature review
      • collection of data: number of hours required
      • date for completion of research

    f.   projected costs for study:
- clerical
- instrumentation
- other

8.   References

9.7 Sample Proposal of a Graduate Research Project

The Sample Proposal of a Graduate Research Project on pages 387–410 is reprinted with the permission of the author.

Survey of the Needs

of

Undergraduate Students with Mobility Impairments

Attending

Public Postsecondary Educational Institutions in the Midwest

Completed by:

Sarah Ruth Schweppe Montgomery

Completed for:

Franklin Stein, Ph.D., OTR/L

Submitted:

March 29, 1994

i

1   TABLE OF CONTENTS

1.0   **THE RESEARCH PROBLEM**

1.1   STATEMENT OF RESEARCH PROBLEM IN QUESTION FORM:

How many undergraduate students with disabilities are currently enrolled in postsecondary educational institutions in the United States? In the Midwest?

How many students with disabilities are classified as having a physical disability?

How does the Americans with Disabilities Act of 1990 (ADA) define the term "disability"?

How does the ADA define "physical" disability?

What are the different types of physical disabilities?

How does the ADA define "mobility impaired"?

What does the ADA state in regards to meeting the needs of the college students with disabilities?

What are the needs of college students with disabilities?

Are postsecondary educational institutions in the Midwest meeting the needs of the population of students with disabilities?

Has there been a recent increase in the number of students with disabilities on college campuses?

If there has been an increase in students with disabilities on campuses, what factors have contributed to this increase?

1.2   JUSTIFICATION AND NEED FOR THE STUDY:

The 1989-90 school year welcomed 12.7 million undergraduate students onto college campuses in the United States. Of those 12.7 million students, approximately 7 percent of the undergraduate population reported having some kind of disability. In other words, almost 900,000 of the students enrolled in undergraduate institutions during the 1989-90 school year had a disability (U.S. Department of Education, 1993).

Over the last decade, the number of students with disabilities on the nation's college campuses has tripled (Rothstein, 1991). The increase in students with disabilities has challenged colleges to create programs which provide access to higher education for students with disabilities without discrimination. The services provided to this population must "help ensure that higher education environments are attitudinally, as well as physically, accessible" (Sergent, Carter, Sedlacek, & Scales, 1988, p. 21).

1

Both able-bodied and students with disabilities enter higher education with the expectation that the time and energy they invest will somehow improve their quality of life in the future. It seems obvious that the more education one receives, the more one learns. According to McLoughlin (1982),

> If the added knowledge obtained through higher education translates into increased economic benefits for minorities, and it seems to have done so, then the physically handicapped, as much as any group and possibly more than most, have a substantial need for these economic benefits because their ordinary living expenses are so great. (p. 241)

Furthermore, Bowman and Marzouk (1992) noted that,

> Data suggest that education may be the route out of the poverty and financial dependency that many Americans with disabilities experience. It is clear, therefore, that colleges and universities have an important role in helping Americans with disabilities attain the same opportunities in higher education as Americans without disabilities, thus helping them to become an integral part of American society. (p. 522)

Therefore, it is necessary that every effort be put forth to create an environment, in higher education, which is equally accessible to persons with disabilities as it is to persons without disabilities. The philosophy of the office of services for students with disabilities at the University of Pennsylvania supports this assumption as it states:

> Society, not the particular individual, creates handicaps. Disabled persons can and should make a positive contribution to society. With a college education, many disabled individuals have been able to make the world better for all people, not just themselves. Because of disability, a particular person will need some assistance in order to survive as a university student. A disabled student must learn more than just an academic discipline while in college. He/she must also learn to function independently and become a productive member of society (Foulk, 1990, p. 6).

2

In 1980, Penn and Dudley conducted a survey which asked college students with disabilities why they valued a higher education. The majority of the participants reported that they considered their college education as a way of "increasing their employability and economic security" (Penn & Dudley, 1980, p. 355). Furthermore, some of those surveyed stated, "that a college education was a means to become more self-supporting and a way to develop a more independent life-style" (Penn & Dudley, 1980, p. 355).

It was not until 1990, under the Americans with Disabilities Act (ADA), that it became required for both public and private postsecondary educational institutions to "make special accommodations and adjustments to insure that students do not experience discrimination which is based on disabling conditions" (Frank & Wade, 1993, p. 26). The ADA was passed into law on July 26, 1990 and prohibits discrimination on the basis of disability. It is currently unknown whether or not all colleges have followed the instructions of this law in order to meet the needs of students with disabilities. Failure to make mandatory modifications to campuses might "result in significant financial liability, costly litigation, loss of public image, and, most important, loss of the valuable contributions that disabled individuals can make to any academic community" (Rothstein, 1991, p. 10).

Unfortunately, a recent increase in disability-related litigation has occurred with the increase of students with disabilities on college campuses (Rothstein, 1991). These law suits have been filed as colleges have not made changes to campuses which are necessary to provide accessibility for students with disabilities. Often times colleges learn, in retrospect, that they should have spent money to modify their campuses in order to prevent law suits from being filed. Law suits cost colleges significantly more money than if they would have initially made the necessary changes to have a fully accessible campus for persons with disabilities. In 1992, for example, a student at Washington University in St. Louis brought up a lawsuit claiming that the campus was inaccessible. Subsequently, Washington University spent $2.5 million to revise buildings on campus to settle the lawsuit (Rothstein, 1991).

In order to avoid discriminating against students with disabilities, colleges should utilize an occupational therapist as an integral part of their student services office for those with disabilities. Occupational therapists are qualified for this position as

3

they are trained to assist both persons with dysfunctional and persons with no dysfunction discover ways to achieve their fullest potential in everyday roles. According to Bowman and Marzouk (1992),

> The most effective programs are usually those that are well planned and designed from a holistic perspective, rather than those that are developed as a reaction to a specific situation or incident, that is programs that are proactive rather than reactive. (p. 521)

Furthermore, Bowman and Marzouk suggested that an occupational therapist can help the college administration and students take a proactive approach to the ADA by assisting with the following:

> (a) the formation of a committee to respond to the needs of students and employees with disabilities, (b) the development of guidelines for work-study programs for students with disabilities, (c) the identification of private sources that provide scholarships for students with disabilities, (d) the formation of an office for students with disabilities, and delineation of its responsibilities, (e) the identification of concrete, abstract, and natural barriers to persons with disabilities. (p. 529)

Currently, it seems surprising that relatively little information exists about the population of college students who have mobility impairments. Past surveys have gathered the opinions of the college administration in regards to the accessibility of education on college campuses, however, none have actually asked the students with mobility impairments about their needs. According, to Gallagher (1992),

> Survey results can be used not only to help set clinical priorities and focus outreach activities for counseling programs but also to sensitize the campus community to the many stresses college students are experiencing and increase community knowledge of available services. (p. 281)

Among the 7 percent of undergraduates who reported having some type of disability, mobility impairment was the most frequently reported disability in 1989-90 (U.S. Department of Education, 1993). Approximately 37 percent of the undergraduate stu-

4

dents with disabilities in the United States are mobility impaired. With almost 335,000 documented undergraduate students with mobility impairments, it is time for colleges to take note of this population. In the United States, higher education is regarded as an idealistic institution—where persons of all backgrounds are able to come together and work toward a common goal. However, in order for the population of students with disabilities to be able to equally benefit from the experience of higher education, this researcher theorizes that changes are necessary for their needs to be satisfactorily met.

2.0   **THE LITERATURE REVIEW**

2.1   How the Literature Was Searched:

MEDLINE

Internet Gopher, University of Alabama

CINAHL

Reliable Source, American Occupational Therapy Association

Psychological Abstracts

ERIC

Expanded Academic Index

PALS

AHEAD

U.S. Department of Education, Kansas City

U.S. Department of Education Center for Statistics, Washington D.C.

International Center on Disabled

National Rehabilitation Information Center

National Office on Disability

National Counsel on Disability

HEATH

Indexes of: American Journal of Occupational Therapy

                 Journal of College Student Development

Franklin Stein, Ph.D., OTR/L, Occupational Therapy Department,

       University of South Dakota

Tim Lillie, Ph.D., Special Education, University of South Dakota

5

Elaine Pearson, Services Coordinator for Students with Disabilities,
University of South Dakota

Randy Christensen, Vocational Rehabilitation, Yankton, South Dakota

Casey Davidson, Prairie Freedom Center, Sioux Falls, South Dakota

Ernetta L. Fox, MA, MFA, Director of Information and Resources,
University Affiliated Program, University of South Dakota

2.2   Underlying Theoretical Assumptions

- There is a deficiency of knowledge regarding the needs of college students with a disability (Rothstein, 1991).
- Students with a disability should be entitled to the same educational experiences as students without a disability.
- There is a gap between student needs and services provided.
- The college should play a critical role in guiding and nurturing all students—those with a disability and those without a disability.
- The actual needs of college students with disabilities, in the 1990s, are unknown by college administrations—and therefore, not being satisfactorily met.
- The needs of college students with disabilities are not being satisfactorily met due to lack of knowledge about the Americans with Disabilities Act of 1990.
- College students with disabilities are not having their needs met due to lack of financial resources for this population.

2.3   History of Students with Disabilities in Higher Education

Persons with disabilities were not given the opportunity for "equal" education until the mid-70s when President Ford signed into law the "Education for All Physically Handicapped Children Act" (PL 94-142). The purpose of PL 94-142 was to provide a free and appropriate education for all children with disabilities. Although PL 94-142 was a crucial step towards providing accessible education for persons with disabilities, it only addressed the issue of accessibility and accommodation of education for children with disabilities (Frinks & McNamara, 1985).

6

The Rehabilitation Act of 1973 provided rights for persons with disabilities of all ages. Section 104.44 of Title 34, Code of Federal Regulations influenced the execution of Section 504 of the Rehabilitation Act. Section 104.44(a) stated that a

> postsecondary institution receiving federal financial assistance shall make such modifications to its academic requirements as are necessary to ensure that such requirements do not discriminate or have the effect of discriminating, on the basis of handicap, against a qualified handi-capped applicant or student. (Frank & Wade, 1993, p. 26)

It was not until July 26, 1990, that the Americans with Disabilities Act (ADA) was signed into law. The ADA requires that both public and private institutions provide persons with disabilities equal access to all education and places of public accommodation. Under the ADA, private colleges had until July 26, 1992 to put the ADA into effect. The implementation date for public colleges was January 26, 1992 (Frank & Wade, 1993).

The ADA has numerous effects on colleges as there are many different places of "public accommodation" within the college environment. According to section 301(7) of the ADA, "places of public accommodation" include those of

> lodging, establishments serving food of drink, entertainment and sports facilities, places of public gathering, service establishments such as offices of health care professionals, stations used for public transporta-tion, places of public display, places of recreation, social service centers, and places of exercise or recreation. (Frank & Wade, 1993, p. 27)

All aspects of the university, not just education, must be equally accessible to students with disabilities as they are to students without disabilities as stated by the ADA.

2.4   Target Population

The ADA defines disability in functional terms. Basically, a person who has a physical, mental, or emotional problem which disrupts any major life activity is quali-fied as disabled. According to the ADA, major life activities include such things as caring for one's self, performing manual tasks, walking, seeing, hearing, speaking, breathing, learning, and working (Americans with Disabilities Act, 1990). Furthermore, the ADA notes that "only those who identify themselves as being disabled can be accommodated" (Bowman & Marzouk, 1992, p. 526). Students with disabilities are required to initiate the process of being identified as "disabled" through documentation of the disability, and by "requesting specific accommodations [from the college] on a timely basis" (Frank & Wade, 1993, p. 29).

The current study focuses on undergraduate college students in the Midwest (Nebraska, Iowa, South Dakota, North Dakota, Kansas & Minnesota) with disabilities, specifically mobility impairments. A person is considered mobility impaired if their disability interferes with the "major life activity" of walking.

The review of literature revealed that members of this population, like most other college students, are somewhat unsure of their future and interested in finding a rewarding job (Penn & Dudley, 1980). Since the ADA passed in 1990, there has been little research published on college students with mobility impairments. Research which has been published, regarding students with disabilities, concentrates on the college administration or the disabled student services office at the institution—instead of the students' opinions. A few studies have surveyed students with disabilities in regards to why they chose a certain college—but not if their needs are being met in regards to obtaining satisfactory access to all aspects of their college education.

The current study proposes to survey students with mobility impairments regarding their needs and the students' satisfaction with how well their needs are being met. In conducting this study, it is proposed that the data collected will be useful in informing postsecondary educational institutions about the needs of students with mobility impairments. Consequently, the colleges may use the data gathered by this study to modify their campuses, if needed, in order to provide the same educational experiences to students with disabilities as to students without disabilities. In order for students to reach their fullest potential, it is necessary that the college equally guide and nurture all students.

3.0   **RESEARCH DESIGN**

The current study will utilize a survey design to determine whether or not the needs of college students with mobility impairments are having their needs satisfactorily

8

met. A survey will be distributed via mail to the services offices for students with disabilities at randomly selected public postsecondary educational institutions in the Midwest (Nebraska, Iowa, Minnesota, South Dakota, North Dakota). These offices will be asked to then distribute the surveys to students with mobility impairment on their campuses. The students will be requested to complete the survey and return it to the researcher in a provided self-addressed, stamped envelope.

3.1 <u>Research Design Questions Proposed</u>

- How many students with disabilities will I sample?
- Where will I obtain a list of colleges?
- From what type of postsecondary educational institutions will I obtain my sample?
- How will I collect my data?

3.2 <u>Statement of Hypothesis</u>

It is hypothesized that the needs of students with mobility impairments, on Midwest college campuses, are not having their needs adequately met. Therefore, students with mobility impairments are not receiving an equal educational experience as students without disabilities.

3.3 <u>Diagrammatical Relationship Between Variables</u>

Target Population: Undergraduate students (between 17 and 25 years of age), with mobility impairments attending public, 4 year, postsecondary educational institutions in the Midwest (NE, SD, ND, IA, MN). Total population of students with disabilities = 1000 students. According to the ADA, a person has a mobility impairment if their disability interferes with the major life activity of walking. Subjects are to be documented by their respective college as having a mobility impairment.

Sample: 1000 students

Projected Return: 50% (500 students)

Survey Characteristics: demographic

educational needs

Survey Characteristics: physical barriers

                                     interpersonal barriers

3.4   Possible Limitations of the Study

Despite an attempt to control all variables, limitations to the study are unavoidable. Possible limitations which may affect the study are:

1. The target population may not complete and return the surveys.
2. The construction of a reliable and valid questionnaire may be difficult.
3. The sample population may be too small to generalize to the entire population of undergraduate students with mobility impairments.

4.0   **METHODOLOGY**

4.1   Screening Criteria for Target Population

One thousand male and female undergraduate students with mobility impairments will be asked, via a mail survey, to participate in the current study. A person is classified as having a mobility impairment if their disability interferes with the "major life activity" of walking. The students surveyed will be attending public, 4 year postsecondary educational institutions in Nebraska, Iowa, South Dakota, North Dakota and Minnesota. The subjects surveyed are to be identified (i.e., through documentation) by their respective college as having a mobility impairment. The subjects will be between the ages of 17 and 25 years.

4.2   Data Collection Procedure

One thousand surveys will be mailed to the office of services for students with disabilities at randomly selected, public, 4 year, postsecondary educational institutions in Minnesota, Nebraska, Iowa, North Dakota and South Dakota. These offices will be asked to distribute the surveys to those students currently enrolled in the college who have a documented mobility impairment.

A cover letter will be attached to each individual survey, explaining the study to the target population. The target population will be asked to complete the survey and return it to the researcher in a provided, self-addressed, stamped envelope.

4.3   Projected Time Schedule for Completing Study

Selection of Topic .... 2.0 hours

Literature Review .... 55.0 hours

Research Proposal .... 20.0 hours

Create Survey .... 10.0 hours

Pretest Survey .... 10.0 hours

Send Survey/Wait for Response .... 3.0 months

Data Analysis .... 15.0 hours

Write discussion .... 5.0 hours

Complete Research .... 5.0 hours

Total time to complete study .... **approx. 4 months**

4.4   Statistical Design for Analyzing Data

Descriptive and non-parametric statistics will be used to analyze the data gathered by the survey. It is proposed that the statistics will be summarized in the text of the
study, as well as in tables and pie graphs.

4.5   Projected Costs of Study

Data collection forms $400.00

Letter of informed consent .... $ 50.00

Collection of Literature Review .... $ 30.00

Telephone calls to obtain data .... $ 75.00

Mileage .... $ 25.00

Presentation materials .... $ 20.00

Postage $310.00

Total Cost of Study **$910.00**

4.6   Informed Consent Form

You are invited to participate in a research project being conducted by Sarah R.S.
Montgomery, a graduate student in occupational therapy at the University of South
Dakota, as part of her master's degree. The purpose of this study is to gather information

11

regarding the needs of undergraduate students with mobility impairments in the Midwest. You are asked to provide information regarding whether or not your university is satisfactorily meeting your needs. The survey which you are being asked to complete should take approximately 15 minutes of your time.

Your identity and answers to the questions will be kept confidential as you are asked not to place your name anywhere on this survey. Completion of this survey will indicate that you have given your consent to participate in this research project. Please return the completed survey to the researcher in the self-addressed and stamped envelope which is provided.

It is the assumption of this researcher that students with disabilities should be entitled to the same educational experiences as students without disabilities. This researcher hopes that colleges will take note of the information gathered through this survey and make changes, if necessary, to their campuses and/or administration in order to provide equal access to all aspects of the college environment for students with disabilities.

If you have any questions specifically about the research project itself, or if you would like to receive results obtained in this study, you are welcome to contact the researcher by phone (605-624-6637) or by mail at the address listed below.

Thank you for your willingness to consider and, hopefully, to participate in this important research project.

Sarah R.S. Montgomery

Occupational Therapy Department

University of South Dakota

Vermillion, SD 57069

4.7   Data Collection Form

Please answer the following question by circling the letter next to the answer you choose.

1. Does your campus offer designated parking spaces for students with disabilities (i.e. "handicapped parking")?

    a. yes

    b. no

    c. don't know

2. Do you feel that there is an adequate number of parking spaces designated for students with disabilities on your campus?

   a. yes

   b. no

   c. don't know

3. Does your campus offer wheelchair repair/maintenance service?

   a. yes

   b. no

   c. don't know

4. Does your campus have a computer lab which enables you to complete your class assignments in an independent manner?

   a. yes

   b. no

   c. don't know

5. Does your campus offer Academic Aides who help you with mechanical or physical tasks which are not possible for you to do without assistance? (For example, Academic Aides may be used in the library where students cannot reach books. Academic aides may also be used as notetakers, or test/quiz writers. Academic aides are not used as tutors or study partners.)

   a. yes

   b. no

   c. don't know

   d. does not apply to me

6. Does your campus have a center or department which allows students with disabilities to learn and practice the skills necessary to live independently and become marketable in the work force following graduation?

   a. yes

   b. no

   c. don't know

   d. Other_____

13

7. Does your campus have an Occupation Therapist available for your assistance?

   a. yes

   b. no

   c. don't know

   d. other_____

8. Does your campus offer van transportation for students with mobility impairments to any of the following: (circle all of those that apply)

   a. classes on campus

   b. special social events affiliated with the campus

   c. other_____

   d. don't know

   e. none of the above

9. Does your campus offer a weight/training room which is accessible to students with mobility impairments?

   a. yes

   b. no

   c. other_____

   d. don't know

10. What organized recreational activities for students with mobility impairments are offered by your campus? (Circle all that apply to your campus):

    a. basketball

    b. swimming

    c. track and field

    d. weight lifting

    e. table tennis

    f. archery

    g. other_____

    h. don't know

11. Do you use the office of student services for those with disabilities on your campus?

    a. yes

    b. no

12. Please rank where you go for assistance with an academic problem. Using "1" for the place you would go to first, "2" for the place you would go to second, "3" for the place you would go to third, and so on.

___Family member

___Counseling Center on campus

___Other students

___Student services for those with disabilities

___Departmental advisor

___Faculty member

___Academic Advisor

___Other_____

___Other_____

___Other_____

13. Are all of your classes in a location which is accessible for you?

a. yes

b. no

14. Which of the following do you have the most difficulty with on your campus?

a. attitudinal barriers

b. physical barriers

c. a & b are equally difficult

d. none of the above

e. other_____

15. Does your campus have an adequate number of restrooms with accessible toilet stalls for persons with a mobility impairment?

a. yes

b. no

c. don't know

16. Does your campus have an adequate number of restrooms with sinks which are accessible for persons with a mobility impairment?

a. yes

b. no

c. don't know

17. Are there an adequate number of drinking fountains on campus which are accessible for persons with mobility impairments?

    a. yes

    b. no

    c. don't know

18. Are there an adequate number of public phones on campus which are accessible for persons with mobility impairments?

    a. yes

    b. no

    c. don't know

19. Does your campus have building entrance and exit doors which open automatically (i.e., by a button or by sensors)?

    a. yes

    b. no

    c. don't know

20. Do all of the campus buildings with more than 1 floor offer accessibility to all floors (i.e., via ramp, elevator, or lift)?

    a. yes

    b. no

    c. don't know

21. I am able to gain access to buildings via the same route as persons without disabilities:

    a. always

    b. sometimes

    c. rarely

    d. never

22. All of the doors on campus are wide enough for a wheelchair to fit through with ease:

    a. yes

    b. no

    c. don't know

    d. does not apply to me

16

For questions 23–29, please answer according to the following scale:

    1 = strongly agree

    2 = somewhat agree

    3 = no opinion

    4 = somewhat disagree

    5 = strongly disagree

23. _____I feel that the student services office for those with disabilities at my college is helpful with preregistration procedures.

24. _____My college is trying to eliminate physical barriers for students with mobility impairments.

25. _____My college is trying to eliminate attitudinal barriers for students with disabilities.

26. _____I feel that the student services office for those with disabilities at my college is helpful with registration procedures.

27. _____I feel that the student services office for those with disabilities at my college has provided services to insure equal opportunity at the school for students with mobility impairments.

28. _____Because of my disability, I feel left out of things at my school.

29. _____As a student with a disability, instructors meet my academic needs.

(Questions 23 through 29 are adapted from Patterson, Sedlacek, & Scales, 1988, p. 91)

Please answer the questions 30–35, according to the following scale:

    1 = strongly agree

    2 = somewhat agree

    3 = no opinion

    4 = somewhat disagree

    5 = strongly disagree

30. _____All of the campus buildings have are accessible for persons with mobility impairments.

31. _____I am able to gain access to all aspects of the campus.

32. _____I am frustrated due to the fact that I am unable to gain access to all aspects of the campus.

33. _____I never need to ask for assistance in order to access a certain part a of campus building.

34. _____The student services office for those with disabilities makes every effort to make all aspects of the college environment accessible to me.

35. _____When I request the college to remove a physical barrier, they do so in a timely manner.

36. Are you: _____male _____female

37. How old are you?_____

38. Are you:

    a. Single

    b. Married

    c. Divorced

    d. Widowed

    e. Other

39. Do you have dependents?

    a. Yes

    b. No

**If you answered "yes," how many dependents do you have?_____

40. Do you live with (circle all that apply):

    a. Your spouse

    b. Your children

    c. Your parents

    d. A roommate

    e. I live alone

    f. Other_____

41. What is your estimated family income:

    a. 0 – $5000 per year

    b. $5000 – $15,000 per year

    c. $15,000 – $25,000 per year

    d. $25,000 or more per year

42. How is the major part of your college expense being financed?

    a. parental support

    b. vocational rehabilitation funds

c. federal aid

d. money earned on part-time and/or summer jobs

e. scholarship

f. savings

g. other (please list)_____

43. How many hours are you currently employed?

   a. 1–10 hours per week

   b. 10–20 hours per week

   c. 20–30 hours per week

   d. 30–40 hours per week

   e. over 40 hours per week

   f. Currently I am not employed

44. How long have you had a mobility impairment?

   a. 0–1 year

   b. 1–3 years

   c. 3–5 years

   d. 5–10 years

   e. 10–15 years

   f. 15–20 years

   g. over 20 years

45. Are you a:

   a. Freshman

   b. Sophomore

   c. Junior

   d. Senior

   e. Other_____

46. What is the average number of credit hours you enroll in per semester?

   a. 1–6 credit hours

   b. 7–12 credit hours

   c. 13–16 credit hours

   d. over 16 credit hours

47. What is your current cumulative GPA?_____

48. How long do you anticipate it taking you to complete the necessary courses to graduate?

    a. under 4 years

    b. 4 years

    c. 4½ years

    d. 5 years

    e. Other_____

5.0   **REFERENCES**

Americans With Disabilities Act of 1990 (Public Law 101–336), 42 U.S.C. 12101.

Bowman, O. J., & Marzouk, D. K. (1992). Implementing the Americans with Disabilities Act of 1990 in higher education. *American Journal of Occupational Therapy, 46*, 521–533.

Foulk, J. B. (1990). *Office of disabled student services*. (Report No. HE 023 656). Washington, D.C.: Edinboro University of Pennsylvania. (ERIC Document Reproduction Service No. ED 321 638)

Frank, K., & Wade, P. (1993). Disabled student services in postsecondary education: Who's responsible for what? *Journal of College Student Development, 34*, 26–30.

Frinks, R. M., & McNamara, D. B. (1985). The wheelchair–bound student in the physics laboratory. *Journal of College Science Teaching, 13–14*, 416–420.

Gallagher, R. P. (1992). Student needs surveys have multiple benefits. *Journal of College Student Development, 33*, 281–282.

McLoughlin, W. P. (1982). Helping the physically handicapped in higher education. *Journal of College Student Personnel, 23*, 240–246.

Patterson, A. M., Sedlacek, W. E., & Scales, W. R. (1988). The other minority: Disabled student backgrounds and attitudes toward their university and its services. *Journal of Postsecondary Education and Disability, 6*, 86–94.

Penn, J. R., & Dudley, D. H. (1980). The handicapped student: Problems and perceptions. *Journal of College Student Personnel, 21*, 354–357.

Rothstein, L. (1991, September 4). Campuses and the disabled. *Chronicle of Higher Education.* pp. B3, B10

20

Sergent, M. T., Carter, R. T, Sedlacek, W. E., & Scales, W. R. (1988). A five year analysis of disabled student services in higher education. *Journal of Postsecondary Education and Disability, 6,* 21–27.

United States Department of Education, Office of Educational Research and Improvement. (1993). *Profile of undergraduates in U.S. postsecondary education institutions: 1989–90.* (NCES Publication No. 93–091). Washington, DC: U.S. Government Printing Office.

6.0 **ANNOTATED BIBLIOGRAPHY**

6.1 Population of Students with Disabilities

Patterson, A. M., Sedlacek, W. E., & Scales, W. R. (1988). The other minority: Disabled student backgrounds and attitudes toward their university and its services. *Journal of Postsecondary Education and Disability, 6,* 86–94.

ABSTRACT: Among disabled students attending colleges of the Washington, D.C., area 100% reported that the main reason they came to their school was that a high school teacher or counselor recommended it; 43% were quite certain of their career goals; 73% reported that they currently use the disabled student services at their campus. Differences by type of disability and implications for faculty and staff are discussed.

Penn, J. R., & Dudley, D. H. (1980). The handicapped student: Problems and perceptions. *Journal of College Student Personnel, 21,* 354–357.

ABSTRACT: As a result of federal legislation and slowly changing social attitudes, institutions of higher education have begun to respond to the needs of handicapped students by modifying their facilities and by providing special services. Yet, handicapped students still face many problems that tend to prohibit their full participation in campus life. The authors present the perceptions of a group of handicapped students and discuss these perceptions in light of their personal goals and campus experiences.

Sergent, M. T., Carter, R. T, Sedlacek, W. E., & Scales, W. R. (1988). A five year analysis of disabled student services in higher education. *Journal of Postsecondary Education and Disability, 6,* 21–27.

21

ABSTRACT: As an increasing number of disabled students exercise their rights to higher education, campus service providers are confronted with the challenge of providing programs and services most needed by this group of students. Providing appropriate services is one way to ensure that campus environments are attitudinally, as well as physically, accessible. Systematic research has been suggested as one means of assessing the needs of disabled students, the programs that are currently offered, and the ways in which service delivery could be improved to become increasingly responsive. This study was undertaken to provide information about the services offered to disabled students over the past 5 years on college and university campuses nationwide. Data were provided by the disabled student services data bank sponsored by the Association on Handicapped Student Service Programs in Postsecondary Education (AHSSPPE). The results of the study and their implications for service providers are discussed.

22

CHAPTER
10

Qualitative Research

Gwynnyth Llewellyn
Senior Lecturer in Developmental Disabilities
Faculty of Health Sciences
University of Sydney, NSW, Australia

It is undesirable to believe a proposition when there is no ground whatever for supposing it is true.—Bertrand Russell, Sceptical Essays (p. 1)

All great truths begin as blasphemies.—George Bernard Shaw, Annajanska, (p. 262)

● ●

Operational Learning Objectives

By the end of this chapter, the reader should be able to

1. identify the characteristics of qualitative research
2. explain the qualitative research process
3. recognize the difference between quantitative and qualitative research designs
4. identify qualitative data collection methods
5. identify the principles of qualitative data analysis
6. critically analyze examples of qualitative research from the allied health literature

● ●

10.1 Defining Qualitative Research

Qualitative research is defined as the study of people and events in their natural setting. In this method researchers use multiple and interconnected methods, seeking to explore

411

perceptions and experiences to understand phenomena in terms of the meanings that people bring to them. These phenomena are examined in context and from the individual's point of view. In rehabilitation settings the phenomena investigated include the experience of disability or of a chronic medical condition. The people involved may be clients, their family members, or medical and allied health personnel.

Among health and rehabilitation personnel, there is a rapidly growing interest in exploring the views of clients and their families (Ferguson, Ferguson, & Taylor, 1992; Llewellyn, 1995; Morse, 1994). This interest is being shaped by two forces. The first is the disability movement. Consumers of health and related services are actively campaigning for a less medical approach to disability and a more positive acceptance of people with disabilities' place in society (French, 1994). The second is the coming together of researchers in medical and social science disciplines. This has led to the demise of the traditional illness-based view of disability. In its place, disability is regarded as a social construction. This view takes into account the ways in which particular societies regard impairments and the influence of situational factors such as poor socioeconomic conditions on the incidence of disability (Oliver, 1991).

Exploring the viewpoint of individuals requires different research designs from those usually employed in the medical and health sciences. Allied health researchers are turning to sociology (the study of groups) and to anthropology (the study of cultures) for more appropriate research models. Investigators in these disciplines have been "unraveling" the complex interactions between individuals since the turn of the century (Parsons, 1964).

Qualitative research models differ from those in the positivist quantitative tradition in three fundamental ways. First, qualitative researchers are interested in "participatory and holistic knowing" (Reason, 1988, p. 12). This contrasts with the distance and objectivity found particularly in experimental research designs. Second, there is a focus on critical subjectivity in qualitative research. This involves researchers acknowledging their primary subjective experience. The researcher becomes his or her own "research instrument." This is in direct contrast to the notion of the objective researcher in experimental research designs. Third, researchers working in the qualitative tradition hold the view "that knowledge is formed in and for action" (p. 12). Action, as it naturally occurs, is viewed as the appropriate context for the development of knowledge.

10.2 Characteristics of Qualitative Research

There are four fundamental characteristics of qualitative research:

- phenomena are investigated and interpreted in their natural settings, taking into account the socio-cultural-historical context
- multiple methods are used to understand and offer interpretations of the meanings held by participants about these phenomena
- the researcher occupies a central place in the qualitative research process
- an inductive process is used to develop general principles from the study of specific instances.

Phenomena are investigated and interpreted in their natural settings, taking into account the socio-cultural-historical context. Qualitative research takes place in the field: Qualitative researchers get involved in the natural setting to understand the meanings held by participants about the phenomena under investigation. From this involvement and understanding, qualitative researchers develop knowledge. This knowledge may be in the form of patterns or themes or a fully developed theory about the phenomena being studied. Whatever the case, the resulting knowledge is grounded in direct field research experience rather than imposed a priori through hypotheses or deductive propositions (Glaser & Strauss, 1967).

Multiple methods are used to understand and offer interpretations of the meanings held by participants about the phenomena under investigation. Qualitative researchers use an array of methods to collect information about, describe, and interpret events and meanings in individuals' lives. The basic methods used for gathering data are interviewing, observation, and documentary analysis. The strategies most commonly used to analyze data include content or theme analysis, grounded theory procedures, and story analysis. These strategies are employed in the search for regularities in the meanings that participants hold about the phenomena under investigation. For some researchers, these regularities are viewed as a form of conceptual order; for others, their interest lies in the repetition of patterns across the data.

The researcher occupies a central place in the qualitative research process. In qualitative research, the researcher is acknowledged as an individual located within a historical context and within a research tradition or traditions. Researchers bring to the research process particular sets of beliefs about the world that guide their actions. However, in contrast to experimentally based research designs, qualitative researchers do not impose preexisting expectations on the phenomena or setting under study. Rather, the researchers' set of beliefs function as an interpretive framework (Guba, 1990). This interpretive framework guides the research purpose and shapes the research questions and the methods employed to address these questions. In addition to an interpretive framework, qualitative researchers become familiar with the literature and develop a guiding question to focus the purpose of the research.

An inductive process is used to develop general principles from the study of specific instances. In qualitative research, the analysis begins with specific instances of data and builds toward general principles. This contrasts with the deductive process employed in the quantitative tradition in which hypotheses are constructed prior to data collection and then tested. In qualitative research, preparing the research text is the final stage of the inductive analysis process. The research text is a construction that integrates and interprets data and researcher understanding of the area of study. The completed product is the public text, which may be delivered either as a research report, journal article, book, or seminar paper.

10.3 Types of Qualitative Research

Qualitative research is a term widely used to indicate methods that subscribe to the characteristics described above. Tesch (1990), for example, lists 46 different research approaches under the rubric of qualitative research. Some research methods more closely fit the characteristics described whereas others are less closely associated. Several qualitative methods have become standard in the medical and related health professional literature (Morse, 1994). These include case study, field study, focus group research, ethnography, and oral history. Other methods, such as ethnoscience, discourse analysis, transformative research, and hermeneutics are not so familiar.

Ethnoscience and discourse analysis are concerned with the study of the characteristics of language as a communication tool and as culture, respectively. Transformative research involves the research subjects as active participants in developing and implementing the research project to overcome the usually passive nature of the research process by turning this into a "transforming" activity. Researchers employing hermeneutics take as their central theme, the understanding of events in relation to the context of which these are part, with special reference to the historical context.

Tesch proposed that working with words is a basic requirement of qualitative research. She developed a continuum of qualitative research types based on the degree of focus on language. At one end of this continuum are research types primarily concerned with the characteristics of language. At the other end are those with an interest solely in reflection. In between some types focus on the discovery of regularities in text; others focus on the comprehension of the meaning of text or action. Those approaches that focus on language are more structured and employ more codified methods of data collection and analysis. In contrast, the approaches that rely mainly on reflection employ more holistic procedures that "build on intuition and on insight that are achieved through deep immersion in and dwelling with the data" (Tesch, 1990, p. 60).

Another way of classifying the different approaches used in qualitative research is by the research purpose. Some approaches are ideal for identifying regularities, patterns, or themes. Others are better suited to generating and refining tentative theoretical propositions. Yet others are more useful for intense, intimate study of a particular phenomenon using personal reflection. There is ongoing debate in the qualitative research literature about this diversity of approaches and associated methodological issues (Denzin & Lincoln, 1994). Each approach has adherents in the core disciplines of psychology, sociology, and anthropology and in the rehabilitation and allied health professions.

10.4 Collecting Qualitative Data

10.4.1 Interviewing

The most common data collection method in qualitative research is interviewing. Using interviews as a research method rests on the assumption that "the perspective of others is meaningful, knowable, and able to be made explicit" (Patton, 1990, p. 270). In short, interviewing is done to find out about those things that cannot be directly observed. Everyday familiarity with conversational or therapeutic interviews can lead novice researchers to regard interviewing for research purposes as quite straightforward. However, to effectively use interviewing as a research method requires knowledge of, and practice with, available techniques.

Research interviews take several forms. Interviews can be done face-to-face, over the telephone, or in a group. The format may be structured, semistructured, or openended. Interviewing may be used to collect personal experiences, or to understand particular phenomena, or to identify the perspective of a particular group of people. Interviews may be brief or lengthy, they may be "one-off," or part of a series.

Oftentimes investigators will employ a combination of interviewing approaches if this suits the purpose of the research and the research questions. For example, an interview may begin with a standardized, structured format, followed by sections made up of semistructured questions. Alternatively, the interview may begin with an unstructured open-ended format and conclude with a set of standardized questions. The type of interview that will best suit the research purpose needs particular care and thought.

Structured Interviewing

In this type of interview the interviewer uses a preestablished set of questions in a uniform manner. Although the questions may be open-ended, the interviewer cannot alter the predetermined format. The aim of this structured approach is to achieve as close as possible a standard format across interviewers and respondents. One disadvantage of this approach is that the interviewer is not able to pursue topics of interest that arise during the interview.

Semistructured Interviewing

This type of interviewing utilizes a general interview guide. The issues to be covered in the interview are predetermined; however, question format and exact content are not pre-specified. Rather, the interviewer uses a guide that can be adapted, as necessary, during the interview. Semistructured interviewing is an effective use of time while still allowing the interviewer to build up rapport and conduct the interview in a flexible way. This approach is particularly appropriate for group interviews where it can be used to encourage all participants to contribute to the topic under discussion.

Unstructured Interviewing

Unstructured interviews are sometimes referred to as informal conversational interviews or in-depth interviews. The purpose of this approach is to interview respondents without imposing any a priori categories on the content or format of the interview. The emphasis is on listening and on understanding each interviewee's individual point of view, not on explaining interviewees' perspectives within a predetermined interpretive framework.

Unstructured interviews often occur as part of observation in field research. Unstructured interviews may also be used with a specific purpose in mind, such as to explore one or more issues in depth. In unstructured interviewing, most of the questions flow from the immediate interview context. Specific questioning techniques are used to elicit, as clearly as possible, the way that each interviewee constructs meaning. For example, Spradley (1979) suggests three types of questions: descriptive, contrast, and structural. Patton (1990) also lists a number of alternative questioning formats. Whichever techniques are used, the researcher's primary task is to understand as fully as possible the interviewee's point of view.

Unstructured interviews are particularly useful for interviewing individuals over a period of time. Later interviews can be used to elaborate information gathered in earlier interviews to help build a comprehensive picture of the topic being investigated. One disadvantage of unstructured interviewing is the time involved. Another is the resources needed to analyze the quantity and variety of information gained.

Group Interviews

Interviewing people in groups is gaining popularity in allied health research. Group interviews are commonly called focus groups. Focus groups may be structured, semistructured, or unstructured. Group interviews are a cost effective and efficient way to gather information. However, interviewers need to be experienced in managing group processes. For example, aspects of group interaction such as the tendency of one or more members to dominate the group or the group members sliding into "group think" may impede the interview process (Frey & Fontana, 1995).

Attentive Listening

The role of self is critical in interviewing. Interviewing requires a commitment to, and an interest in, understanding another's point of view. Developing skills as an attentive listener are as important, if not more so, than becoming a skilled questioner. To resist the temptation to fit individuals into predetermined response categories requires careful listening and skillful questioning. Questions need to be unambiguous, focused, and as value-free as humanly possible. Compiling such questions and learning how to create a context in which interviewees are willing to answer openly and honestly require effort and practice. The time spent is well worth the rewards.

Using a Tape Recorder

Using a tape recorder is an efficient and accurate method to record an interview, although this needs to be done unobtrusively so as not to inhibit interviewees' responses. Researchers can easily become dependent on using a tape recorder: Disaster then strikes if for any reason a taped account is not possible. Not using a tape recorder requires a methodical approach and self-discipline to make sure that the researcher's notes are adequate. This is essential if the researcher is to gather the richest possible information in as many situations as possible.

There are instances where tape recording is not a suitable means of documenting information. In some situations using a tape recorder may invade the privacy of the participant by drawing attention to the interviewee. Circumstances may mitigate against adequate sound recording. This is particularly troublesome in open and crowded public places such as a shopping center. Tape recording may be inappropriate when the aim is to keep interviews as informal as possible

Experience suggests that interviewees frequently share valuable information when tape recording is not possible, for example, on the sidewalk or just after the machine is turned off! No matter how relaxed interviewees become with a tape recorder, occasions still occur when information is withheld for privacy reasons or because of personal embarrassment. It is, therefore, most unwise to rely on taped interviews. Alternative procedures are described in the section on field notes (Section 10.4.3) discussed later in the chapter.

10.4.2 Observation

Observation is essential to understanding human and natural phenomena. As Adler and Adler (1994) noted, "as long as people have been interested in studying the social and natural world around them, observation has served as the bedrock source of human knowledge" (p. 377). Observation in qualitative inquiry goes by several terms: participant observation, direct observation, field research, or qualitative observation. Whatever the term employed, the essence of observation "lies in the prolonged and unobtrusive presence of a *sensitive* and *trained* observer among the people being studied" (Edgerton & Langness, 1978, p. 339, emphasis added). All observational methods require disciplined training and rigorous preparation.

The primary purpose of observation in qualitative research is to describe. Description includes the setting, the activities taking place, the participants, and the meaning of the setting and its activities from the perspective of the participants. Observing activities as they take place provides the researcher with direct first-hand experience. This is essential to a full understanding of the phenomena under investigation. There are a number of sources of data in fieldwork settings. These include the physical setting, social interactions and activities (both planned and informal), the language used, nonverbal communication, unobtrusive indicators, program documents and "notable nonoccurrences" (Patton, 1990). In any setting, however, there is far more happening than can be accurately observed and documented. Therefore, qualitative researchers usually employ a framework to guide their fieldwork observations.

Several dimensions to observing need careful consideration in the research design phase. These are the role of the observer, portrayal of role and purpose, and duration and focus of observation.

Role of the Observer

The first dimension relates to the extent to which the observer not only observes but participates in the setting. There are several typologies of observer involvement in research settings. For example, Gold (1958) outlined four modes: the complete participant, the participant-as-observer, the observer-as-participant, and the complete observer. The latter is now rarely used owing to the ethical concerns about covert observation.

Recently, Adler and Adler (1994) suggested three roles for researchers as observers. These are: the complete-member-researcher, the active-member-researcher, and the peripheral-member-researcher. These roles fall along a continuum. The role chosen will depend on the purpose and nature of the research study. The peripheral-member-researcher is part of a setting while remaining removed from the core activities. The active-member-researcher participates in the core activities of the setting. The complete-member-researcher is one who already has full membership in the setting or converts to genuine membership during the study.

Portrayal of Role and Purpose

Researchers may explicitly explain their observer role and purpose, or may choose not to disclose any information about their observational role, or may portray their role somewhere in between these two extremes. The nature of the research questions and the access the researcher has to the setting and their position within that setting will influence how much others are told about the researcher role. For example, in primarily evaluative research, there will usually be full and complete explanation of the observational component. As Patton succinctly noted, "People are seldom deceived or reassured by false or partial explanations—at least not for long" (1990, p. 212). In contrast, in research of a more public nature, there may be little need to describe exactly what will be observed, when, how, and why.

Duration and Focus of Observation

Observation may occur once only, happen for a limited period, or be of varying duration carried out multiple times over an extended period. The duration of the observational period relies heavily on the purpose of the research. For example, research investigating complex processes that change over time, such as adaptation to acquired disability, require prolonged observation. In contrast, the timeliness and resources available for evaluation research often determine how much—or how little—observation occurs.

Not everything in a single research project warrants observation. The focus and scope of the observation need to be considered when framing the research question. Decisions will need to be made, for example, about whether to observe a small number of occasions in great depth or many occasions in less depth.

10.4.3 Field Notes

Field notes are the basic tool of the qualitative researcher. As Patton noted, "There are many options in the mechanics of taking field notes. . . . *What is not optional is the taking of field notes*" (Patton, 1990, p. 239, italics in original). Taking field notes can be used to substitute for tape-recording interviews. Note taking can also be used to expand the taped account, for example, with enriching descriptions of visual "pictures" of participants' facial expressions, gestures, and other nonverbal behaviors. Taking notes also expands the opportunities to collect data. For example, taking notes can provide a documented account of participants' reactions and interactions.

As noted above, researchers need to learn to observe methodically. Similarly, learning to systematically document observations requires the researcher to develop disciplined methods. The first step in this process is to decide on a format. Field notes can be in one notebook or can be contained in a file system. The second step is to organize the different types of field notes according to their content. The content of field notes will vary according to their purpose. The purposes of field notes include maintaining a transcript file, a personal log, or an analytical log (Minichiello, Aroni, Timewell, & Alexander, 1990).

The transcript file contains descriptive data about the observation or interview setting. This includes where the observation took place, who was present, and what social interactions and activities took place. This file may also contain a diagram of the setting. The transcript file also contains either a transcription of the interview or a written account of the observation. The secret of making good field notes for the transcript file is to be descriptive, concrete, and detailed. The researcher needs to avoid interpretation or judgment, loosely defined comparisons, and abbreviations that although making sense at the time of documenting may mean nothing at all when reviewing the file. This file should also contain direct quotations of what the research participants say. The quotations may be documented in the actual transcript of a recorded interview. If not, it is critical that the researcher record relevant information in the participants' own words. Participants' words can be differentiated from the researcher's descriptions by using quotation marks.

The personal log is the repository for the researcher's thoughts on the field research. This log includes personal feelings, reactions to the fieldwork experience, and personal and methodological reflections during the study. Writing this log needs to be done as soon as possible after each encounter in the field. It is not possible at the end of a study to go back and capture the feelings, reactions, and reflections that occurred during fieldwork. Keeping the personal log in the form of a journal may be helpful. Using headings and subheadings will help to organize the material and make it easier to review the contents in the analysis stage. The headings will vary according to research focus. For example, headings can be used to organize the material according to the sequence of events.

The analytical log contains the researcher's insights and reflections on data collection and analysis in the context of the theoretical framework of the study. Minichiello et al. (1990) suggest that this is where the researcher asks and answers questions such as What is it that I know so far? What do I not know? What do I need to know? How do I collect this information? This log also provides a record or audit trail of the analysis and theoretical propositions as these develop throughout the study.

10.4.4 Political and Ethical Context for Research

The political context sets the background for any research project. This context ranges from the micropolitical of personal relationships to the macropolitical of government sponsorship of research. Feminist research and research about race and ethnicity have highlighted the potential nature of research as a political activity. Grappling with the political context may seem overwhelmingly daunting to the beginning researcher. This is more so because little is written about how experienced researchers understand and deal with the political dimensions of the contexts in which they are working (Shaffir & Stebbins, 1991). Consideration of the political context is crucial in the research design phase.

Much has been written about the stages of field work, particularly strategies for entering and leaving the field (see, for example, Schatzman & Strauss, 1973, and Shaffir & Stebbins, 1991). Personal factors such as age, race, and gender of both the researcher and the research participants affect field work. Other influences on fieldwork include the nature and status of the researcher's institution and the institution where the research occurs, for example, a prestigious teaching hospital compared to a community health center. Gatekeeping—the term used to describe institutional power holders blocking access to people served by their institution—does occur in the health and welfare fields. For example, family workers may be unwilling to inform client families about a proposed research project or may tell only some families and not others. This may be done on the grounds that some families are more likely to be willing to participate, are more articulate, or are more able to withstand yet another intrusion into their lives. Frequently, however, those families not informed are less well educated, from minority ethnic groups, or are disadvantaged parents. Professional gatekeeping of these families may result in nonrepresentative samples for the research.

Professional associations, academic institutions, funding bodies, and medical facilities have ethical standards and convene human ethics committees. These have a mandate to permit or disallow proposed research according to federal and state regulations. Traditionally, the ethical precepts of biomedical research have been applied to social science research, although this research is more likely to be of a qualitative nature. These regulations, although providing a useful framework, may offer little guidance for the proper and ethical conduct of research in the field. Of primary interest to field researchers are issues of consent, privacy, confidentiality, trust, and betrayal (Bulmer, 1982).

Gaining the informed consent of research participants is essential to the ethical conduct of any research. Informed consent, however, is not as straightforward as it first appears. What happens, for example, to individuals' behaviors if they are informed a priori that they will be observed? What constitutes "informed" consent under circumstances such as mental illness, cognitive limitations, extreme youth, and extreme age? Research in the medical, rehabilitation and allied health fields is often carried out with individuals identified as vulnerable subjects on ethics clearance forms. Obtaining informed consent from research participants in these groups may require special procedures (Booth & Booth, 1994; Llewellyn, 1995).

A major aim for ethical researchers is to protect the privacy and confidentiality of research participants. Typical ways that this is done include keeping data in locked storage, destroying identifying material, and using pseudonyms in research reports. Safeguards also need to be in place against less obvious intrusions on participant privacy and confidentiality. For example, the researcher's institutional affiliation, the description of the research context, or the bibliography of the research report may give away the research location and the likely participants.

Finishing a field research study presents a further ethical concern. At the beginning of a research study, intense effort, possibly over weeks, months, or even years will have gone into building trust with the research participants. At the end of the study, the researcher leaves while the participants remain. After a period of engagement the participants may feel betrayed or, at the very least, let down. There are no simple rules to deal with this possibility. Each researcher must find a way to leave the field in an acceptably ethical manner. Fontana and Frey (1994) suggest a three-point guide to exercising moral responsibility toward research participants. They suggest responsibility "to our subjects first, to the study next and to ourselves last" (Fontana & Frey, 1994, p. 373).

10.5 Analyzing Qualitative Data

There is a diverse variety of methods for analyzing qualitative data (for example, see Bryman & Burgess, 1994; Miles & Huberman, 1994; Strauss & Corbin, 1990; Tesch, 1990). Qualitative data analysis methods are based on the following general principles.

10.5.1 Principles

The first principle is that the analysis is conducted concurrently with data collection. This means that, as analysis occurs, the researcher develops further questions that guide ongoing data collection. The researcher analyzes the data, proposes new questions or tentative propositions and then "checks these out" by returning to the data. This proposing and verifying process illustrates the movement between inductive and deductive procedures typical of qualitative analysis procedures.

The second principle is that the analysis process is systematic. Methods vary according to schools of thought and the researcher's interpretive framework. All methods make use of systems that involve reflection, are open to examination, and can be applied to more than one researcher. Miles and Huberman (1994) describe their system as follows: "Margin notes are made on the field notes, more reflective passages are reviewed carefully, and some kind of summary sheet is drafted. At the next level are coding and memo writing" (p. 432). These memos are analytic in nature and result from reflection on the data. Memos help the process of generating an increasingly more abstract conceptualization from the concrete field data (Miles & Huberman, 1994).

The third principle is that, during the analytic process, the data is "divided" into segments. These segments of data, however, remain part of the whole. Dividing the data into segments is carried out by using content analysis procedures. The researcher reviews the data from transcribed interviews or questionnaire responses or field notes and gives a name or code to each unit of meaning. This process is called *open coding* (Strauss & Corbin, 1990). The names or codes given to these units of meaning are developed directly from the text data, or are generated from previous studies, from the relevant literature, or from a combination of all these sources.

The fourth principle is that comparison is the main intellectual tool employed by the researcher in doing the analysis. Comparison is used to "discern conceptual similarities, to refine the discriminative power of categories, and to discover patterns" (Tesch, 1990, p. 96). Glaser and Strauss (1967) developed the term *constant comparative analysis* to describe the process whereby the researcher compares and contrasts elements of data in a search for recurring regularities. These regularities are further compared and contrasted to develop concepts. These concepts are then compared and contrasted to form internally consistent and mutually exclusive categories.

The fifth principle is that the researcher refines the category organizing system as familiarity with the data develops. Using the comparative process, the researcher clusters together categories that are alike. The organizing system remains flexible, becoming more conceptually sound and parsimonious as the researcher develops a deeper understanding of the phenomena under study. This occurs as the categories are expanded and elaborated. This elaboration is done by building on existing information, making links between items of information, and proposing and verifying new information. Category organization is continually refined until "theoretical saturation" is reached (Glaser & Strauss, 1967). Theoretical saturation is said to occur when new data lead to redundancy and the categories appear to be conceptually sound.

The sixth and final principle is that the goal of qualitative analysis is synthesis of the data into a higher level of conceptualization. In this process, a qualitative researcher has dual roles. The first is to describe phenomena as they exist—the what, how, when, and where. The second is to interpret and explain these phenomena as concepts. Patton (1990) suggests that this involves "discovering" and "uncovering." *Discovering* involves elaborating concepts that are obvious to participant and researcher alike. *Uncovering* requires clarifying or elaborating already existing sociological concepts or building new concepts from the research setting. In summary, the aim in qualitative research designs is not casual determination, prediction, or generalization as in quantitative research. Rather, qualitative researchers aim to elucidate relationships, and investigate and interpret connections and, by so doing, develop an understanding about particular phenomena and their place within existing theoretical knowledge about the social world.

10.5.2 Practice

Qualitative data is, most frequently, text derived from interview transcripts, questionnaire responses, field notes, and documents such as case records. The researcher may also use photographs and video (Harper, 1989). The volume of text data gathered can create a data management challenge. Miles and Huberman (1994) provide a useful summary of storage and retrieval requirements (see Table 10–1).

Qualitative researchers need to develop a data management system that suits their own style or that of the research team and the purpose of the research. Traditional methods for organizing data using notebooks, file folders, card systems, filing cabinets, and the like. Newer methods include word processing programs, databases, spreadsheets, and other computer-based programs. Storage and retrieval of data can be done quickly and efficiently using computer software.

Table 10–1   *What to Store, Retrieve From, and Retain*

- Raw material: field notes, tapes, site documents
- Partially processed data: write-ups, transcriptions. Initial version and subsequent corrected, "cleaned," "commented-on" versions
- Coded data: write-ups with specific codes attached
- The coding scheme or thesaurus, in its successive iterations
- Memos or other analytic material: the researcher's reflections on the conceptual meaning of the data
- Search and retrieval records: information showing which coded chunks or data segments the researcher looked for during analysis, and the retrieved material; records of links made among segments
- Data displays: matrices or networks used to display retrieved information, along with the associated analytic text. Revised versions of these
- Analysis episodes: documenting what you did, step by step, to assemble the displays and write the analytic text
- Report text: successive drafts of what is written on the design, methods, and findings of the study
- General chronological log or documentation of data collection and analytic work
- Index of all the above material

Note. From Miles, M. B., & Huberman, A. M. (1994). *Qualitative Data Analysis. An Expanded Sourcebook* (2nd ed., p. 48). Thousand Oaks: Sage.

Recent developments in computer software mean that researchers can also get help with data analysis. Several computer-based text analysis programs are available. The researcher needs to be aware of the assumptions underlying the design of the software and to decide whether such assumptions are congruent with the research purpose and design. For example, a common assumption is that concepts are of a hierarchical nature (such that A is an instance of a higher-order concept B, and so on). Three widely known programs are NUD.IST (Richards & Richards, 1990), Ethnograph (Seidel, 1989) and ATLAS/ti (Muhr, 1991). Comprehensive reviews of available programs, their functions, advantages, and shortcomings are available (Miles & Huberman, 1994; Weitzman & Miles, 1995).

10.6 Credibility in Qualitative Research

In qualitative research designs, the aim is to make sense of the meanings that people bring to phenomena in the social world. Qualitative researchers therefore want to make sure that their research findings are credible in the everyday sense of being plausible, believable, and trustworthy (Morse, 1994). Researchers using experimental designs and quantitative methods for collecting and analyzing data use constructs of reliability and validity. Many investigators have written on ways to address credibility in qualitative research. These range from applying the experimental concepts of reliability and validity to suggesting alternative concepts better suited to qualitative designs (see, for example, Kirk & Miller, 1986, and Lincoln & Guba, 1985). Among these writers, there is general agreement that three elements of the inquiry process must be addressed. These are the research techniques used, the researcher's credibility, and the assumptions underpinning the study.

Credibility of the research techniques can be checked by testing rival explanations, searching for negative cases, and triangulation. The first, testing rival explanations, requires the researcher to consider and "test out" alternative explanations to that proposed and then to report the results. Searching for negative cases is a related process. In this instance, the researcher searches for cases that do not fit the proposed patterns or themes identified from the data. Identifying negative or outlier cases increases understanding of the commonly occurring cases and, therefore, the totality of the phenomenon under investigation. The last way to check credibility is by a process called triangulation.

Triangulation has come to mean the use of multiple methods, sources, analysts, or theoretical perspectives to verify the information gained in different arenas. The aim of triangulation is "to guard against the accusation that a study's findings are simply an artifact of a single method, a single source, or a single investigator's bias" (Patton, 1990, p. 470). Triangulation of methods may involve collecting both quantitative and qualitative data for comparison and potential reconciliation. This helps to expand and elaborate the quality of information gained by one method alone.

Triangulation of sources involves comparing the consistency of information derived from varying sources, for example, comparing the data gathered from interviews and observations, from public and private documents, or from informants making the same claim independently. Triangulation across analysts is becoming more common. This can take the form, for example, of agreement between the field notes of one observer and the observations made by another. Lastly, some investigators have suggested triangulation of theoretical perspectives. This means applying more than one theoretical perspective to the research findings to reveal any differences and similarities (Patton, 1990).

As mentioned at the beginning of this chapter, the researcher is an integral part of the qualitative research process. Concern for researcher credibility is therefore an inherent part of the verification process. Researcher credibility is dependent on training, experience, and acknowledgment of the researcher role in the research process. Most of all, credibility requires a clear and concise explanation of the researcher role and contribution to the study findings. It is the researcher's responsibility to explain the extent of possible researcher effect on the study and whether changes in perceptions or responses occurred during the study or whether any predispositions or biases influenced the study findings.

The final element is the need for concise clarification by the researcher of the philosophical orientation underpinning the study. For example, there is continuing debate about the place of objectivity in scientific inquiry. This often takes the form of competition between the two paradigms of quantitative and qualitative research (Guba, 1990). Clear explanation by the researcher of the philosophical orientation of the study helps to place the study findings within a particular interpretive framework and allows the reader to judge for him- or herself the authenticity of the study results. Frank and open explanation in reporting research enhances credibility (Miles & Huberman, 1994).

Readers of qualitative research need a method to evaluate study credibility and the contribution to knowledge of the study findings. The following questions proposed by Schwandt and Halpern (1988) and cited in Miles and Huberman (1994, p. 439) provide useful criteria for readers in the medical and rehabilitation research literature:

- Are findings grounded in the data? (Is sampling appropriate? Are data weighted correctly?)
- Are inferences logical? (Are analytic strategies applied correctly? Are alternative explanations accounted for?)
- Is the category structure appropriate?
- Can inquiry decisions and methodological shifts be justified? (Were sampling decisions linked to working hypotheses?)
- What is the degree of researcher bias (premature disclosure, unexplored data in field notes, lack of search for negative cases, feelings of empathy?)
- What strategies were used for increasing credibility (second readers, feedback to informants, peer review, adequate time in the field?)

In summary, qualitative research offers a diversity of methods well suited to the interests of researchers in the medical and rehabilitation fields. The increasing popularity of these methods in these fields is evident in the growing number of qualitative studies reported in the allied health literature and the appearance of journals devoted specifically to qualitative research studies.

Until recently, however, the positivist experimental tradition was predominant in the medical profession, and rehabilitation and related health professions. Several authors have noted that the pendulum appears to be in danger of swinging to an exclusive focus on using quantitative research designs in health-related research (for example, Ottenbacher, 1992). As this book makes clear, both quantitative and qualitative research approaches contribute to the development of scientific inquiry in clinical research. The challenge for researchers in the health fields is to incorporate qualitative and quantitative approaches into their research practice.

APPENDIX
A
Allied Health Professions

What constitutes an allied health profession? Is there a distinction between the traditional health professions, such as medicine, dentistry, and nursing, and the newer health professions? Does educational level, clinical involvement with patients, or the degree of administrative responsibility in health care enter into a definition of allied health? If we examine the history of medicine we find that the physician and dentist about 70 years ago were the only independent health practitioners having formal educational requirements and licensing standards. The third health profession, nursing, has traditionally been practiced under the supervision of a medical doctor. The other health practitioners historically competing with other physicians were the homeopath, osteopath, chiropractor, and acupuncturist, among others. In the past, these fields were on the fringe of public acceptance and only recently have had internal and external regulation standards and levels for practicing. Presently, the health fields contain both independent practitioners licensed by governmental agencies and supportive health workers who practice under the supervision of a primary care professional. However, there is a growing trend in the health fields toward professional autonomy. For example, nurse practitioners, optometrists, clinical psychologists, nutritionists, and audiologists in certain instances have been granted virtually full responsibility for individual patient care.

The distinction between a primary care health professional and those in a supplementary role is becoming blurred. With the increased specialization among health workers it will become even more difficult in the future to determine who the primary and secondary care workers are. Those responsible for diagnosing an illness, prescribing treatment, and implementing the recommendations can all be different individual health workers. As the complexity for treatment grows, there will probably be a need for a coordinator who has an overall perspective of the patient's medical history and treatment procedures.

In view of the rapid changes and trends in health care, it seems to us that a definition of allied health should be inclusive and take into consideration the multitude of personnel who have a direct or indirect relationship to preventive medicine, health maintenance, treatment, rehabilitation, and habilitation. An allied health profession comprises any health services occupation that has a formal education program, a body of knowledge applicable to health care, and specified credentials for practice. The list of allied health professions recognized by the council on medical education is shown below. Address of selected professional health associations are listed in Chapter 6, Table 6–4.

Anesthesiologist's Assistant
Athletic Trainer

Cardiovascular Technologist
Clinical Laboratory Scientist

Clinical Laboratory Technician
(Associate Degree)
Clinical Laboratory Technician
(Certificate)
Cytotechnologist
Diagnostic Medical
Sonographer
Electroneurodiagnostic
Technologist
Emergency Medical Technician—
Paramedic
Health Information
Administrator
Health Information Technican
Histologic Technician/
Technologist
Medical Assistant

Medical Illustrator
Nuclear Medicine Technologist
Occupational Therapy Assistant
Occupational Therapist
Ophthalmic Medical
Technician/Technologist
Orthotist/Prosthetist
Pathologists' Assistant
Perfusionist
Physician Assistant
Radiation Therapist
Radiographer
Respiratory Therapist
Respiratory Therapy Technician
Specialist in Blood Bank
Technology
Surgical Technologist

APPENDIX
B

Nobel Prize For
Medicine or Physiology

NOBEL FOUNDATION, Nobel House, Sturegatan 14, 11436-Stockholm, Sweden

One of six Nobel Prizes given annually, the Nobel Prize for Medicine or Physiology is generally recognized as the highest honor that can be bestowed on a physician or scientist for an exceptionally significant contribution in medicine or physiology. The award, which consists of a gold medal diploma and large honorarium, is given at a ceremony on December 10 of each year in Stockholm's City Hall. The award itself is presented and administered by the Karolinska Institute, in Stockholm, which selects the recipients of the award. The amount of cash honorarium fluctuates. In 1995, it was approximately $1,000,000.

1901   Emil A. von Behring (Germany): Serum therapy, specifically for diphtheria.

1902   Sir Ronald Ross (Great Britain): Investigation on how malaria parasites enter the body.

1903   Niels R. Finsen (Denmark): Treatment of tubercular skin diseases, such as lupus vulgaris, with concentrated light radiation.

1904   Ivan P. Pavlov (Russia): Physiological studies on digestion.

1905   Robert Koch (Germany): Research on tuberculosis.

1906   Camillo Golgi (Italy) and Santiago Roman y Cajal (Spain): Studied structure of the nervous system.

1907   Charles A. Laveran (France): Research on the role protozoa play in cause of disease.

1908   Paul Edich (Germany) and Elie Metchnikoff (France, born in Russia): Immunity research.

1909   Emil Theodor Kocher (Switzerland): Study of thyroid, including pathology, physiology and surgery.

1910   Albrecht Kossel (Germany): Research in proteins, specifically in the area of cell chemistry.

1911   Alvar Gullstrand (Sweden): Research on eye dioptics.

1912   Alexis Carrel (USA, born in France): Transplantation and suture of blood vessels and organ.

1913   Charles R. Richet (France): Research on allergies and anaphylaxis.

1914   Robert Barany (Hungary): Physiology and pathology of inner ear.

1915   No award.

1916   No award.

1917   No award.

1918   No award.

1919   Jules Bordet (Belgium): Immunity research.

1920   August Krogh (Denmark): Discovered the motor regulation mechanism of capillaries.

1921   No award.

1922   Archibald V. Hill (Great Britain): Work on production of heat in muscles.

Otto Meyerhof (Germany): Recognized relationship between oxygen consumption and lactic acid production in muscles.

1923   Frederick G. Banting and John J. R. MacLeod (Canada): Discovered insulin.

1924   Willem Einthoven (Netherlands): Discovered electrocardiogram mechanism.

1925   No award.

1926   Johannes A. G. Fibiger (Denmark): Experiments on producing cancerlike growths in rats.

1927   Julius Wagner-Jauregg (Austria): Used inoculations against malaria to treat paralysis and mental deterioration from syphilis.

1928   Charles J. H. Nicolle (France): Typhus research.

1929   Christiaan Eijkman (Netherlands): Discovered effects of vitamin B deficiency.

Sir Frederick Hopkins (England): Discovered growth-producing vitamins.

1930   Karl Landsteiner (USA, born in Austria): Discovered blood groups of humans.

1931   Otto H. Warburg (Germany): Work in function of respiratory enzyme.

1932   Edgar D. Adrian and Sir Charles S. Sherrington (Great Britain): Discoveries about nerve-cell functioning.

1933   Thomas H. Morgan (USA): Research on role of chromosomes in heredity.

1934   George R. Minot, William P. Murphy, and George H. Whipple (USA): Research on liver therapy for anemia.

1935   Hans Spemann (Germany): Discovered "organizer effect" of development of embryo.

1936   Otto Loewi (Germany) and Sir Henry H. Dale (Great Britain): Research on chemical transmission of nerve impulses.

1937   Albert Szent-Györgyi von Nagyrapolt (Hungary): Work in body metabolism, especially regarding vitamin C and fumaric acid.

1938   Corneille Heymanns (Belgium): Discovered role of sinus and aortic mechanisms in regulation of respiration.

1939   Gerhard Domagk (Germany): Work on antibacterial properties of prontocilate.

1940   No award.

1941   No award.

1942   No award.

1943   Henrik C. R. Dam (Denmark): Discovered vitamin K.

Edward A. Doisy (USA): Work in chemistry of vitamin K.

1944   Joseph Erlanger (USA) and Herbert S. Gasser (USA): Discoveries on differentiated functions of single nerve fibers.

1945   Sir Alexander Fleming (Great Britain, born in Scotland), Ernst B. Chain (Great Britain, born in Germany), and Sir Howard W. Florey (Great Britain, born in Australia): Discovered penicillin and its effect on curing certain infectious diseases.

1946   Herman J. Muller (USA): Discovered mutations of genes caused by X-Ray use.

1947   Carl F. and Gerty T. Cori (USA, born in Czechoslovakia): Research on catalytic conversion of glycogen.

Bernardo A. Houssay (Argentina): Work in role of anterior pituitary lobe hormone in metabolizing sugar.

1948   Paul H. Müeller (Switzerland): Discovered DDT as an efficient insecticide.

1949   Walter Rudolf Hess (Switzerland): Discovered role of interbrain as a "co-ordinator" of internal organ activity.

Antonio Egas Moniz (Portugal): Developed brain operation of prefrontal lekotomy.

1950   Philip S. Hench (USA), Edward C. Kendall (USA), and Tadeus Reichstein (Switzerland, born in Poland): Work on adrenal cortex hormones, including their structural and biological effects.

1951   Max Theiler (USA, born in South Africa): Work combating yellow fever.

1952   Selman A. Waksman (USA, born in Russia): Discovered streptomycin for tuberculosis treatment.

1953   Hans A. Krebs (Great Britain, born in Germany): Discovered cycle of citric acid.

Fritz A. Lipmann (USA, born in Germany): Work in studying living cells.

1954   John F. Enders, Frederick C. Robbins, and Thomas H. Weller (USA): Discovered how poliomyelitis viruses grow in various tissue cultures.

1955   Alex H. Theorell (Sweden): Work on oxidation enzymes.

1956   Andre E. Cournand (USA, born in France): Werner Forssmann (Germany), and Dickinson W. Richards, Jr. (USA): Work on heart catherization and changes in circulatory system.

1957   Daniel Bovet (Italy, born in Switzerland): Work on synthetic compounds that curtail action of some body substances.

1958   George W. Beadie and Edward L. Tatum (USA): Discovered that genes regulate certain chemical events.

Joshua Lederberg (USA): Work with mechanisms involved in gene transmission.

1959   Arthur Kornberg (USA) and Severo Ochoa (USA, born in Spain): Discovered biological synthesis of RNA and DNA.

1960   Sir E. Macfarlane Burnet (Australia) and Peter B. Medawar (Great Britain): Work in acquired immunological tolerance.

1961   George von Békésy (USA, born in Hungary): Discovered physical mechanism of stimulation of the cochlea of the inner ear.

1962   Francis H. C. Crick (Great Britain), James D. Watson (USA), and Maurice H. E. Wilkins (Great Britain): Research on molecular structure of nuclear acids and its importance in information transfer in living material.

1963   Sir John Carew Eccles (Australia), Alan Lloyd Hodgkin, and Andrew Fielding Huxley (Great Britain): Work in nerve cell membrane.

1964   Konrad E. Bloch (USA, born in Germany) and Feodor Lynen (Germany): Work on mechanism and regulation of cholesterol and metabolism of fatty acids.

1965   François Jacob, André Lwoff, and Jacques Monod (France): Discovered regulatory processes of body cells contributing to genetic control of enzymes and virus synthesis.

1966   Charles B. Huggins (USA): Work on hormonal treatment of prostate gland cancer.

Francis Peyton Rous (USA): Discovered tumor-inducing viruses in chickens.

1967   Ragnar Granit, (Sweden, born in Finland), Haldan Keffer Hartline (USA), and George Wald (USA): Work on primary chemical and physiological processes in the eye.

1968   Robert W. Holley (USA), Har Gobind Khorana (USA, born in India), and Marshall W. Nirenberg (USA): Described genetic code that determines cell functions.

1969   Max Delbrück (USA, born in Germany), Alfred H. Hershey (USA), and Salvador E. Luria (USA, born in Italy): Work on reproduction and genetic structure of viruses.

1970   Julius Axelrod (USA), Ulf S. von Euler (Sweden), and Sir Bernard Katz (Great Britain): Basic research in nerve-transmission chemistry.

1971   Earl W. Sutherland, Jr. (USA): Work on mechanisms of hormonal actions.

1972   Gerald M. Edelman (USA) and Rodney Porter (Great Britain): Determined nature of an antibody.

1973   Karl von Frisch (Germany, born in Austria), Konrad Lorenz (Austria), and Nikolaas Tinbergen (Great Britain, born in the Netherlands): Work on individual and social behavior patterns of birds and bees, specifically related to selection and survival of the species.

1974   Albert Claude (Belgium), Christian Rene de Duve (USA, born in Belgium) and George Emil Palade (USA, born in Rumania): Founded cell-biology science, pioneered use of electron microscope to study living cells and discovered certain cell parts.

1975   David Baltimore (USA), Howard Martin Temin (USA), and Renato Dulbecco (USA, born in Italy): Research on tumor viruses and the genetic material of the living cell.

1976   Baruch S. Blumberg (USA): Research on the hepatitis viris in donated blood and on a health vaccine.

        D. Carlton Gajdusek (USA): Discovered kuru disease virus among cannibals.

1977   Rosalyn Yalow (USA), Roger C.L. Guillemin (USA, born in France), and Andrew V. Schalley (USA, born in Poland): Research in hormones in human body.

1978   Werner Arber (Switzerland), Daniel Nathans (USA), and Hamilton Smith (USA): Research and restriction enzymes used in DNA.

1979   Allan M. Cormack (USA, born in South Africa) and Godfrey N. Hounsfield (Great Britain): Developed revolutionary X-Ray technique known as computed axial tomography (CAT).

1980   Baruj Benacerraf (USA, born in Venezuela), George D. Snell (USA), and Jean Dausset (France): Explanation of the ways in which cell structure relates to organ transplants and disease.

1981   Roger W. Sperry (USA), Daniel H. Hubel (USA, born in Canada), and Torsten N. Wiesel (Sweden): Research on how the brain processes visual signals and left and right brain functioning.

1982   Sune Bergström (Sweden), Bengt Ingemar Samuelsson (Sweden), John R. Vane (England): Discoveries concerning prostaglandins and related biologically active substances.

1983   Barbara McClintock (USA): Understanding of the organization and function of genes.

1984   Niels K. Jerne (Great Britain), Georges J. F. Koehler (West Germany), and César Milstein (Argentina/Great Britain): Pioneering contributions to the theory and techniques of immunology.

1985   Michael Stuart Brown (USA) and Joseph Leonard Goldstein (USA). Regulation of cholesterol metabolism and the treatment of diseases related to elevated blood cholesterol.

1986   Rita Levi-Montalcini (USA/Italy) and Stanley Cohen (USA): Understanding of substances that influence all growth.

1987   Susumu Tonegawa (Japan): Structure of the immune defense.

1988   Gertrude B. Elion (USA), George H. Hitchings (USA), and Sir James Black (Great Britain): Discovery of important principles in drug treatment.

1989   J. Michael Bishop (USA) and Harold E. Varmus (USA): Proposed a theory of cancer development.

1990   Joseph E. Murray (USA) and E. Donnall Thomas (USA): Pioneered work in organ transplants.

1991   Erwin Neher (Germany) and Bert Sakmann (Germany): Research and development of the patch clamp.

1992   Edmond H. Fischer (USA) and Edwin G. Krebs (USA): Discovery of the cellular regulatory mechanism.

1993   Philip A. Sharp (USA) and Richard J. Roberts (Great Britain): Independently discovered "split genes."

1994   Alfred G. Gilman, (USA) and Martin Rodbill, (USA): discovery of the G-protein and the role of these proteins in the signal tranduction in cells.

1995   Edward B. Lewis (USA), Christiane Nusslein-Volhard (Germany), and Eric F. Wieschaus (USA): genetic control of early embryonic development.

APPENDIX
C
Statistical Tables

Table C-1   *Random Numbers*

42633	85191	32547	32269	10908	35182	00284	99873	95254	40027
06209	88389	48024	95890	13292	16221	27782	09404	40189	48909
85898	48518	01214	37532	90850	17004	38953	45438	71640	84200
17400	40484	58975	03822	00198	62540	08208	82205	89763	44359
51364	07817	74822	95198	34819	25405	83700	05230	69497	61566
34213	08216	46959	13598	89666	28787	66484	82557	48150	81122
70400	43058	48979	96808	25443	34465	20115	42316	34080	41474
84299	66933	75092	83971	93540	05376	65480	75168	17532	63121
78898	16916	73510	63004	50028	20628	69911	83874	87816	79883
41147	30346	83101	00871	60805	91507	83296	18837	19083	77353
69188	42697	29250	11798	51714	62164	43985	70541	33481	30840
22989	80881	71584	41438	05866	37535	09563	42476	07407	91274
40099	81818	05353	98309	06652	34581	86018	52315	37575	79671
02452	17310	90430	14091	83717	99672	95237	79317	88585	80219
46530	90762	26018	96366	24901	16410	56321	00532	06681	12892
44577	11687	48201	99119	40613	09780	73211	22183	21860	24967
64872	97263	57319	39577	05130	36644	29826	94473	03378	10981
56857	78071	16266	99378	33372	14342	08779	49183	00800	07549
99752	05537	86961	06577	12200	05373	93315	11706	27400	01408
39304	76855	56687	29105	10115	23621	58117	65234	13430	36956
73023	80267	60894	25405	86174	77846	40441	04687	82391	67259
98011	28318	34823	05844	04665	24591	83957	90698	86199	36384
42788	15532	41566	31167	86497	93622	91529	32847	30910	43211
75472	52144	60842	11490	45700	03259	51719	03704	49174	37430
89811	97066	95603	16941	51187	08668	54111	91978	73757	93861
04777	69628	82825	68993	23145	77347	13748	29433	35462	99406
02313	39086	77605	25713	47946	13783	14899	41976	61464	83912
58476	04674	79654	75772	65232	56555	70766	18024	66966	52512
49864	49565	70584	31605	92906	39582	02907	25963	30476	47285
69315	87419	87510	51040	14911	03129	50254	79739	67229	14317
81086	71619	02829	13270	92828	65769	63155	29682	96185	41238
29540	79599	46241	19956	31435	44347	49646	44797	16704	10947
78091	53339	11535	79479	58427	81372	49797	68726	00013	55003
89736	90234	44334	88512	37652	31853	93140	50757	67760	65361
08245	09009	11510	84653	30109	33482	14014	20335	41614	78466

Source: The table was generated by Y. L. Lio, Department of Mathematics, University of South Dakota, using the software in IMSL statistical library.

Table C–2 *Proportion of Areas Under the Normal Curve (Percentile Rank)*

z	0.00	0.01	0.02	0.03	0.04	0.05	0.06	0.07	0.08	0.09
0.00	.5000	.5040	.5080	.5120	.5160	.5199	.5239	.5279	.5319	.5359
0.10	.5398	.5438	.5478	.5517	.5557	.5596	.5636	.5675	.5714	.5753
0.20	.5793	.5832	.5871	.5910	.5948	.5987	.6026	.6064	.6103	.6141
0.30	.6179	.6217	.6255	.6293	.6331	.6368	.6406	.6443	.6480	.6517
0.40	.6554	.6591	.6628	.6664	.6700	.6736	.6772	.6808	.6844	.6879
0.50	.6915	.6950	.6985	.7019	.7054	.7088	.7123	.7157	.7190	.7224
0.60	.7257	.7291	.7324	.7357	.7389	.7422	.7454	.7486	.7517	.7549
0.70	.7580	.7611	.7642	.7673	.7704	.7734	.7764	.7794	.7823	.7852
0.80	.7881	.7910	.7939	.7967	.7995	.8023	.8051	.8078	.8106	.8133
0.90	.8159	.8186	.8212	.8238	.8264	.8289	.8315	.8340	.8365	.8389
1.00	.8413	.8438	.8461	.8485	.8508	.8531	.8554	.8577	.8599	.8621
1.10	.8643	.8665	.8686	.8708	.8729	.8749	.8770	.8790	.8810	.8830
1.20	.8849	.8869	.8888	.8907	.8925	.8944	.8962	.8980	.8997	.9015
1.30	.9032	.9049	.9066	.9082	.9099	.9115	.9131	.9147	.9162	.9177
1.40	.9192	.9207	.9222	.9236	.9251	.9265	.9279	.9292	.9306	.9319
1.50	.9332	.9345	.9357	.9370	.9382	.9394	.9406	.9418	.9429	.9441
1.60	.9452	.9463	.9474	.9484	.9495	.9505	.9515	.9525	.9535	.9545
1.70	.9554	.9564	.9573	.9582	.9591	.9599	.9608	.9616	.9625	.9633
1.80	.9641	.9649	.9656	.9664	.9671	.9678	.9686	.9693	.9699	.9706
1.90	.9713	.9719	.9726	.9732	.9738	.9744	.9750	.9756	.9761	.9767
2.00	.9772	.9778	.9783	.9788	.9793	.9798	.9803	.9808	.9812	.9817
2.10	.9821	.9826	.9830	.9834	.9838	.9842	.9846	.9850	.9850	.9857
2.20	.9861	.9864	.9868	.9871	.9875	.9878	.9881	.9884	.9887	.9890
2.30	.9893	.9896	.9898	.9901	.9904	.9906	.9909	.9911	.9913	.9916
2.40	.9918	.9920	.9922	.9925	.9927	.9929	.9931	.9932	.9934	.9936
2.50	.9938	.9940	.9941	.9943	.9945	.9946	.9948	.9949	.9951	.9952
2.60	.9953	.9955	.9956	.9957	.9959	.9960	.9961	.9962	.9963	.9964
2.70	.9965	.9966	.9967	.9968	.9969	.9970	.9971	.9972	.9973	.9974
2.80	.9974	.9975	.9976	.9977	.9977	.9978	.9979	.9979	.9980	.9981
2.90	.9981	.9982	.9982	.9983	.9984	.9984	.9985	.9985	.9986	.9986
3.00	.9987	.9987	.9987	.9988	.9988	.9989	.9989	.9989	.9990	.9990
3.10	.9990	.9991	.9991	.9991	.9992	.9992	.9992	.9992	.9993	.9993
3.20	.9993	.9993	.9994	.9994	.9994	.9994	.9994	.9995	.9995	.9995
3.30	.9995	.9995	.9995	.9996	.9996	.9996	.9996	.9996	.9996	.9997
3.40	.9997	.9997	.9997	.9997	.9997	.9997	.9997	.9997	.9997	.9998
3.50	.9998	.9998	.9998	.9998	.9998	.9998	.9998	.9998	.9998	.9998
3.60	.9998	.9998	.9999	.9999	.9999	.9999	.9999	.9999	.9999	.9999
3.70	.9999	.9999	.9999	.9999	.9999	.9999	.9999	.9999	.9999	.9999
3.80	.9999	.9999	.9999	.9999	.9999	.9999	.9999	.9999	.9999	.9999

Note: z Score values are given for two places after the decimal point. For example, a z score of 1.03 represents .8485 proportion of the normal curve or percentile rank.

Source: Adapted from Table 1.1 The Normal Distribution and Related Functions, by D. B. Owen, *Handbook of Statistical Tables* (pp. 3–10), © 1962 by Addison-Wesley, Publishing Company, Inc. Reprinted by permission of Addison-Wesley Publishing Company, Inc.

Table C–3   *Critical Values for t Test*

	Level of significance for one-tailed test				
	.10	.05	.025	.01	.005
	Level of significance for two-tailed test				
df	.20	.10	.05	.02	.01
1	3.0777	6.3138	12.7062	31.8207	63.6574
2	1.8856	2.9200	4.3027	6.9646	9.9248
3	1.6377	2.3534	3.1824	4.5407	5.8409
4	1.5332	2.1318	2.7764	3.7469	4.6041
5	1.4759	2.0150	2.5706	3.3649	4.0322
6	1.4398	1.9432	2.4469	3.1427	3.7074
7	1.4149	1.8946	2.3646	2.9980	3.4995
8	1.3968	1.8595	2.3060	2.8965	3.3554
9	1.3830	1.8331	2.2622	2.8214	3.2498
10	1.3722	1.8125	2.2281	2.7638	3.1693
11	1.3634	1.7959	2.2010	2.7181	3.1058
12	1.3562	1.7823	2.1788	2.6810	3.0545
13	1.3502	1.7709	2.1604	2.6503	3.0123
14	1.3450	1.7613	2.1448	2.6245	2.9768
15	1.3406	1.7531	2.1315	2.6025	2.9467
16	1.3368	1.7459	2.1199	2.5835	2.9208
17	1.3334	1.7396	2.1098	2.5669	2.8982
18	1.3304	1.7341	2.1009	2.5524	2.8784
19	1.3277	1.7291	2.0930	2.5395	2.8609
20	1.3253	1.7247	2.0860	2.5280	2.8453
21	1.3232	1.7207	2.0796	2.5177	2.8314
22	1.3212	1.7171	2.0739	2.5083	2.8188
23	1.3195	1.7139	2.0687	2.4999	2.8073
24	1.3178	1.7109	2.0639	2.4922	2.7969
25	1.3163	1.7081	2.0595	2.4851	2.7874
26	1.3150	1.7056	2.0555	2.4786	2.7787
27	1.3137	1.7033	2.0518	2.4727	2.7707
28	1.3125	1.7011	2.0484	2.4671	2.7633
29	1.3114	1.6991	2.0452	2.4620	2.7564
30	1.3104	1.6973	2.0423	2.4573	2.7500
40	1.3031	1.6839	2.0211	2.4233	2.7045
50	1.2987	1.6759	2.0086	2.4033	2.6778
60	1.2958	1.6706	2.0003	2.3901	2.6603
70	1.2938	1.6669	1.9944	2.3808	2.6479
90	1.2910	1.6620	1.9867	2.3685	2.6316
120	1.2886	1.6577	1.9799	2.3578	2.6174
–	1.2816	1.6449	1.9600	2.3263	2.5758

Note: Adapted from Table 2.1 Critical Values for Student's *t* Distribution, by D. B. Owen, *Handbook of Statistical Tables* (pp. 3–10), ©1962 by Addison-Wesley Publishing Company, Inc. Reprinted by permission of Addison-Wesley Publishing Company, Inc.

Steps in Determining Critical Values for *t* for Table C–3.

1.   Calculate the degrees of freedom (*df*):

- In one-sample *t* test it is number of cases of the sample minus 1
- In paired-data of correlated *t* test it is number of pairs minus 1
- In independent *t* test it is number of cases in $_n1 + _n2$ minus 2

2. Determine if hypothesis is one-tailed or two-tailed test.
3. Establish level of significance (.05 or .01)
4. Locate *t* critical (crit) value:

> e.g., 10 df, two-tailed test, .05 level
> $t_{crit} = 2.2281$

5. Note that these critical values are the same for negative or positive numbers.
6. Calculate *t* observed (obs) from formulas for three *t* tests.
7. Decision rule:

- If t_{obs} is equal to or above t_{crit} then reject the null hypothesis.
- If t_{obs} is below t_{crit} then accept the null hypothesis.

Table C–4   *Critical Values for F (Analysis of Variance, NOVA)*

df Associated with the Denominator		*df* Associated with the Numerator								
		1	2	3	4	5	6	7	8	9
1	5%	161	200	216	225	230	234	237	239	241
	1%	4052	5000	5403	5625	5764	5859	5928	5982	6022
2	5%	18.5	19.0	19.2	19.2	19.3	19.3	19.4	19.4	19.4
	1%	98.5	99.0	99.2	99.2	99.3	99.3	99.4	99.4	99.4
3	5%	10.1	9.55	9.28	9.12	9.01	8.94	8.89	8.85	8.81
	1%	34.1	30.8	29.5	28.7	28.2	27.9	27.7	27.5	27.3
4	5%	7.71	6.94	6.59	6.39	6.26	6.16	6.09	6.04	6.00
	1%	21.2	18.0	16.7	16.0	15.5	15.2	15.0	14.8	14.7
5	5%	6.61	5.79	5.41	5.19	5.05	4.95	4.88	4.82	4.77
	1%	16.3	13.3	12.1	11.4	11.0	10.7	10.5	10.3	10.2
6	5%	5.99	5.14	4.76	4.53	4.39	4.28	4.21	4.15	4.10
	1%	13.7	10.9	9.78	9.15	8.75	8.47	8.26	8.10	7.98
7	5%	5.59	4.74	4.35	4.12	3.97	3.87	3.79	3.73	3.68
	1%	12.2	9.55	8.45	7.85	7.46	7.19	6.99	6.84	6.72
8	5%	5.32	4.46	4.07	3.84	3.69	3.58	3.50	3.44	3.39
	1%	11.3	8.65	7.59	7.01	6.63	6.37	6.18	6.03	5.91
9	5%	5.12	4.26	3.86	3.63	3.48	3.37	3.29	3.23	3.18
	1%	10.6	8.02	6.99	6.42	6.06	5.80	5.61	5.47	5.35
10	5%	4.96	4.10	3.71	3.48	3.33	3.22	3.14	3.07	3.02
	1%	10.0	7.56	6.55	5.99	5.64	5.39	3.20	5.06	4.94
11	5%	4.84	3.98	3.49	3.26	3.11	3.00	2.91	2.85	2.80
	1%	9.65	7.21	6.22	5.67	5.32	5.07	4.89	4.74	4.63
12	5%	4.75	3.89	3.49	3.26	3.11	3.00	2.91	2.85	2.80
	1%	9.33	6.93	5.95	5.41	5.06	4.82	4.64	4.50	4.39

(continued)

Table C–4   *Critical Values for F (Analysis of Variance, NOVA) (continued)*

df Associated with the Denominator		df Associated with the Numerator								
		1	2	3	4	5	6	7	8	9
13	5%	4.67	3.81	3.41	3.18	3.03	2.92	2.83	2.77	2.71
	1%	9.07	6.70	5.74	5.21	4.86	4.62	4.44	4.30	4.19
14	5%	4.60	3.74	3.34	3.11	2.96	2.85	2.76	2.70	2.650
	1%	8.86	6.51	5.56	5.04	4.70	4.46	4.28	4.14	4.03
15	5%	4.54	3.68	3.29	3.06	2.90	2.79	2.71	2.64	2.59
	1%	8.68	6.36	5.42	4.89	4.56	4.32	4.14	4.00	3.89
16	5%	4.49	3.63	3.24	3.01	2.85	2.74	2.66	2.59	2.54
	1%	8.53	6.23	5.29	4.77	4.44	4.20	4.03	3.89	3.78
17	5%	4.45	3.59	3.20	2.96	2.81	2.70	2.61	2.55	2.49
	1%	8.40	6.11	5.18	4.67	4.34	4.10	3.93	3.79	3.68
18	5%	4.41	3.55	3.16	2.93	2.77	2.66	2.58	2.51	2.46
	1%	8.29	6.01	5.09	4.58	4.25	4.01	3.84	3.71	3.60
19	5%	4.38	3.52	3.13	2.90	2.74	2.63	2.54	2.48	2.42
	1%	8.18	5.93	5.01	4.50	4.17	3.94	3.77	3.63	3.52
21	5%	4.32	3.47	3.07	2.84	2.68	2.57	2.49	2.42	2.37
	1%	8.02	5.78	4.87	4.37	4.04	3.81	3.64	3.51	3.40
22	5%	4.30	3.44	3.05	2.82	2.66	2.55	2.46	2.40	2.34
	1%	7.95	5.72	4.82	4.31	3.99	3.76	3.59	3.45	3.35
23	5%	4.28	3.42	3.03	2.80	2.64	2.53	2.44	2.37	2.32
	1%	7.88	5.66	4.76	4.26	3.94	3.71	3.54	3.41	3.30
24	5%	4.26	3.40	3.01	2.78	2.62	2.51	2.42	2.36	2.30
	1%	7.82	5.61	4.72	4.22	3.90	3.67	3.50	3.36	3.26
25	5%	4.24	3.39	2.99	2.76	2.60	2.49	2.40	2.34	2.28
	1%	7.77	5.57	4.68	4.18	3.86	3.63	3.46	3.32	3.22
26	5%	4.23	3.37	2.98	2.74	2.59	2.47	2.39	2.32	2.27
	1%	7.72	5.53	4.64	4.14	3.82	3.59	3.42	3.29	3.18
27	5%	4.21	3.35	2.96	2.73	2.57	2.46	2.37	2.31	2.25
	1%	7.68	5.49	4.60	4.11	3.78	3.56	3.39	3.26	3.15
28	5%	4.20	3.34	2.95	2.71	2.56	2.45	2.36	2.29	2.24
	1%	7.64	5.45	4.57	4.07	3.75	3.53	3.36	3.23	3.12
29	5%	4.18	3.33	2.93	2.70	2.55	2.43	2.35	2.28	2.22
	1%	7.60	5.42	4.54	4.04	3.73	3.50	3.33	3.20	3.09
30	5%	4.17	3.32	2.92	2.69	2.53	2.42	2.33	2.27	2.21
	1%	7.56	5.39	4.51	4.02	3.70	3.47	3.30	3.17	3.07
40	5%	18.5	19.0	19.2	19.2	19.3	19.3	19.4	19.4	19.4
	1%	7.31	5.18	4.31	3.83	3.51	3.29	3.12	2.99	2.89
60	5%	4.00	3.15	2.76	2.53	2.37	2.25	2.17	2.10	2.04
	1%	7.08	4.98	4.13	3.65	3.34	3.12	2.95	2.82	2.72
120	5%	3.92	3.07	2.68	2.45	2.29	2.18	2.09	2.02	1.96
	1%	6.85	4.79	3.95	3.48	3.17	2.96	2.79	2.66	2.56

Note: Adapted from "Tables of Percentage Points of the Inverted Beta (F) Distribution," by M. Merrington and C.M. Thompson, 1943, *Biometrika, 33*, pp. 73–88, and *Elementary Statistics*, by R.J. Underwood, C.P. Duncan, J.A. Taylor, and J.W. Cotton, 1954, New York: Appleton-Century-Crofts, with permission of the publisher.

Steps in Determining Critical Values for *F* for Table C–4.

1. Calculate the degrees of freedom (*df*) for numerator and denominator:

    *   The *df* for numerator is derived from the number of groups in the study minus 1. For example, if three treatment methods are being compared, then *df* equals 3 minus 1, or 2 *df*, for numerator.
    *   The *df* for denominator is derived from the total number of subjects in all groups being compared minus the number of groups. For example for three treatment methods with 6 subjects in each group the *df* for the denominator will equal 18 minus 3, or 15 *df*.

2. Apply the level of significance, such as .05 or .01.
3. Locate critical value of *F*.

    e.g., *df* equals 2/15 at .05 level then $F_{crit} = 3.68$.

4. Calculate F_{obs} for data.
5. Decision rule:

    *   If F_{obs} is equal to or above F_{crit} then reject the null hypothesis.
    *   If F_{obs} is below F_{crit} accept the null hypothesis.

Table C–5   *Critical Values for the Pearson Product–Moment Correlation Coefficient*

		Level of significance for one-tailed test			
.25	.10	.05	.025	.01	.005
		Level of significance for two-tailed test			
df	.50	.20	.10	.05	.02	.01
1	0.7071	0.9511	0.9877	0.9969	0.9995	0.9999
2	0.5000	0.8000	0.9000	0.9500	0.9800	0.9900
3	0.4040	0.6870	0.8054	0.8783	0.9343	0.9587
4	0.3473	0.6084	0.7293	0.8114	0.8822	0.9172
5	0.3091	0.5509	0.6694	0.7545	0.8329	0.8745
6	0.2811	0.5067	0.6215	0.7067	0.7887	0.8343
7	0.2596	0.4716	0.5822	0.6664	0.7498	0.7977
8	0.2423	0.4428	0.5493	0.6319	0.7155	0.7646
9	0.2281	0.4187	0.5214	0.6021	0.6851	0.7348
10	0.2161	0.3981	0.4973	0.5760	0.6581	0.7079
11	0.2058	0.3802	0.4762	0.5529	0.6339	0.6835
12	0.1968	0.3646	0.4575	0.5324	0.6120	0.6614
13	0.1890	0.3507	0.4409	0.5140	0.5923	0.6411
14	0.1820	0.3383	0.4259	0.4973	0.5742	0.6226
15	0.1757	0.3271	0.4124	0.4822	0.5577	0.6055
16	0.1700	0.3170	0.4000	0.4683	0.5426	0.5897

(continued)

Table C–5   *Critical Values for the Pearson Product–Moment Correlation Coefficient*
(continued)

		Level of significance for one-tailed test			
.25	.10	.05	.025	.01	.005
		Level of significance for two-tailed test			
df	.50	.20	.10	.05	.02	.01
17	0.1649	0.3077	0.3887	0.4555	0.5285	0.5751
18	0.1602	0.2992	0.3783	0.4438	0.5155	0.5614
19	0.1558	0.2914	0.3687	0.4329	0.5034	0.5487
20	0.1518	0.2841	0.3598	0.4227	0.4921	0.5368
21	0.1481	0.2774	0.3515	0.4132	0.4815	0.5256
22	0.1447	0.2711	0.3438	0.4044	0.4716	0.5151
23	0.1415	0.2653	0.3365	0.3961	0.4622	0.5052
28	0.1281	0.2407	0.3061	0.3610	0.4226	0.4629
33	0.1179	0.2220	0.2826	0.3338	0.3916	0.4296
38	0.1098	0.2070	0.2638	0.3120	0.3665	0.4026
43	0.1032	0.1947	0.2483	0.2940	0.3457	0.3801
48	0.0976	0.1843	0.2353	0.2787	0.3281	0.3610
58	0.0888	0.1678	0.2144	0.2542	0.2997	0.3301
68	0.0820	0.1550	0.1982	0.2352	0.2776	0.3060
78	0.0765	0.1448	0.1852	0.2199	0.2597	0.2864
88	0.0720	0.1364	0.1745	0.2072	0.2449	0.2702
98	0.0682	0.1292	0.1654	0.1966	0.2324	0.2565

Note: Adapted from Table 19.1 Critical Values for the Product–Moment Correlation Coefficient, by D. B. Owen, *Handbook of Statistical Tables* (pp. 509–510), ©1962 by Addison-Wesley Publishing Company, Inc. Reprinted by permission of Addison-Wesley Publishing Company, Inc.

Steps in Determining Critical Values for Pearson *r* for Table C–5.

1. Determine the number of variables being correlated.
2. Determine if hypothesis calls for a one-tailed or two-tailed test. Usually a null hypothesis indicates a one-tailed test and a directional hypothesis indicates a two-tailed test of significance.
3. Apply level of significance, for example, .05 or .01.
4. Locate critical value of *r* from statistical table. For example, with $n = 20$, two-tailed test, .05 level, then $r_{crit} = .4227$.
5. Calculate r_{obs} from data.
6. Decision Rule:

   - If r_{obs} is equal to or greater then r_{crit}, then reject null hypothesis.
   - If r_{obs} *is below* r_{crit} then accept null hypothesis.

Table C–6   *Spearman Rank Order Correlation Coefficient*

	Level of significance for one-tailed test			
	.05	.025	.01	.005
	Level of significance for two-tailed test			
n*	.10	.05	.02	.01
5	.900	1.000	1.000	—
6	.829	.886	.943	1.000
7	.714	.786	.893	.929
8	.643	.738	.833	.881
9	.600	.683	.783	.833
10	.564	.648	.746	.794
12	.506	.591	.712	.777
14	.456	.544	.645	.715
16	.425	.506	.601	.665
18	.399	.475	.564	.625
20	.377	.450	.534	.591
22	.359	.428	.508	.562
24	.343	.409	.485	.537
26	.329	.392	.465	.515
28	.317	.377	.448	.496
30	.306	.364	.432	.478

*n = number of pairs

Note: Adapted from "The 5 percent significance levels of sums of squares of rank differences and a correction," by E. G. Olds, 1949, *Annals of Mathematical Statistics, 20*, pp. 117–118; and "Distribution of the sum of squares of rank differences for small numbers of individuals," by E. G. Olds, 1938, *Annals of Mathematical Statistics, 9*, pp. 133–148; and *Fundamentals of Behavioral Statistics*, by R. P. Runyon and A. Haber, 1967, Reading, MA: Addison-Wesley, with permission of the publishers.

Steps in Determining Critical Values for Spearman r_s (formerly rho) for Table C–6.

1. Determine the number of pairs of variables being correlated.
2. Determine if hypothesis calls for a one-tailed or two-tailed test.
3. Apply level of significance, .05 or .01
4. Locate critical value of r_s from statistical table. For example, with n = 12, two-tailed test, .05 level, then r_s critical = .591.
5. Calculate $r_{s\text{-obs}}$ from data.
6. Decision Rule:

   - If $r_{s\text{-obs}}$ is equal to or greater then $r_{s\ crit}$, then reject the null hypothesis.
   - If $r_{s\text{-obs}}$ is below $r_{s\ crit}$ then accept the null hypothesis.

Table C–7A Critical Values for the Mann–Whitney U Test [a]

n_B \ n_A	1	2	3	4	5	6	7	8	9	10	11	12	13	14	15	16	17	18	19	20
1	—	—	—	—	—	—	—	—	—	—	—	—	—	—	—	—	—	—	—	—
2	—	—	—	—	—	—	—	0 16	0 18	0 20	0 22	1 23	1 25	1 27	1 29	1 31	2 32	2 34	2 36	2 38
3	—	—	—	—	0 15	1 17	1 20	2 22	2 25	3 27	3 30	4 32	4 35	5 37	5 40	6 42	6 45	7 47	7 50	8 52
4	—	—	—	0 16	1 19	2 22	3 25	4 28	4 32	5 35	6 38	7 41	8 44	9 47	10 50	11 53	11 57	12 60	13 63	13 67
5	—	—	0 15	1 19	2 23	3 27	5 30	6 34	7 38	8 42	9 46	11 49	12 53	13 57	14 61	15 65	17 68	18 72	19 76	20 80
6	—	—	1 17	2 22	3 27	5 31	6 36	8 40	1 44	11 49	13 53	14 58	16 62	17 67	19 71	21 75	22 80	24 84	25 89	27 93
7	—	—	1 20	3 25	5 30	6 36	8 41	10 46	12 51	14 56	16 61	18 66	20 71	22 76	24 81	26 86	28 91	30 96	32 101	34 106
8	—	0 16	2 22	4 28	6 34	8 40	10 46	13 51	15 57	17 63	19 69	22 74	24 80	26 86	29 91	31 97	34 102	36 108	38 111	41 119
9	—	0 18	2 25	4 32	7 38	10 44	12 51	15 57	17 64	20 70	23 76	26 82	28 89	31 95	34 101	37 107	39 114	42 120	45 126	48 132
10	—	0 20	3 27	5 35	8 42	11 49	14 56	17 63	20 70	23 77	26 84	29 91	33 97	36 104	39 111	42 118	45 125	48 132	52 138	55 145
11	—	0 22	3 30	6 38	9 46	13 53	16 61	19 69	23 76	26 84	30 91	33 99	37 106	40 114	44 121	47 129	51 136	55 143	58 151	62 158
12	—	1 23	4 32	7 41	11 49	14 58	18 66	22 74	26 82	29 91	33 99	37 107	41 115	45 123	49 131	53 139	57 147	61 155	65 163	69 171
13	—	1 25	4 35	8 44	12 53	16 62	20 71	24 80	28 89	33 97	37 106	41 115	45 124	50 132	54 141	59 149	63 158	67 167	72 175	76 184
14	—	1 27	5 37	9 47	13 51	17 67	22 76	26 86	31 95	36 104	40 114	45 123	50 132	55 141	59 151	64 160	67 171	74 178	78 188	83 197
15	—	1 29	5 40	10 50	14 61	19 71	24 81	29 91	34 101	39 111	44 121	49 131	54 141	59 151	64 161	70 170	75 180	80 190	85 200	90 210
16	—	1 31	6 42	11 53	15 65	21 75	26 86	31 97	37 107	42 118	47 129	53 139	59 149	64 160	70 170	75 181	81 191	86 202	92 212	98 222
17	—	2 32	6 45	11 57	17 68	22 80	28 91	34 102	39 114	45 125	51 136	57 147	63 158	67 171	75 180	81 191	87 202	93 213	99 224	105 235
18	—	2 34	7 47	12 60	18 72	24 84	30 96	36 108	42 120	48 132	55 143	61 155	67 167	74 178	80 190	86 202	93 213	99 225	106 236	112 248
19	—	2 36	7 50	13 63	19 76	25 89	32 101	38 114	45 126	52 138	58 151	65 163	72 175	78 188	85 200	92 212	99 224	106 236	113 248	119 261
20	—	2 38	8 452	13 67	20 80	27 93	34 106	41 119	48 132	55 145	62 158	69 171	76 184	83 197	90 210	98 222	105 235	112 248	119 261	127 273

[a]Test for a one-tailed test at .025 or a two-tailed test at .05. If the U_{obs} value falls within the two values in the table for n_A and n_B, do not reject the null hypothesis. If the U_{obs} is less than or equal to the lower value in the table or greater than or equal to the larger value in the table then reject the null hypothesis.

Table C–7B Critical Values for the Mann–Whitney U Test [b]

n_B \ n_A	1	2	3	4	5	6	7	8	9	10	11	12	13	14	15	16	17	18	19	20
1	—	—	—	—	—	—	—	—	—	—	—	—	—	—	—	—	—	—	0- 19	0 20
2	—	—	—	—	0 10	0 12	0 14	1 15	1 17	1 19	1 21	2 22	2 24	2 26	3 27	3 29	3 31	4 32	4 34	4 36
3	—	—	0 9	0 12	1 14	2 16	2 19	3 21	3 24	4 26	5 28	5 31	6 33	7 35	7 38	8 40	9 42	9 45	10 47	11 49

(continued)

Table C–7B   Critical Values for the Mann–Whitney U Test[b] (continued)

nB \ nA	1	2	3	4	5	6	7	8	9	10	11	12	13	14	15	16	17	18	19	20
4	–	–	0	1	2	3	4	5	6	7	8	9	10	11	12	14	15	16	17	18
		12	15	18	21	24	27	30	33	36	39	42	45	48	50	53	56	59	62
5	–	0	1	2	4	5	6	8	9	11	12	13	15	16	18	19	20	22	23	25
		10	14	18	21	25	29	32	36	39	43	47	50	54	57	61	65	68	72	75
6	–	0	2	3	5	7	8	10	12	14	16	17	19	21	23	25	26	28	30	32
		12	16	21	25	29	34	38	42	46	50	55	59	63	67	71	76	80	84	88
7	–	0	2	4	6	8	11	13	15	17	19	21	24	26	28	30	33	35	37	39
		14	19	24	29	34	38	43	48	53	58	63	67	72	77	82	86	91	96	101
8	–	1	3	5	8	10	13	15	18	20	23	26	28	31	33	36	39	41	44	47
		15	21	27	32	38	43	49	54	60	65	70	76	81	87	92	97	103	108	113
9	–	1	3	6	9	12	15	18	21	24	27	30	33	36	39	42	45	48	51	54
		17	24	30	36	42	48	54	60	66	72	78	84	90	96	102	108	114	120	126
10	–	1	4	7	11	14	17	20	24	27	31	34	37	41	44	48	51	55	58	62
		19	26	33	39	46	53	60	66	73	79	86	93	99	106	112	119	125	132	138
11	–	1	5	8	12	16	19	23	27	31	34	38	42	46	50	54	57	61	65	69
		21	28	36	43	50	58	65	72	79	87	94	101	108	115	122	130	137	144	151
12	–	2	5	9	13	17	21	26	30	34	38	42	47	51	55	60	64	68	72	77
		22	31	39	47	55	63	70	78	86	94	102	109	117	125	132	140	148	156	163
13	–	2	6	10	15	19	24	28	33	37	42	47	51	56	61	65	70	75	80	84
		24	33	42	50	59	67	76	84	93	101	109	118	126	134	143	151	159	167	176
14	–	2	7	11	16	21	26	31	36	41	46	51	56	61	66	71	77	82	87	92
		26	35	45	f54	63	72	81	90	99	108	117	126	135	144	153	161	170	179	188
15	–	3	7	12	18	23	28	33	39	44	50	55	61	66	72	77	83	88	94	100
		27	38	48	57	67	77	87	96	106	115	125	134	144	153	163	172	182	191	200
16	–	3	8	14	19	25	30	36	42	48	54	60	65	71	77	83	89	95	101	107
		29	40	50	61	71	82	92	102	112	122	132	143	153	163	173	183	193	203	213
17	–	3	9	15	20	26	33	39	45	51	57	64	70	77	83	89	96	102	109	115
		31	42	53	65	76	86	97	108	119	130	140	151	161	172	183	193	204	214	225
18	–	4	9	16	22	28	35	41	48	55	61	68	75	82	88	95	102	109	116	123
		32	45	56	68	80	91	103	114	123	137	148	159	170	182	193	204	215	226	237
19	0	4	10	17	23	30	37	44	51	58	65	72	80	87	94	101	109	116	123	130
	19	34	47	59	72	84	96	108	120	132	144	156	167	179	191	203	214	226	238	250
20	0	4	11	18	25	32	39	47	54	62	69	77	84	92	100	107	115	123	130	138
	20	36	49	62	75	88	101	113	126	138	151	163	176	188	200	213	225	237	250	262

[b]Test for a one-tailed test at .05 or a two-tailed test at .10. If the U_{obs} value falls within the two values in the table for n_A and n_B, do not reject the null hypothesis. If the U_{obs} is less than or equal to the lower value in the table or greater than or equal to the larger value in the table then reject the null hypothesis.

Table C–7C   Critical Values for the Mann–Whitney U Test[c]

nB \ nA	1	2	3	4	5	6	7	8	9	10	11	12	13	14	15	16	17	18	19	20
1	–	–	–	–	–	–	–	–	–	–	–	–	–	–	–	–	–	–	–	–
2	–	–	–	–	–	–	–	–	–	–	–	–	0	0	0	0	0	0	1	1
													26	28	30	32	34	36	37	39
3	–	–	–	–	–	–	0	0	1	1	1	2	2	2	3	3	4	4	4	5
							21	24	26	29	32	34	37	40	42	45	47	50	52	55
4	–	–	–	–	0	1	1	2	3	3	4	5	5	6	7	7	8	9	9	10
					20	23	27	30	33	37	40	43	47	50	53	57	60	63	67	70
5	–	–	–	0	1	2	3	4	5	6	7	8	9	10	11	12	13	14	15	16
				20	24	28	32	36	40	44	48	52	56	60	64	68	72	76	80	84

(continued)

Table C–7C *Critical Values for the Mann–Whitney U Test^c (continued)*

n_B \ n_A	1	2	3	4	5	6	7	8	9	10	11	12	13	14	15	16	17	18	19	20
6	–	–	–	1	2	3	4	6	7	8	9	11	12	13	15	16	18	19	20	22
				23	28	33	38	42	47	52	57	61	66	71	75	80	84	89	94	93
7	–	–	0	1	3	4	6	7	9	11`	12	14	16	17	19	21	23	24	26	28
			21	27	32	38	43	49	54	59	65	70	75	81	86	91	96	102	107	112
8	–	–	0	2	4	6	7	9	11	13	15	17	20	22	24	26	28	30	32	34
			24	30	36	42	49	55	61	67	73	79	84	90	96	102	108	114	120	126
9	–	–	1	3	5	7	9	11	14	16	18	21	23	26	28	31	33	36	38	40
			26	33	40	47	54	61	67	74	81	87	94	100	107	113	120	126	133	140
10	–	–	1	3	6	8	11	13	16	19	22	24	27	30	33	36	38	41	44	47
			29	37	44	52	59	67	74	81	88	96	103	110	117	124	132	139	146	153
11	–	–	1	4	7	9	12	15	18	22	25	28	31	34	37	41	44	47	50	53
			32	40	48	57	65	73	81	88	96	104	112	120	128	135	143	151	159	167
12	–	–	2	5	8	11	14	17	21	24	28	31	35	38	42	46	49	53	56	60
			34	43	52	61	70	79	87	96	104	113	121	130	138	146	155	163	172	180
13	–	0	2	5	9	12	16	20	23	27	31	35	39	43	47	51	55	59	63	67
		26	37	47	56	66	75	84	94	103	112	121	130	139	148	157	166	175	184	193
14	–	0	2	6	10	13	17	22	26	30	34	38	43	47	51	56	60	65	69	73
		28	40	50	60	71	81	90	100	110	120	130	139	149	159	168	178	187	197	207
15	–	0	3	7	11	15	19	24	28	33	37	42	47	51	56	61	66	70	75	80
		30	42	53	64	75	86	96	107	117	128	138	148	159	169	179	189	200	210	220
16	–	0	3	7	12	16	21	26	31	36	41	46	51	56	61	66	71	76	82	87
		32	45	57	68	80	91	102	113	124	135	146	157	168	179	190	201	212	222	233
17	–	0	4	8	13	18	23	28	33	38	44	49	55	60	66	712	77	82	88	93
		34	47	60	72	84	96	108	120	132	143	155	166	178	189	201	212	224	234	247
18	–	0	4	9	14	19	24	30	36	41	47	53	59	65	70	76	82	88	94	100
		36	50	63	76	89	102	114	126	139	151	163	175	187	200	212	224	236	248	260
19	–	1	4	9	15	20	26	32	38	44	50	56	63	69	75	82	88	94	101	107
		37	53	67	80	94	107	120	133	146	159	172	184	197	210	222	235	248	260	273
20	–	1	5	10	16	22	28	34	40	47	53	60	76	73	80	87	93	100	107	114
		39	55	70	84	98	112	126	140	153	167	180	193	207	220	233	247	260	273	286

^{c}Test for a one-tailed test at .01 or a two-tailed test at .02. If the U_{obs} value falls within the two values in the table for n_A and n_B, do not reject the null hypothesis. If the U_{obs} is less than or equal to the lower value in the table or greater than or equal to the larger value in the table then reject the null hypothesis.

Note: Adapted from "On a Test of Whether One of Two Random Variables Is Stochastically Larger Than the Other," by H. B. Mann and D. R. Whitney, 1947, *Annals of Mathematical Statistics*, (pp. 18, 52–54); Extended tables for the Mann–Whitney statistic, *Bulletin of the Institute of Educational Research at Indiana University*, 1, No. 2; and *Fundamentals of Behavioral Statistics*, by R. P. Runyon and A. Haber, 1967. © 1967 by Addison-Wesley Publishing Company, Inc. Reprinted by permission of Addison-Wesley Publishing Company, Inc.

Table C–8 *Critical Values of T for Wilcoxon's Signed Ranks Test*[a]

	Level of significance for one-tailed test					Level of significance for one-tailed test			
	.05	.025	.01	.005		.05	.025	.01	.005
	Level of significance for two-tailed test					Level of significance for two-tailed test			
N	.10	.05	.02	.01	N	.10	.05	.02	.01
5	0	–	–	–	28	130	116	101	91
6	2	0	–	.	29	140	126	110	100
7	3	2	0	–	30	151	137	120	109
8	5	3	1	0	31	163	147	130	118
9	8	5	3	1	32	175	159	140	128
10	10	8	5	3	33	187	170	151	138
11	13	10	7	5	34	200	182	162	148
12	17	13	9	7	35	213	195	173	159
13	21	17	12	9	36	227	208	185	171
14	25	21	15	12	37	241	221	198	182
15	30	25	19	15	38	256	235	211	194
16	35	29	23	19	39	271	249	224	207
17	41	34	27	23	40	286	264	238	220
18	47	40	32	27	41	302	279	252	233
19	53	46	37	32	42	319	294	266	247
20	60	52	43	37	43	336	310	281	261
21	67	58	49	42	44	353	327	296	276
22	75	65	55	48	45	371	343	312	291
23	83	73	62	54	46	389	361	328	307
24	91	81	69	61	47	407	378	345	322
25	100	89	76	68	48	426	396	362	339
26	110	98	84	75	49	446	415	379	355
27	119	107	92	83	50	466	434	397	373

[a]The T_{crit} value indicates the smaller sum of ranks associated with differences that are all of the same sign. For any given N (number of ranked differences), the T_{obs} is significant at a given level if it is equal to or less than the critical value in the table.

Note: From D. B. Owen, *Handbook of Statistical Tables* (pp. 325–362), ©1962 by Addison-Wesley Publishing Company, Inc. and adapted from *Fundamentals of Behavioral Statistics* (p. 266), by R. P. Runyon and A. Haber, ©1967 by Addison-Wesley Publishing Company, Inc. Reprinted by permission of Addison-Wesley Publishing Company, Inc. We acknowledge the assistance of Y. L. Lio Mathematics Department, University of South Dakota, in interpreting the tables.

Table C-9 *Student Range Statistic for Tukey's Honestly Significantly Difference Test (HSD)*

df for Error Term	k = Number of Treatments										
	2	3	4	5	6	7	8	9	10	11	12
5	3.64	4.60	5.22	5.67	6.03	6.33	6.58	6.80	6.99	7.17	7.32
	5.70	**6.98**	**7.80**	**8.42**	**8.91**	**9.32**	**9.67**	**9.97**	**10.24**	**10.48**	**10.70**
6	3.46	4.34	4.90	5.30	5.63	5.90	6.12	6.32	6.49	6.65	6.79
	5.24	**6.33**	**7.03**	**7.56**	**7.97**	**8.32**	**8.61**	**8.87**	**9.10**	**9.30**	**9.48**
7	3.34	4.16	4.68	5.06	5.36	5.61	5.82	6.00	6.16	6.30	6.43
	4.95	**5.92**	**6.54**	**7.01**	**7.37**	**7.68**	**7.94**	**8.17**	**8.37**	**8.55**	**8.71**
8	3.26	4.04	4.53	4.89	5.17	5.40	5.60	5.77	5.92	6.05	6.18
	4.75	**5.64**	**6.20**	**6.62**	**6.96**	**7.24**	**7.47**	**7.68**	**7.86**	**8.03**	**8.18**
9	3.20	3.95	4.41	4.76	5.02	5.24	5.43	5.59	5.74	5.87	5.98
	4.60	**5.43**	**5.96**	**6.35**	**6.66**	**6.91**	**7.13**	**7.33**	**7.49**	**7.65**	**7.78**
10	3.15	3.88	4.33	4.65	4.91	5.12	5.30	5.46	5.60	5.72	5.83
	4.48	**5.27**	**5.77**	**6.14**	**6.43**	**6.67**	**6.87**	**7.05**	**7.21**	**7.36**	**7.49**
11	3.11	3.82	4.26	4.57	4.82	5.03	5.20	5.35	5.49	5.61	5.71
	4.39	**5.15**	**5.62**	**5.97**	**6.25**	**6.48**	**6.67**	**6.84**	**6.99**	**7.13**	**7.25**
12	3.08	3.77	4.20	4.51	4.75	4.95	5.12	5.27	5.39	5.51	5.61
	4.32	**5.05**	**5.50**	**5.84**	**6.10**	**6.32**	**6.51**	**6.67**	**6.81**	**6.94**	**7.06**
13	3.06	3.73	4.15	4.45	4.69	4.88	5.05	5.19	5.32	5.43	5.53
	4.26	**4.96**	**5.40**	**5.73**	**5.98**	**6.19**	**6.37**	**6.53**	**6.67**	**6.79**	**6.90**
14	3.03	3.70	4.11	4.41	4.64	4.83	4.99	5.13	5.25	5.36	5.46
	4.21	**4.89**	**5.32**	**5.63**	**5.88**	**6.08**	**6.26**	**6.41**	**6.54**	**6.66**	**6.77**
15	3.01	3.67	4.08	4.37	4.59	4.78	4.94	5.08	5.20	5.31	5.40
	4.17	**4.84**	**5.25**	**5.56**	**5.80**	**5.99**	**6.16**	**6.31**	**6.44**	**6.55**	**6.66**
16	3.00	3.65	4.05	4.33	4.56	4.74	4.90	5.03	5.15	5.26	5.35
	4.13	**4.79**	**5.19**	**5.49**	**5.72**	**5.92**	**6.08**	**6.22**	**6.35**	**6.46**	**6.56**
17	2.98	3.63	4.02	4.30	4.52	4.70	4.86	4.99	5.11	5.21	5.31
	4.10	**4.74**	**5.14**	**5.43**	**5.66**	**5.85**	**6.01**	**6.15**	**6.27**	**6.38**	**6.48**
18	2.97	3.61	4.00	4.28	4.49	4.67	4.82	4.96	5.07	5.17	5.27
	4.07	**4.70**	**5.09**	**5.38**	**5.60**	**5.79**	**5.94**	**6.08**	**6.20**	**6.31**	**6.41**
19	2.96	3.59	3.98	4.25	4.47	4.65	4.79	4.92	5.04	5.14	5.23
	4.05	**4.67**	**5.05**	**5.33**	**5.55**	**5.73**	**5.89**	**6.02**	**6.14**	**6.25**	**6.34**
20	2.95	3.58	3.96	4.23	4.45	4.62	4.77	4.90	5.01	5.11	5.20
	4.02	**4.64**	**5.02**	**5.29**	**5.51**	**5.69**	**5.84**	**5.97**	**6.09**	**6.19**	**6.28**
24	2.92	3.53	3.90	4.17	4.37	4.54	4.68	4.81	4.92	5.01	5.10
	3.96	**4.55**	**4.91**	**5.17**	**5.37**	**5.54**	**5.69**	**5.81**	**5.92**	**6.02**	**6.11**
30	2.89	3.49	3.85	4.10	4.30	4.46	4.60	4.72	4.82	4.92	5.00
	3.89	**4.45**	**4.80**	**5.05**	**5.24**	**5.40**	**5.54**	**5.65**	**5.76**	**5.85**	**5.93**
40	2.86	3.44	3.79	4.04	4.23	4.39	4.52	4.63	4.73	4.82	4.90
	3.82	**4.37**	**4.70**	**4.93**	**5.11**	**5.26**	**5.39**	**5.50**	**5.60**	**5.69**	**5.76**
60	2.83	3.40	3.74	3.98	4.16	4.31	4.44	4.55	4.65	4.73	4.81
	3.76	**4.28**	**4.59**	**4.82**	**4.99**	**5.13**	**5.25**	**5.36**	**5.45**	**5.53**	**5.60**
120	2.80	3.36	3.68	3.92	4.10	4.24	4.36	4.47	4.56	4.64	4.71
	3.70	**4.20**	**4.50**	**4.71**	**4.87**	**5.01**	**5.12**	**5.21**	**5.30**	**5.37**	**5.44**

(continued)

Table C–9   *Student Range Statistic for Tukey's Honestly Significantly Difference Test (HSD)*
(continued)

df for Error Term	**k = Number of Treatments**										
	2	**3**	**4**	**5**	**6**	**7**	**8**	**9**	**10**	**11**	**12**
∞	2.77	3.31	3.63	3.86	4.03	4.17	4.29	4.39	4.47	4.55	4.62
	3.64	**4.12**	**4.40**	**4.60**	**4.76**	**4.88**	**4.99**	**5.08**	**5.16**	**5.23**	**5.29**

Note that critical values in the table for (q) the boldface type represents values at the $p = .01$ level and the regular type represents values at the $p = .05$ level.

Note: Biometrika Tables for Statisticians (3rd. ed.), Table 29, by E. Pearson and H. Hartley, 1966, London: Cambridge University Press, and reprinted by permission from the Biometrika Trustees.

Table C–10   *Critical Values for the Chi-Square Distribution*

df	.25	.10	.05	.025	.01	.005
1	1.323	2.706	3.841	5.024	6.635	7.879
2	2.773	4.605	5.991	7.378	9.210	10.597
3	4.108	6.251	7.815	9.348	11.345	12.838
4	5.385	7.779	9.488	11.143	11.277	14.860
5	6.626	9.236	11.071	12.833	15.086	16.750
6	7.841	10.645	12.592	14.449	16.812	18.548
7	9.037	12.017	14.067	16.013	18.475	20.278
8	10.219	13.362	15.507	17.535	20.090	21.955
9	11.389	14.684	16.919	19.023	21.666	23.589
10	12.549	15.987	18.307	20.483	23.209	25.188
11	13.701	17.275	19.675	21.920	24.725	26.757
12	14.845	18.549	21.026	23.337	26.217	28.299
13	15.984	19.812	22.362	24.736	27.688	29.819
14	17.117	21.064	23.685	26.119	29.141	31.319
15	18.245	22.307	24.996	27.488	30.578	32.801
16	19.369	23.542	26.296	28.845	32.000	34.267
17	20.489	24.769	27.587	30.191	33.409	35.718
18	21.605	25.989	28.869	31.526	34.805	37.156
19	22.718	27.204	30.144	32.852	36.191	38.582
20	23.828	28.412	31.410	34.170	37.566	39.997
21	24.935	29.615	32.671	35.479	38.932	41.401
22	26.039	30.813	33.924	36.781	40.289	42.796
23	27.141	32.007	35.172	38.076	41.638	44.181
24	28.241	33.196	36.415	39.364	42.980	45.559
25	29.339	34.382	37.652	40.646	44.314	46.928
26	30.435	35.563	38.885	41.923	45.642	48.290
27	31.528	36.741	40.113	43.194	46.963	49.645
28	32.620	37.916	41.337	44.461	48.278	50.993
29	33.711	39.087	42.557	45.722	49.588	52.336
30	34.800	40.256	43.773	46.979	50.892	53.672
31	35.887	41.422	44.985	48.232	52.191	55.003
32	36.973	42.585	46.194	49.480	53.486	56.328
33	38.058	43.745	47.400	50.725	54.776	57.648
34	39.141	44.903	48.602	51.966	56.061	58.964

(continued)

Table C–10   *Critical Values for the Chi-Square Distribution (continued)*

df	.25	.10	.05	.025	.01	.005
35	40.223	46.059	49.802	53.203	57.342	60.275
36	41.304	47.212	50.998	54.437	58.619	61.581
37	42.383	48.363	52.192	55.668	59.892	62.883
38	43.462	49.513	53.384	56.896	61.162	64.181
39	44.539	50.660	54.572	58.120	62.428	65.476
40	45.616	51.805	55.758	59.342	63.691	66.766
41	46.692	52.949	56.942	60.561	64.950	68.053
42	47.766	54.090	58.124	61.777	66.206	69.336
43	48.840	55.230	59.304	62.990	67.459	70.616
44	49.913	56.369	60.481	64.201	68.710	71.893
45	50.985	57.505	61.656	65.410	69.957	73.166

Note: Adapted from Table 3.1 Critical Values for the Chi-square Distribution, by D. B. Owen, *Handbook of Statistical Tables* (pp. 49–55), ©1962 by Addison-Wesley Publishing Company, Inc. Reprinted by permission of Addison-Wesley Publishing Company, Inc.

Steps in Determining Critical Values for Chi-Square for Table C–10.

1. Calculate the degrees of freedom (*df*). The formula is $df = (r - 1)(c - 1)$. *r* = number of rows in the matrix and *c* = number of columns in the matrix. For example, in a 2 × 3 matrix, 2 rows and 3 columns, $df = (2 - 1)(3 - 1) = 2$ *df*.
2. Apply level of significance such as .05 or .01.
3. Locate critical value for chi-square from statistical table. For example, *df* = 2, .05 level, chi-square $_{crit}$ = 5.99.
4. Calculate chi-square $_{obs}$ from data.
5. Decision rule:

   - If chi-square $_{obs}$ is equal to or above chi-square $_{crit}$ reject the null hypothesis.
   - If chi-square $_{obs}$ is below chi-square $_{crit}$ accept the null hypothesis.

Glossary

a priori: reasoning from cause to effect. A *priori* criteria are criteria that an investigator states before collecting data.

A-B research design: single subject research where the A phase represents the collection of baseline data and the B phase represents the treatment phase. Variations of this include A-B-A, A-B-A-B, and other related research designs. *See also* single subject case study design.

abscissa: the horizontal coordinate or X axis in a distribution.

abstract: a summary of a published article that contains the important points and results of each section, such as literature review, methodology, results, and conclusions.

achievement test: assessment tool measuring an individual's knowledge or learning. Generally this test is believed to measure school learning.

alpha: the probability of a Type I error in research. It is usually defined as .05 or .01 in the social sciences. It is also referred to as significance level and p value.

alternative hypothesis (H_1): the hypothesis that is the opposite of the stated hypothesis and is not predicted to be true.

attitude scale: a measure of an individual's feeling, belief, or opinion towards a subject or topic.

analysis of covariance **(ANCOVA):** a statistical test arising from an analysis of variance that adjusts for a priori differences in comparable groups.

analysis of variance **(ANOVA):** an inferential statistical test that is applied to data when comparing two or more independent group means. An F score is derived. The formula for F in a one-way ANOVA is:

$$F = \frac{\text{Variance between group means}}{\text{Variance within groups}}$$

annotated bibliography: includes the bibliographical citation and the abstract.

applied research: the direct application of research to improving the quality of life in areas such as reduction of work injuries, prevention of alcoholism, and evaluation of clinical treatment methods. *See also* problem-oriented research.

aptitude: inherent, natural ability of individual; underlying capacity to learn or perform in a specific area.

artifact: an unexplained result in an experiment not caused by the independent variable.

associational relationship: the degree of correlation between two variables.

biased sample: a sample that is not representative of a target population from which it is drawn. It does not reflect the major characteristics of the target population and therefore results from a biased sample that cannot be generalized.

bar graph: a histogram with unattached bars.

baseline data: the results of initial testing of a subject before intervention.

basic research: investigations in areas related to processes, functions, and attributes that can lead to applied research. An example of basic research is examining how serotonin, a neurochemical transmitter, operates in the brain. The results of basic research often have important significance for clinical researchers.

before-and-after-design: an experimental research design in which performance or characteristics are measured before and after a treatment intervention.

beta: the probability of a Type II error in research.

bibliographical citation: the exact reference for a journal, book, or article referred to in the research paper or manuscript. The citation includes the author, title of article, journal, or book, volume and page numbers, and in books, the place of publication and the publisher.

bimodal: a frequency distribution showing two highest points.

box and whisker plots, box plots, box graphs: descriptive figures that display the maximum and minimum scores and the median and quartiles in a rectangular box. Useful in demonstrating graphically the degree of skewness of data.

case study: intensive study of individual either through an experimental prospective design or through retrospective research.

central tendency: a summary measure of a distribution indicated by the mean, median, or mode. Frequently referred to as measures of central tendency.

chi-square: a nonparametric statistical technique that tests the probability between observed and expected frequencies using nominal level measurement.

clinical observation research: the systematic and objective investigation in normal development, course of a disease, cultural ethnography, field studies, and naturalistic observations.

closed-ended questions: questions that can be answered with either *yes* or *no.* This type of question is not considered useful in survey research.

cohort: a study population that has common characteristics, such as the residents of a community or an occupational group.

concurrent validity: a measure of a test's correlation with an established instrument to test its accuracy in measuring a variable. For example, a new test for intelligence will be frequently correlated with the Wechsler Intelligence Scales because it has a high reliability and established validity. New tests are developed to include updated concepts, improved administration, and costs, and time considerations.

confidence interval: the area in a distribution that contains a population parameter. The confidence interval is related to the level of statistical confidence in results.

confounding variable: the effect of extraneous variables on research results. For example, test anxiety, fatigue, and lack of control are confounding variables.

content validity: the most elementary type of validity. It is determined by a logical analysis of test items to see whether the items are consistent and measure what they purport to measure. Sometimes referred to as face validity.

contingency table: a table of values that includes observed and expected frequencies such as in a chi-square table.

continuous variable: a quantitative value that has infinite number of measures between any two points. Examples of continuous variables are height, weight, and heart rate.

control group: a comparative group to control for the Hawthorne effect. Both the experimental and comparative groups receive equal time or attention.

correlation coefficient: a statistical value that indicates the degree of relationship between two variables. It can range from +1.00 to 0 to –1.00.

correlation matrix: a statistical table describing the degree of correlation between two variables. The correlation matrix indicates the correlation coefficient index for each pair of correlates.

correlational research: retrospective investigations into the relationship between variables. Variables are not manipulated by the researcher, such as in experimental research.

criterion: standard of performance which is the basis or yardstick for comparisons.

criterion-referenced test: a test based on standards of performance, competence, or mastery, rather than on comparison to a normative group.

critical value: the statistical value displayed in tables that is used to accept or reject the null hypothesis.

cross-validation: a method to measure test validity by extending testing from the initial target population to other groups.

culture-free test: a test that is not culturally biased and can be administered across cultures.

data: the numerical results of a study. The term is always plural (e.g., data are. . .).

decile: a point in a distribution where ten percent of the cases fall at or below that point.

deductive reasoning: inference to particulars from a general principle. For example, proposing a theory and then hypothesizing specific results from an experiment.

degrees of freedom (df): a mathematically derived value that is used in reading statistical tables.

demography: the application of statistical methods to describe human populations regarding, for example, mortality, morbidity, birth and marriage rates, gender differences, physical and intellectual characteristics, socioeconomic status and religious beliefs. In general, demography can be defined as the statistical study of human populations regarding their size, their structure and development (United Nations, 1958).

demographic variables: relate to the statistical characteristics of a target population such as distribution of ages, gender, income, presence of disease (morbidity), death rates (mortality), occupation, accident and injury rates, health status, and nutritional input.

dependent variable: resultant effect of the independent variable. In clinical research it represents the desired outcome, such as decrease in anxiety, increase in range of motion, or increase in reading achievement.

descriptive statistics: statistical tests or procedures to describe a population, sample, or variable. Examples of descriptive statistics include measures of central tendency, measures of variability, frequency distribution, vital statistics, scatter diagram, polygons, and histograms.

developmental test: a measure of a child's performance in age-related tasks such as language, perceptual–motor, social, emotional, and ambulation.

"devil effect": a negative prejudging of subject's performance based on the rater's bias.

directional hypothesis: a statement by the researcher that predicts that there will be a statistically significant difference or relationship between variables for example, a clinical researcher states, "Aerobic exercise is more effective than antidepressive medication in reducing anxiety in individuals with clinical depression."

discourse analysis: the study of language as communication through the forms and mechanisms of verbal interaction.

discrete variable: a variable that is distinct and does not have an infinite number of values between categories. Examples of discrete variables are gender, diagnostic categories, or eye color.

double blind control: a research design in which the researcher and subjects do not know whether the subjects are in the experimental or control group.

dyslexia: inability to understand written language or difficulty to read.

effect size: the degree of differences between two means or the degree of relationship between two variables in the results of a study. Effect size index is related to statistical power, which is the probability of not making a Type II error (e.g., accepting the null hypothesis when it should be rejected). (See Cohen, 1977, for a further discussion of effect size and statistical power.)

empiricism: the philosophy that advocates knowledge based on controlled observation and experiment.

error variance: the presence of error factors in the subject, researcher, test instrument, and environment that threatens internal validity. These factors include poor motivation, fatigue, and test anxiety in the subject, researcher bias, unreliability in the test instrument, and a distracting or noisy testing environment in conducting a research study.

ethnoscience: the study of the characteristics of language as culture in terms of lexical and/or semantic relations.

evaluation research: the qualitative and systematic evaluation of systems and organizations such as hospitals and educational programs by applying a priori criteria or standards.

experimental group: the group identified that is manipulated by the researcher. For example, the experimental group receives an innovative method of teaching.

experimental research: a prospective study where the investigator seeks to discover cause and effect relationships by manipulating the independent variable and observing the effects on the dependent variable.

ex post facto design: a retrospective study where the investigator examines the relationships of variables that have already occurred.

external validity: the degree to which the results of a study can be generalized to a target population. External validity depends on the representativeness of a sample and the rigor of an experiment. Replication of a study producing consistent results increases the external validity.

extraneous variable: a variable other than the independent variable that can potentially affect the results of a study. Extraneous variables can include such factors as gender, intelligence, severity of disability, or socioeconomic status. These variables, if they are uncontrolled, can threaten the internal validity of a study.

extraneous historical factors: threats to internal validity when unexpected events take place during an experiment that affect the results. These unpredictable events in the subject are extraneous variables.

historical research: the systematic and objective investigation, through primary sources, into the events and people that shaped history.

factor analysis: a statistical method to categorize data into identifiable factors. The procedure is an extension of a correlation matrix where a set of variables are correlated with each other.

factorial design: a research study exploring the interaction between variables such as in a two-factor analysis of variance.

feasible research study: a study where the investigator has examined in detail and provided solutions for the practical aspects of implementing a research study, such as costs, time, setting for study, availability of subjects, human ethics, selection of outcome measures, and procedure for collecting data.

forced choice test items: items that require the subject to make a choice when completing a questionnaire, rating scale, or attitude inventory. The subject selects items generated by the researcher.

frequency distribution table: a descriptive statistic summarizing data by showing the number of times each score value occurs in a set category or interval.

frequency polygon: a line graph depicting the number of cases that fall into designated categories. It is composed of an X and a Y axis.

functional capacity evaluation (FCE): a comprehensive and systematic approach that measures the client's overall physical capacity such as muscle strength and endurance. Examples are the Isernhagen Work Systems and BTE.

grounded theory analysis: the search for regularities consistuting a conceptual order by constantly comparing and contrasting similarities and differences in incidents to form categories with distinctive properties and conceptual relationships.

Guttman scale: a cumulative attitude scale that indicates an individual's feelings toward a specific issue. The respondent usually answers *yes* or *no* to a statement.

"halo effect": A carry-over effect from previous knowledge of an individual, resulting in a bias on the part of a tester or rater. Halo effects typically occur when raters positively prejudge a subject's performance based on the rater's previous experience with the subject. It is a bias in testing.

Hawthorne effect: a confounding variable that creates a positive result that is not due to the independent variable. The Hawthorne effect is eliminated by introducing a control group or by using the subject as one's own control.

hermeneutics: the study and interpretation of text in which each event is understood by reference to the whole of which it is part, especially the broader historical context.

heterogeneous: of different origin or characteristic, such as male and female or mixed ages.

heuristic research: investigations that seek to discover relationships between variables through pilot studies and factor analysis. The major purpose is to generate further research.

histogram: a descriptive statistic describing a frequency distribution using attached bars.

homogeneous: of like characteristic such as age, gender, or intelligence.

honeymoon effect: a confounding variable that produces a short-term beneficial effect. It is created by the initial optimism of the researcher desiring to show the positive effects of a specific treatment method and the patient or subject wanting the treatment method to work. The subject rejects the initial effects of treatment and disregards side effects or negative results. It is controlled by long-term follow-up and reducing researcher bias.

hypothesis: a statement that predicts results and can be tested. An example of a hypothesis is: Aerobic exercise lower blood pressure in middle-aged sedentary males.

idiographic approach: intensive study of an individual or dynamic case study.

incidence rate: the rate of the initial occurrence or new cases of a disease over a period of time. For example, the incidence of AIDS in the United States for the year 1994 includes all the new cases of AIDS diagnosed during 1994.

independent living evaluation: an assessment tool used to measure a client's ability to perform the activities of daily living. An example is the Barthel Self Care Index.

independent variable: a variable manipulated by the researcher. In clinical research it represents the treatment method, such as sensory integration therapy, or cognitive-behavioral therapy.

inductive reasoning: inferences from particulars or experiments to the general. For example, integrating the results of research studies to a general theory or conclusion.

inferential statistics: statistical tests used for making inferences from a sample to a population based on objectively derived data. They include t tests, analysis of variance, chi-square, correlation coefficients, factor analysis, and multiple regression.

informed consent form: a voluntary consensual agreement between the investigator and the subject that details the procedures in the study and the possible psychological and physical risks that could result in harm to the subject.

institutional review board: An interdisciplinary committee established in a university, hospital, or private industry to protect the rights of human subjects from possible harm that could occur by participating in a research study. It is recommended that all research with human subjects should be approved for ethical consideration before data are collected or the research is initiated.

intelligence test: a measure of an individual's capacity to store, evaluate, and retrieve verbal, spatial, and numerical data.

intra-rater reliability: the degree of consistency within single raters.

internal validity: the degree of rigor in an experiment in controlling for extraneous variables and error variance. Potential sources of internal validity have been identified as extraneous historical factors, maturation, instrumentation, and lack of random sampling. Internal validity is an indication of the trustworthiness of the results. Well-designed studies with good control of variables that can potentially distort the results have high internal validity. The quality of a research study is increased by eliminating the threats to internal validity.

inter-rater reliability: the degree of agreement between two independent raters in measuring a variable.

interval scale of measurement: quantification of a variable where there are infinite points between each measurement as well as equal intervals. Examples include the measurement of systolic blood pressure, and intelligence scores as measured by the Wechsler scales. An absolute zero is not assumed in measuring a variable, nor are comparative statements such as X is twice as large as Y assumed.

kappa test (k): a statistical procedure to detect the degree of interrater agreement based on probability.

key word: an important word or concept in a study that is identified by the researcher. It is used to retrieve a study when it is part of a database.

Kruskal–Wallis test: a nonparametric test, is an alternative to the one-way ANOVA for comparing significant differences between several groups.

Likert scale: a measurement scale used in questionnaires to assess a subject's agreement or disagreement with a statement. Likert scales usual come with five to seven descriptors, such as totally agree, agree, neutral, disagree, or totally disagree.

logical positivism: a philosophical approach to verifying reality. Logical positivists assert that reality is a result of sensory data.

matched group: a control group selected to use as a comparable group to experimental group. Variables matched typically include age, gender, intelligence, socioeconomic status, and degree of disability.

MANCOVA: multiple analysis of covariance is a statistical technique that is based on the analysis of variance where multiple variables are being analyzed and corrected for differences in initial scores.

Mann–Whitney test: a nonparametric test, is an alternative to the independent t test when testing significant differences between two independent means. The normality assumptions and equal variances assumptions need not be satisfied when applying the Mann–Whitney test.

maturation: a threat to internal validity that occurs when the researcher does not account for the subject's maturity during an experiment. For example, in testing children, the researcher must consider the age variable in measuring changes from pre- to posttest evaluation. Maturation can also refer to a practice effect, and development in the subject during the experiment.

mean: the arithmetical average derived from all scores in a distribution.

measures of central tendency: the mean, mode, and median.

measures of variability: the range, variance, and standard deviation.

median: the score at the 50th percentile or midpoint where all the cases in a distribution are divided in half.

meta-analysis: a qualitative analysis of a group of related research studies to determine if the results of the study are consistent and therefore lend support to their conclusions. Meta-analysis is based on the effect size estimation. (See Rosenthal & Rosnow, 1991, for a detailed discussion of meta-analysis).

methodological research: objective and systematic investigation for designing instruments, tests, procedures, curriculum, software programs, and treatment programs.

mode: the most frequent score or numerical value in a frequency distribution.

multiple regression: a statistical method that is used to predict the individual effects of independent variables on a designated dependent variable. Multiple regression has been used in medical research to identify the multiple risk factors in a certain disease such as cardiovascular disease, stroke, or emphysema. For example, multiple regression is used to predict the effect of designated risk factors (presumed independent variables) on a dependent variable (such as heart disease).

nominal scale of measurement: classification of variables into discrete categories, such as diagnostic groups, professions, or gender. There is no specific order in the categories; no category is more important than any other category. Likewise, each category is mutually exclusive from any other category.

nomothetic approach: research leading to general laws in science or universal knowledge.

nonparametric statistical tests: inferential statistical procedures that calculate data from samples that are distribution-free and not based on the normal curve. These tests include Mann–Whitney, Kruskall–Wallis, chi-square, Spearman correlational coefficient, and Wilcoxon.

norm-referenced test: a test used to assess the degree of achievement, aptitude, capacity, interest, or attitude compared to established norms or standard scores based on population.

normal curve: a bell-shaped polygon that describes a mathematical probability distribution of a variable where most scores cluster around the mean.

null hypothesis (H_0): a statement by the researcher that predicts no statistically significant differences or relationships between variables. For example, a clinical researcher states, "There is no statistically significant difference between exercise and splinting in reducing spasticity in children with cerebral palsy."

objective psychological test: standardized test that contains comparative norms for interpreting individual raw scores.

observed statistical value: the value obtained from applying a statistical formula to statistical results. These values such as t or F observed are compared to the critical value that is derived from a statistical table to accept or reject the null hypothesis.

open-ended questions: used in survey research. The investigator elicits attitudes, beliefs, and emotions from subjects by asking nonobjective questions, or questions that cannot be answered by *yes* or *no.* The opposite of open-ended questions are closed-ended questions.

operational definition of variable: specific test, procedure, or set of criteria that defines independent or dependent variables and target population. It is important in replicating a study or in evaluating a group of studies such as through a meta-analysis.

ordinal scale of measurement: classification of variables into rank order, such as the degree of anxiety, or academic achievement, or grade level. The classification defines which group is first, second, third, etc.; however, it does not define the distance between classifications.

outcome measure: the specific test or procedure to measure the dependent variable. For example an outcome measure for pain is the *McGill–Melzack Pain Inventory.*

outlier: a test result or score outside the normal range of values.

p value: the risk of making a *Type I error,* or the level of significance. In the social sciences, it is usually established at the $p < .05$ or $p < .01$ level.

parameter: a descriptive value assigned to a condition or population. Parameters are constant—like the characteristics of a specified population.

parametric statistical tests: inferential statistics that are based on certain assumptions such as the normally distributed population variable, random selection of subjects, and homogeneity of variance and independence of samples.

Pearson product–moment correlation coefficient: an inferential test used to test whether there is a statistically significant relationship between two variables. An r score is derived: r can range from +1.00 (a perfect correlation), to 0.00 (no correlation), to –1.00 (a perfect negative or inverse correlation). A computational formula is used in calculating r.

percentage: the number of cases per hundred.

percentile: a point in a distribution that defines where a given percentage of the cases fall. For example the 80th percentile is the point where 80 percent of the cases are at that point or below.

performance test: a test of an individual's skill or capacity such as grip strength, range of motion, manual dexterity, or driving skills.

personal equation in measurement: the effect of the mere presence of tester on subject's performance. The tester, per se, as the evaluator is a variable in the test situation, and if uncontrolled, could distort the test results.

pilot study: a research study with usually a small number of subjects, that is innovative, but that does not control for all extraneous variables. The primary advantage of a pilot study is that it generates further research.

placebo effect: a confounding variable that occurs when the subject shows signs of improvement or the reduction of symptoms that are not due to a treatment effect. It is due to the subject's belief that a treatment method is causing improvement even though the subject is receiving a "dummy" or "sham" treatment. The placebo effect was initially observed in drug studies where an experimental drug was compared to a placebo or non-active drug. Researchers observed that some of the subjects receiving a placebo improved. The current explanation of the placebo effect is that the subject produces a psychophysiological response that results in more relaxed and less stressed individual. In a way, the subject wills him- or herself to health in a placebo effect. The placebo effect is controlled by comparing baseline measures to posttreatments in the experimental and control groups.

positive correlation: a relationship between two variables when scores on both variables tend to be in the same direction such as high values for cholesterol and obesity.

posttesting: the results of testing after the intervention has taken place.

postulate: a principle or hypothesis presented without supporting evidence.

predictive validity: the degree to which a test or measuring instrument can predict future performance, functioning, or behavior. For example, the Scholastic Aptitude Test is evaluated for predictive validity in its ability to predict academic success in college.

pretesting: the results of testing before intervening with an independent variable or treatment.

prevalence rate: the number of individuals with a disability or disease divided by the total individuals in a population. For example the prevalence rate of spinal cord injury in the United States in 1994 is the number of individuals with spinal cord injury living in the United States in 1994 divided by the total population in the United States in 1994.

primary prevention: the prevention of the initial onset of a disease, such as the prevention of polio with a vaccination.

primary source: a published article or conference proceedings that include original data, such as a research study or theoretical paper.

probability: the mathematical or statistical likelihood that an event will occur.

problem-oriented research: applied research initiated by the investigator identifying a significant problem, such as the rapid increase in attention deficit disorders in children, or the dramatic rise of homeless men in urban areas. The research design addresses the problem directly.

"Procrustean bed": applying a treatment method such as a panacea to all patients regardless of individual differences and needs. For example, applying a treatment procedure to all patients with arthritis, as well as to all patients with cancer, without regard to the individual and specific needs of the patient. In this method, the patient is fitted to the treatment method rather than, in good treatment, where the best and most effective treatment method is applied.

prospective study: research that is future oriented and attempts to discover causes and effect relationships between variables. In prospective studies the investigator manipulates or observes an independent variable that is predicted to affect function or performance and then collects data. Experimental or longitudinal research are examples of prospective designs.

qualitative research: unbiased evaluation of the effectiveness, quality, and standards of performance of health care, educational programs, or systems.

quartile: a point in a distribution where 25% of the cases fall at or below that point.

quasi-experimental designs: a term defined by Campbell and Stanley (1966) to identify research studies where subjects are not randomly assigned to equivalent groups, or single case studies are employed. In general, most clinical research studies are within the quasi-experimental model because it is almost impossible to truly select a random sample from a target population or to have truly equivalent experimental and control groups.

random assignment: assigning subjects to experimental or control groups with every subject having an equal chance of being selected.

random errors: the effect of uncontrolled variables in an experiment such as unexpected events, test procedural errors, and anxiety within the subject. These errors are unpredictable and unsystematic.

random sample: an unbiased portion of a target population that has been selected by chance such as through random numbers.

range: a measure of variability, is the difference between the highest and lowest values in a distribution of scores.

rank order variables: examples of ordinal scale measurement where ranks are assigned in measuring a variable. Most personality tests such as the Minnesota Multiphasic Personality Inventory (MMPI) measure rank order variables.

rating scale: an individual's appraisal regarding such variables as competence, nonacademic qualities in students, or patient behavior in a psychiatric hospital.

ratio scale of measurement: quantification of a variable which includes equal intervals and an absolute zero point, such as in measuring heart rate, height, and weight. Comparative statements using "twice as" or "half" are possible with ratio scales.

referral source: a database that lists journal articles and books, such as Psychological Abstracts, Index Medicus, as well as information retrieval systems that are accessed by computer (e.g., PsychLit, ERIC, MedLine), or e-mail and newslists.

regression line: a figure that best describes the linear relationship between the X and Y variables. In a high correlation, the researcher is able to predict the unknown value of Y from the known value of X.

regression to the mean: the observation by statisticians that outlier scores will affect the value of the mean disproportionately especially when there are small numbers of cases. It is also apparent when we remeasure a variable and find that the initial score was unexpectedly very high or very low as compared to the group mean. On the second measure the score usually comes closer to the group mean.

reliability: a measure of the consistency of a test instrument. For example, a test has high reliability if it produces consistent results when measuring a variable. Threats to test reliability include ambiguity in the questions and poor test procedures. Reliability is indicated by the correlation coefficient (r). An acceptable test reliability is usually an r of .7 or above.

repeated measures designs: the replication of observations of the effects of treatment methods over a period of time. For example, measuring the effects of biofeedback in reducing anxiety after meditation or exercise.

replicate a research design: to carry out a research design for the second time by replicating the research methodology. The purpose is to strengthen generalizability of the findings and to insure external validity.

representative sample: an unbiased portion of a target population that is representative of the target population as far as demographic characteristics.

research: the systematic and objective investigation into a topic by stating a hypothesis or guiding question and collecting primary data. It includes quantitative and qualitative designs.

retrospective study: research based on variables that have already occurred. For example, in a correlational study the researcher may want to examine the relationship between the onset of emphysema and previous smoking behavior. Both variables are history and have already occurred. The researcher in a way tries to reconstruct events and to hypothesize regarding a presumed cause and effect relationship. Retrospective research can be used to generate experimental designs to further investigate cause and effect relationships.

risk benefit ratio: The estimation by the investigator of the possible risks to the research subject and the benefits accrued for the study. The researcher reveals the potential risks and benefits to the subject taking part in the study through an informed consent form.

sampling error: the error that results from estimating a population value from a sample.

scales of measurement: the level at which a test or instrument measures a specific variable such as intelligence, behavior, personality, muscle strength, or academic achievement. Traditionally, scales of measurement are classified into four levels: nominal, ordinal, interval, and ratio.

scattergram/scatter diagram/scatterplot: a figure depicting the relationship between the X and Y variables.

scientific law: consistent and uniform occurrences that are predictable. Mendelian law of genetic determination predicts characteristics of offspring when genetic traits of parents are known.

scientific method: objective systematic investigation into a subject by stating a hypothesis and collecting empirical data.

secondary prevention: the prevention of the recurrence of a disease such as preventing a second stroke in an individual.

secondary source: a published article of book that reviews primary sources, such as a literature review.

self-evaluation method: subjects in a clinical research study assess their own progress. Self- evaluation is an important factor in assessing treatment effectiveness. Other factors used in assessing treatment effectiveness include objective tests, psychophysiological measures, and mechanical procedures.

self-fulfilling prophesy: the expectation by the researcher or rater that a subject will perform at a certain level based on prejudice or bias towards the group to which the subject belongs.

semantic differential: an attitude scale where the respondent rates concepts such as good–bad, fast–slow and hard–soft.

significance level: in testing a hypothesis, it is the critical level between accepting or rejecting the null hypothesis.

single subject or case study design: See case study

skewness: an indication in a frequency polygon of the asymmetry of a distribution. A distribution can be skewed to the right or left side of the polygon.

slope: the linear direction and angle of a line. It is calculated in the regression line.

Spearman rank correlation coefficient (formerly rho [ρ]): a nonparametric test measured by ordinal scales used in determining the degree of relationship between two variables. It is an alternative to the Pearson product–moment coefficient (r).

split-half reliability: a method to estimate the degree of consistency in a test by correlating one half of the test items, such as even number items, with the other half of the test, such as the odd number items.

standard error of measurement (SEM): a statistical value that indicates the band of error surrounding a test score. For example, a raw score of 90 with a SEM of 4 represents a score ranging from 86 to 94.

standard deviation (SD): a statistical measure of the variability of scores from the mean.

standardized test: a test that has been administered to a target population and for which norms are available.

standard error of the mean (SE_m): a pooled standard deviation of samples of group means drawn randomly from a target population.

statistical assumptions: conditions in research required for a specific statistical test. These assumptions relate to randomness, scale of measurement, sample size, and independence of samples.

statistical pie: a descriptive statistic using the circumference of a circle to describe the percentage of cases for each category within a frequency distribution.

statistical sample: a portion of a target population comprising a specific variable such as gender, age, geographical location, income, or occupation.

statistical significance: the statistical evidence that an observed value is equal to or more than the critical value derived from a statistical table in rejecting the null hypothesis.

stem and leaf display: descriptive figure that displays raw scores from high to low values, organizing scores into leading digits (stems) and secondary digits (leaves). Useful in displaying trends or patterns in data.

survey research: a systematic and objective investigation into the characteristics, attitudes, opinions, and behaviors of target populations through questionnaires and interviews.

t test: inferential statistics that are used to determine whether the difference between two means are statistically significant or are due to chance. They include one-sample *t* test, independent *t* test, and correlated or paired-data *t* test. For testing two independent groups with approximately the same variance, the formula is:

$$t = \frac{Mean_1 - Mean_2}{\text{Standard error of the differences between the means}}$$

target population: an identified group where a representative or random sample of subjects are selected.

tertiary prevention: the prevention of secondary problems that can result from a disability, such as preventing decubiti in individuals with spinal cord injury.

test battery: a group of tests selected to comprehensively measure an individual's capacity such as in performance, vocational interests, attitudes, and intelligence.

test–retest reliability: a method to estimate the degree of consistency of a test. In this method a test is administered to the same group of subjects over a short period of time. Maturation and changes in the subjects can affect the results and must be controlled by the investigator.

theory: a comprehensive body of writings that attempts to explain, for example, how individuals contract and resist disease, learn motoric tasks, and develop cognitive and language functions.

time series research: in experimental research it indicates the measurement of the dependent variable over time intervals such as two weeks or three months. Its purpose is to evaluate the effect of a number of interventions or treatment techniques with the same subject or group.

transformational research: the use of research as a personal-political activity whereby the research participants become empowered by active engagement in the research process.

triangulation: the use of multiple approaches in collecting data and measuring variables. For example, in measuring a variable such as functional independence, the investigator would use a standardized ADL scale, use a functional capacity evaluation, and apply a self-report measure where the patient evaluates his or her performance in self-care activities.

Type I error: rejection of the null hypothesis when it should be accepted. Analogous to a false positive in medicine when a physician detects a disease when, in fact, no disease exists.

Type II error: acceptance of the null hypothesis when it should be rejected. Analogous to a false negative in medicine when a physician fails to detect a disease when in fact a disease is present in the patient.

unobtrusive methodology: a research method where the investigator collects data from indirect sources, such as patient records, historical documents, letters, and relics.

validity: as pertaining to measurement, it refers to the degree to which a test or measuring instrument actually measures what it purports to measure. Validity can also refer to the rigor of an experiment in controlling extraneous variables and the generalizability of the results of a study to a target population. *See also* external and internal validity.

variables: characteristics, factors, or attributes that can be measured qualitatively or quantitatively. Variables can be homogeneous groups such as physical therapy students, individuals with stroke, or hospital administrators. Variables can also be treatment methods such as exercise or biofeedback, or outcomes such as muscle strength, spasticity, functional capacity, or academic achievement.

variability: See measures of variability.

variance: the average of each score's deviation from the mean. Variance is an intermediate value that is used in calculating the standard deviation. The variance is the square of the standard deviation.

vocational interest test: a measure of an individual's preferences toward occupation-related tasks or jobs.

Wilcoxon signed rank test for correlated samples: a nonparametric test and an alternative to the correlated *t* test when comparing matched subjects or two sets of scores from the same subjects. Before-and-after studies are examples of correlated groups.

work samples: well defined activities that are similar to an actual job. Examples include Valpar and Micro-Tower.

z score: a score based on standard deviation units from the mean. For example a *z* score of +1 is one standard deviation unit above the mean.

References

Achenbach, T. M. (1981). *Child Behavior Checklist for Ages 4–16*. San Antonio, TX: The Psychological Corporation.

Achenbach, T. M. (1991). *Manual for the Child Behavior Checklist, 4–18*. Burlington, VT: University of Vermont Department of Psychiatry.

Ackoff, R. L., & Rivett, P. (1963). *A manager's guide to operation research*. New York: Wiley.

Americans with Disabilities Act of 1990, Pub. L. No. 101–336, § 2, 104 Stat. 328 (1991).

Adler, P. A., & Adler, P.(1994). Observational techniques. In N. K. Denzin & Y. S. Lincoln (Eds.), *Handbook of qualitative research* (pp. 377–392). Thousand Oaks: Sage.

Adler, L., & Attwood, M. (1987). *Poor readers: What do they really see on the page: A study of a major cause of dyslexia.* (Available from the Los Angeles County Office of Education, Los Angeles, CA.).

Aleltzoff, J., & Kornreich, M. (1970). *Research in psychotherapy*. New York: Atherton Press.

American Occupational Therapy Association (1991). *OT for the injured worker*. Rockland, MD: Author.

American Psychiatric Association (1994). *Diagnostic and statistical manual* (4th ed.). Washington, DC: Author.

American Psychological Association (1994). *Publication manual of the American Psychological Association*, (4th ed.). Washington, DC: APA.

Anastasi, A. (1988). *Psychological Testing* (6th ed.). New York: MacMillian.

Anderson, G. M., & Lomas, J. L. (1988). Monitoring the difusion of technology: Coronary artery bypass surgery in Ontario. *American Journal of Public Health, 78*, 251–254.

Anderson, K. L. (1961). Respiratory recovery from exercise of short duration. In *Health and fitness in the modern world* (pp. 105–118). Athletic Institute and American College of Sports Medicine.

Anderson, M. H., Bechtol, C. O., & Sollars, R. E. (1959). *Clinical prosthetics for physicians and therapists*. Springfield: IL: Charles C. Thomas.

Applegate, W., Blass, J., & Williams, F. (1990, April 26). Instruments for the functional assessment of older patients. *New England Journal of Medicine. 322*(17), 1207-1214.

Armstrong, C. J. (Ed.). (1993). *World databases in medicine*. London: Bowker-Saur.

Arthur, G. (1949). The Arthur Adaptation of the Leiter International Performance Scale. *Journal of Clinical Psychology, 5*, 345–349.

Atwater, E. C. (1973). The medical profession in a new society, Rochester, York (1811-60). *Bulletin of the History of Medicine, 47*, 221–235.

Auble, D. (1953). Extended tables for the Mann-Whitney statistic. *Bulletin of the Institute of Educational Research at Indiana University, 1*, No. 2.

Baltimore Therapeutic Equipment Company (1992). *Clinical application model: A clinically-oriented reference model for users of the BTE work simulator*. Baltimore, MD: Author.

Barnhard, C. L. (Ed.). (1948). *American College Dictionary*. New York: Random House.

Barzun, J. (1974). *Clio and the doctors: Psycho-history, quanto-history and history*. Chicago, Illinois: The University of Chicago Press.

Barzun, J., & Graff, H. (1970). *The modern researcher*. New York: Harcourt, Brace and World.

Bayley, N. (1993). *Manual: Bayley Scales of Infant Develoment* (2nd ed.). San Antonio, TX: The Psychological Corporation.

Becker, R. L. (1988). *Reading-Free Vocational Interest Inventory.* Columbus, OH: Elbern.

Beery, K. E. (1989). *The Developmental Test of Visual-Motor Integration.* Cleveland: Modern Curriculum Press.

Bender, L. (1938). A visual motor Gestalt test and its clinical use. *American Orthopsychiatric Association Research Monograph,* No. 3.

Benison, S. (1972). The history of polio research in the United States: Appraisal and lessons. In G. Holton (Ed.), *The twentieth-century sciences: Studies in the biography of ideas* (pp. 308–343). New York: W. Norton.

Bergner, M., Bobbitt, R. A., Carter, W. B., & Gilson, B. S. (1981). The sickness impact profile: Development and final revision of a health status measure. *Medical Care, 19,* 787–805.

Bernard, C. (1957). *An introduction to the study of experimental medicine* (H. C. Greene, Trans.). New York: Dover. (Original work published 1865)

Best, J. W. (1977). *Research in education* (3rd ed.). Englewood Cliffs, NJ: Prentice-Hall.

Bettelheim, B. (1967). *The empty fortress: Infantile autism and the birth of the self.* New York: The Free Press.

Bettleheim, B. (1969). *Children of the dream.* New York: Macmillan.

Binet, A. (1899/1912). *The psychology of reasoning: Based on experimental researches in hypnotism* (2nd ed.). (A.G. Whyte, Trans.). Chicago: Open Court.

Blake, J. B., & Roos, C. (Eds.). (1967). *Medical reference works 1679-1966: A selected bibliography.* Chicago: Medical Library Assoc.

Blankenship, K. (1984). *Individual rehabilitation: Procedure manual.* Mason, GA: American Therapeutics.

Blaskey, P., Scheiman, M., Parisi, M., Ciner, E. B., Gallaway, M., & Selznick, R. (1990). The effectiveness of Irlen filters for improving reading performance: A pilot study. *Journal of Learning Disabilities, 23,* 604–612.

Blumberg, D. F. (1972). The city as a system. In J. Beishon & G. Peters (Ed.), *Systems behavior.* New York: Harper and Row.

Boehm, A. E. (1986). *Boehm Test of Basic Concepts—Revised.* San Antonio, TX: The Psychological Corporation.

Booth, T., & Booth, W. (1994). The use of in-depth interviewing with vulnerable subjects: Lessons from a research study of parents with learning difficulties. *Social Science and Medicine, 39,* 415–424.

Borowitz, G. H., Costello, J., & Hirsch, J. G. (1971). Clinical observation of ghetto 4-year-olds: Organization, involvement, interpersonal responsiveness and psychosexual content of play. *Journal of Youth and Adolescence 1,* 59–71.

Botterbusch, K.F. (1980). *A comparison of commercial vocational evaluations systems.* Menomonie, WI: Stout Vocational Rehabilitation Institute.

Bowker Company (1995). *Medical and health care books and serials in print: An index to literature in the health sciences.* New York: R. R. Bowker.

Brown, L., & Hammill, D.D. (1990). *Behavior Rating Profile—2. Austin,* TX: PRO–ED.

Bruininks, R.H. (1978). *Bruininks–Oseretsky Test of Motor Proficiency.* Circle Pines, MN: American Guidance Service.

Bryman, A., & Burgess, R. G. (Eds.). (1994). *Analyzing qualitative data.* London: Routledge.

Bulgren, J. A., Schumaker, J. B., & Deshler, D. D. (1994). The effects of a recall enhancement routine on the test performance of secondary students with and without learning diabilities. *Learning Disabilities Research, 9,* 1–11.

Bulmer, M. (Ed.). (1982). *Social research ethics.* London: Macmillan.

Burgemeister, B. B., Blum, L. H., & Lorge, I. (1972). *Columbia Mental Maturity Scale* (3rd. ed.). The Psychological Corporation.

Burks, H. (1968). *Burks' Behavior Rating Scales.* Los Angeles: Western Psychological Services.

Buros Institute of Mental Measurements (1992). *The mental measurements yearbook, (11th ed.), mental measurements supplement, or tests in print,* Lincoln: NE: Author, The University of Nebraska Press.

Campbell, D. T., & Stanley, J. (1963). *Experimental and quasi-experimental design for research*. Chicago: Rand-McNally.

Campione, J. C., & Brown, A. L. (1978). Toward a theory of intelligence: Contributions from research with retarded children. *Intelligence, 2*, 279–304.

Cannon, W. B. (1932). *The wisdom of the body*. New York: W. W. Norton.

Carey, R. G., & Posavac, E. J. (1980). *Manual for the Level of Rehabilitation Scale II*. Park Ridge II: Lutheran General Hospital.

Cartwright, L. R., & Ruscello, D. M. (1979). A survey on parent involvement practices in the speech clinic. *Journal of the American Speech and Hearing Association, 21*, 275–279.

Cattell, R. B. (1950). *Culture Fair Intelligence Test*. Champaign, IL: Institute for Personality and Ability Testing.

Cattell, R. B. (1963).Theory of fluid and crystalized intelligence: A critical experiment. *Journal of Educational Psychology, 54*, 615–618.

Cattell, R. B., Cattell, A. K., & Cattell, H. E. P. (1993). *Sixteen Personality Factor Questionaire* (5th ed.). San Antonio, TX: The Psychological Corporation.

Church, G., & Bender, M. (1989). *Teaching with computers! A curriculum for special educators*. Boston: Little, Brown.

Cohen, J. (1960). A coefficient of agreement for nominal scales. *Educational and Psychological Measurement, 20*, 37–46.

Cohen, J. (1977). *Statistical power analysis for the behavioral sciences* (rev. ed.). New York: Academic Press.

Cole, B., Finch, E., Gowland, C., & Mayo, N. (1994). *Physical rehabilitation outcome measures*. Toronto, ON: Canadian Physiotherapy Association

Colton, T.(1974). *Statistics in medicine*. Boston: Little, Brown.

Conant, J. B. (1951). *Science and common sense*. New Haven: Yale University Press.

Conners, C. K. (1989a). *Conners Parent Rating Scales*. North Tonawanda, NY: Multi- Health Systems.

Conners, C. K. (1989b). *Conners Teacher Rating Scales*. North Tonawanda, NY: Multi-Health Systems.

Connolly, A. J. (1988). *Keymath—Revised: A Diagnostic Inventory of Essential Mathematics*. Circle Pines, MN: American Guidance Service.

Conoley, J. C., Kramer, J. J., & Murphy, L. I. (1992). *The mental measurements yearbook, (11th ed.), mental measurements supplement, or tests in print*, Lincoln: NE: The University of Nebraska Press.

Copi, I. (1953). *Introduction to logic*. New York: Macmillan.

Corcoran, K., & Fischer, J. (1987). *Measures for clinical practice: A source book*. New York: The Free Press.

Cronbach, L.J. (1984). *Essentials of psychological testing* (4th ed.). New York: Harper and Row.

Crowther, J. G., & Whiddington, R. (1948). *Science at war*. New York: Philosophical Library.

Cunningham, P. H., & Bartuska, T. (1989). The relationship between stress and leisure satisfaction among therapeutic recreation personnel. *Therapeutic Recreation Journal 23*, 65–70.

Cutler, S. K., Keyes, D. W., & Urquhart, M. (1993). [Effects of teaching methods on understanding collaboration concepts]. Unpublished raw data.

Daniels, L., Williams, M., & Worthingham, C. (1956). *Muscle testing: Techniques of manual examination* (2nd ed.). Philadephia: W.B. Saunders.

Das, J. P., Kirby, J., & Jarman, R. (1975). An alternative model for cognitive abilities. *Psychological Bulletin, 82*, 87–103.

Das, J. P., & Molloy, G.N. (1975). Varieties of simultaneous and successive processing in children. *Journal of Educational Psychology, 67*, 213–220.

Davis, A. M., & Findley, T. W. (1990). Research in physical medicine and rehabilition: X. Information resources. *American Journal of Physical Medicine and Rehabilitation, 69*, 266–278.

Davis, F. B. (Chair). (1974). *Standards for education and psychological tests*. Prepared by a joint committee of the American Psychological Association, American Educational Research Assocation, and National Council on Measurement in Education. Washington, DC: American Psychological Assocation.

Dawber, T. R., Meaders, G. F., & Moore, F. E. Jr., (1951). Epidemiological approaches to heart disease: The Framingham study. *American Journal of Public Health, 41*, 279–286.

Dean, C., & Gadd, E. M. (1990). Home treatment for acute psychiatric illness. *British Medical Journal, 301*, 1021–1023.

Deno, S. L. (1985). Curriculum-based assessment: The emerging alternative. *Exceptional Children, 52*, 219–232.

Denzin, N. K., & Lincoln, Y. S. (Eds.). (1994). *Handbook of qualitative research.* Thousand Oaks: Sage.

DiSimoni, F. (1978). *Token Test for Children.* Austin, TX: PRO–ED.

Directory of Online Databases. (1994). New York: Cuadra / Elsevier.

Donaldson, S. W., Wagner, C. C., & Gresham, G. E. (1973). Unified ADL evaluation form. *Archives of Physical Medicine and Rehabilitation, 54*, 175–179, 185.

Downer, A. H. (1970). *Physical therapy techniques.* Springfield, IL: Charles C. Thomas.

Dukes, W. F. (1965). N = 1 . *Psychological Bulletin, 64*, 73–79.

Dunn, L. M. (1968). Special education for the mildly retarded—Is much of it justifiable? *Exceptional Children, 35*, 5–22.

Dunn, L. M. & Dunn, L. (1981). *Peabody Picture Vocabulary Test—Revised.* Circle Pines, MN: American Guidance Service.

Dykes, M. K. (1980). *Developmental assessment for the severely handicapped.* Austin, TX: Exceptional Resources.

Easton, D. (1961). *A framework for political analysis.* Englewood Cliffs, NJ: Prentice-Hall.

Edgerton, R. B., & Langness, L. L. (1978). Observing mentally retarded persons in community settings: An anthropological perspective. In G. P. Sackett (Ed.), Observing behavior. *Theory and applications in mental retardation* (pp. 335–348). Baltimore: University Park Press.

Edwards, A. L. (1959). *Edwards Personal Preference Schedule.* San Antonio, TX: The Psychological Corporation.

Edwards, D. R., & Bristol, M. M. (1991). Autism: Early identification and management in family practice. *AFP, 44*, 1755–1764.

Enders, A., & Hall, M. (Eds.). (1990). *Assistive technology sourcebook.* Washington, DC: RESNA Press.

Englehart, M. D. (1972). *Methods of educational research.* Chicago: Rand McNally.

Epps, S., & Tindall, G. (1987). The effectiveness of differential programming in serving students with mild handicaps: Placement options and instructional programming. In M.C. Wang, M.C. Reynolds, & H.J. Walberg, (Eds.). (1987). *Handbook of special education: Research and practice.* (Vol. 1) (pp. 213–248). Oxford, England: Pergamon Press.

Ferber, R., & Verdoorn, P. J. (1962). *Research methods in economics and business.* New York: Macmillian.

Ferguson, P. M., Ferguson, D. L., & Taylor, S. J. (Eds.). (1992). *Interpreting disability. A qualitative reader.* New York: Teachers College Press.

Festinger, L., & Katz, O. (1953). *Research methods in the behavioral sciences.* NewYork: Holt, Rinehart and Winston.

Fifteenth Annual Report to Congress on the Implementation of the Education of the Handicapped Act, United States Office of Education, 1993.

Finley, T. W. (1989). Research in physical medicine and rehabilitation: II. The conceptual review of the literature or how to read more articles than you ever want to see in your entire life. *American Journal of Physical Medicine & Rehabilitation, 68*, 97–102.

Flexner, A. (1910). *Medical education in the United States and Canada: A report to the Carnegie Foundation for the Advancement of Teaching,* Bulletin Number Four. New York: Carnegie Foundation.

Folio, M. R., & Fewell, R. R. (1983). *Peabody Developmental Motor Scales.* Allen, TX: DLM Teaching Resources.

Fontana, A., & Frey, J. H. (1994). Interviewing: The art of science. In N. K. Denzin & Y. S. Lincoln (Eds.), *Handbook of qualitative research* (pp. 361–376). Thousand Oaks: Sage.

Forness, S. R., & Kavale, K. A. (1984). Education of the mentally retarded: A note on policy. *Education and Training of the Mentally Retarded, 19*, 239–245.

Frankenburg, W. K., Dodds, J. B., Archer, P., Shapiro, H., & Bresnick, B. (1990). *Denver Developmental Screening Test—II.* Denver: Denver Developmental Materials.

Frederic, M. (1928). *Thrasher, the gang: A study of 1,313 gangs in Chicago.* Chicago: University of Chicago Press.

French, J. L. (1964). *Manual: Pictorial Test of Intelligence.* Chicago: Riverside Publishing.

French, S. (Ed.). (1994). *On equal terms. Working with disabled people.* Oxford: Butterworth/ Heinemann.

Frey, J. J., & Fontana, A. (1995). *The group interview.* Newbury Park, CA: Sage.

Friedman, G. D. (1980). *Primer of epidemiology.* New York: McGraw-Hill.

Fruchter, B. (1954). *Introduction to factor analysis.* Princeton, N.J.: D. Van Nostrand

Galen, C. (1972). On the natural faculties. In W.P.D. Wightman, *The emergence of scientific medicine.* Edinburgh: Oliver and Boyd. (Original work published ca. 192)

Gardner, H. (1983). *Frames of mind: Theories of multiple intelligences.* New York: Basic Books.

Gardner, M. F. (1982). *Test of Visual Perceptual Skills (non–motor).* Burlingame, CA: Psychological and Educational Publications.

Gardner, M. F. (1985). *Test of Auditory Perceptual Skills.* Burlingame, CA:Psychological and Educational Publications.

Gardner, M. F. (1990). *The One-Word Expressive Picture VocabularyTest—Revised.* Novato, CA: Academic Therapy Publications.

Gee, W. (1950). *Social science research methods.* New York: Appleton-Century Crofts.

Gesell, A. (1928). *Infancy and human growth.* New York: McGraw-Hill.

Gesell, A., & Thompson, H. (1923). *Infant behavior: Its genesis and growth.* New York: McGraw-Hill.

Gibaldi, J. (1995). *MLA handbook for writers of research papers* (4th ed.). New York: MLA.

Gilson, B. S., Gilson, J. S., Bergner, M., Bobbitt, R., Kressel, S., Pollard, W.E., & Vesselago, M. (1975). The sickness impact profile: Development of an outcome measure of health care. *American Journal of Public Health, 65,* 1304–1310.

Glaser, B. G., & Strauss, A. L. (1967). *The discovery of grounded theory: Strategies for qualitative research.* Chicago: Aldine.

Glaser, R. (1963). Instructional technology and the measurement of learning outcomes. *American Psychologist, 18,* 510–522.

Goffman, E. (1961). *Asylums: Essays on the social situation of mental patients and other inmates.* Garden City, NJ: Anchor Books.

Gold, R. L. (1958). Roles in sociological field observations. *Social Forces, 36,* 217–223.

Goldberg, R. T. (1974). Rehabilitation research, new directions. *Journal of Rehabilitation, 40(3),* 12–14.

Goldberger L, & Breznitz, S. (Eds.). (1993). *Handbook of stress: Theoretical and clinical aspects* (2nd ed.). New York: The Free Press.

Golden, C. J., Purisch, A. D., & Hammeke, T. A. (1985). *Luria–Nebraska Neuropsychological Battery: Forms I and II (Manual).* Los Angeles: Western Psychological Services.

Gordon, E. E. (1968). A view of the target population. In A. J. Tannenbaum (Ed.), *Special education programs for disadvantaged children and youth* (pp. 5–18). Washington, DC: The Council for Exceptional Children.

Gough, H. G. (1987) *California Psychological Inventory.* New York: Consulting Psychologists Press.

Gould, S. J. (1981). *The mismeasure of man.* New York: Norton.

Gould, J., & Kolb, J. G. (Eds.). (1964). *A dictionary of the social sciences.* (Compiled under the auspices of the United Nations Educational, Scientific and Cultural Organizations). New York: The Free Press.

Granger, C. V., & Greer, D. S. (1976). Functional status measurement and medical rehabilitation outcomes. *Archives of Physical Medicine and Rehabilitation, 57,* 103–109.

Granger, C. V., & Wright, B. (1993). Looking ahead to the use of functional assessment in ambulatory physiatric and primary care. *Physical Medicine and Rehabilitation Clinics of North America, 4(3),* 1-11.

Gravette, F. J., & Wellnau, L. B. (1985). *Statistics for the behavioral sciences.* St. Paul: West.

Guba, E. G. (1990). Carrying on the dialog. In E. G. Guba (Ed.), *The paradigm dialog* (pp. 368–378). Newbury Park, CA: Sage.

Guilford, J. P.(1967). *The nature of human intelligence.* New York: McGraw Hill.

Hahn, M. E. (1969). *California Life Goals Evaluation Schedules*. Los Angeles: Western Psychological Services.

Hall, E. T. (1966). *The hidden dimension*. New York: Doubleday.

Hallahan, D. P., & Kauffman, J. M. (1993). *Exceptional children: Introduction to special education* (6th ed.). Boston: Allyn and Bacon.

Hammill, D. D. (1991). *Detroit Tests of Learning Aptitude—3*. Austin, TX: PRO–ED.

Haring, N., White, O. R., Edgar, E. B., Affleck, J. O., Hayden, A. H., Munson, R. G., & Bendersky, M. (1981). *Uniform Performance Assessment System*. Colunbus, OH: Merrill.

Harper, D. (1989). Visual sociology: Expanding sociological vision. In G. Blank et al. (Eds.), *New technology in sociology: Practical applications in research and work* (pp. 81–97). New Brunswick, NJ: Transaction Books.

Harvey, W. (1938). On the motion of the heart and blood in animals (R. Willis, Trans.). In C. W. Eliot (Ed.), *The Harvard classics scientific papers*. New York: P. E Collier and Sons. (Original work published 1628)

Harvey, W. (1952). An anatomical disquisition on the motion of the heart and blood in animals. In R. M. Hutchins (Ed.; R. Willis., Trans.). *Great books of the western world* (Vol. 28, pp. 267–304). Chicago: Encyclopedia Britannica. (Original work published ca. 1628)

Hatch, M. C., Wallenstein, S., Beyen, J., Nieves, J. W., & Susser, M. (1991). Cancer rates after the Three Mile Island nuclear accident and proximity of residents to the plan. *American Journal of Public Health, 81*, 719–724.

Hathaway, S. & McKinley, C. (1970). *Minnesota Multiphasic Personality Inventory*. Minneapolis, MI: National Computer Systems.

Havighurst, R. J. (1952). *Developmental tasks and education*. New York: Longmans, Green.

Hayes, S. P. (1942). Alternative scales for the mental measurement of the visually handicapped. *Outlook for the Blind, 36*, 249—251.

Hayes, S. P. (1943). A second test scale for the mental measurement of the visually handicapped. *Outlook for the Blind, 37*, 37–41.

Haynes, M. C., & Jenkins, J. R. (1986). Reading instruction in special education resource room. *American Educational Research Journal, 23*, 161–190.

Hemphill, B. J. (Ed.). (1982). *The evaluative process in psychiatric occupational therapy*. Thorofare NJ: Slack.

Hemphill, B. J. (Ed.). (1988). *Mental health assessment in occupational therapy: An integrative approach to the evaluative process*. Thorofare, NJ: Slack.

Henry, J. (1971). *Pathways to madness*. New York: Random House.

Hinshelwood, J. (1917). *Congenital word blindness*. London: Lewis.

Hippocratic writings (1952). On the articulations. In R.M. Hutchins (Ed.; F. Adams, Trans.), *Great books for the western world* (Vol. 10; pp. 91–121). Chicago: Encyclopedia Britannica. (Original work published ca. 5th century)

Hiskey, M. (1966). *Hiskey–Nebraska Test of Learning Aptitude*. Lincoln, NE: Author.

Hoaglin, C. C., Mosteller, F., & Tukey, J. N. (1991). *Fundamentals of exploratory analysis of variance*. New York: Wiley.

Hoover, H. D., Hieronymus, A. N., Frisbie, D. A., & Dunbar, S. B. (1993). *Iowa Test of Basic Skills*. Chicago: Riverside.

Horn, J. L. (1968). Organization of abilities and the development of intelligence. *Psychological Review, 75*, 242–259.

Huberman, A. M., & Miles, M. B. (1994). Data management and analysis methods. In N. K. Denzin & Y. S. Lincoln (Eds.), *Handbook of qualitative research* (pp. 428–444). Thousand Oaks: Sage.

Hunt, N., & Marshall, K. (1994). *Exceptional children and youth*. Geneva, IL: Houghton Mifflin.

Hutchins, R. M. (Ed.). (1952). *Great books of the western world*. Chicago: Encyclopedia Britannica.

Iliff, A., & Lee, V. A. (1952). Pulse rate, respiratory rate and body temperature of children between two months and eighteen years of age. *Child Development, 23*, 237–245.

Illingworth, W. H. (1910). *History of the education of blind*. London: Marston.

Individuals With Disabilities Education Act (1990). Public Law 101–476.

Isernhagen, S. J. (1988). *Work injury management and prevention*. Rockville, MD: Aspen.

Iverson, C. (Chair). (1989). *American Medical Association manual of style* (8th ed.). Baltimore: Williams and Wilkins.

Jacobson, M. L., Mercer, M. A., Miller, L .K., & Simpson, T. W. (1987). Tuberculosis risk among migrant farm workers on the Relmarva Peninsula. *American Journal of Public Health, 77*, 29–32.

Jahoda, M., Deutsch, M., & Cook, S.W. (1951).*Research methods in social relations*. New York: Dryden Press.

Juul, D. (1981). Special education in Europe. In J. M. Kauffman & D. P. Hallahan (Eds.), *Handbook of special education*. Englewood Cliffs, NJ: Prentice Hall.

Kamhi, A., & Catts, H.(Eds.). (1989). *Reading disabilities: A developmental language perspective*. Boston: Little, Brown.

Kaplan, E., Fein, D., Morris, R., & Delis, D.C. (1991). *WAIS–R as a neuropsychological instrument*. San Antonio, TX: The Psychological Corporation.

Katz, S., Ford, R. Q., Moskowitz, R. W., Jackson, B. A., & Jaffe, M. W. (1963). Studies of illness in the aged, the index of ADL: A standardized measure of biological and psychosocial functions. *Journal of American Medical Association, 185*, 914–918.

Kaufman, A. S., & Kaufman, N. L. (1983a). *K-ABC: Kaufman Assessment Battery for Children*. Circle Pines, MN: American Guidance Service.

Kaufman, A. S., & Kaufman, N. L. (1983b). *Kaufman Assessment Battery for Children, interpretative manual*. Circle Pines, MN: American Guidance Service.

Kaufman, A. S., & Kaufman, N. L. (1985). *Kaufman Test of Educational Achievement*. Circle Pines, MN: American Guidance Service.

Kaufman, A. S., & Kaufman, N. L. (1993). *Kaufman Adolescent and Adult Intelligence Test*. Circle Pines, MN: American Guidance Service.

Kazdin, A. E. (1992). *Research design in clinical psychology* (2nd ed.). Boston: Allyn & Bacon.

Keith, R. A. (1984). Functional assessment measures in medical rehabilitation: Current status. *Archives of Physical Medicine and Rehabilitation, 65*, 74–78.

Keith, R. A., Granger, C. V., Hamilton, B. B., & Sherwins, F. S. (1987). The functional independence measure. *Advances in Clinical Rehabilitation, 1*, 6–18.

Kendall, H. O., & Kendall, F. M. P. (1949). *Muscles, testing and function*. Baltimore: Williams and Wilkins.

Kerlinger, F. N. (1986). *Foundations of behavioral research*, (3rd ed.). New York: Holt, Rinehart, and Winston.

Key, K. (1988). *Functional capacity testing*. Proceedings from the Third Annual Symposium for Physical Therapy Educators.

Kirk, J., & Miller, M. L. (1986). *Reliability and validity in qualitative research*. Thousand Oaks: Sage.

Kirk, S.A. (April, 1963). Behavioral diagnosis and remediation of learning disabilities. In *Proceedings of the conference on exploration into the problems of the perceptually handicapped child: First Annual Meeting, Vol. 1*. Chicago, IL.: Association for Children with Learning Disabilities.

Kirk, S. A., & Gallagher, J. J. (1989). *Educating exceptional children*, (5th ed.). Boston: Houghten Mifflin.

Kluge, J. B. (1982). The Walldius prosthesis: A total treatment program. *Physical Therapy 52*, 26-33.

Kohs, S. (1923). *Intelligence measurements*. New York: Macmillan.

Kopolow, M. S., & Jensen, B. M. (1975). *Psychosocial adjustment to quadriplegia: A double case study*. Unpublished Master's Thesis, Sargent College, Boston University.

Koppitz, E. M. (1963). *The Bender Gestalt Test for Young Children*. New York: Grune & Stratton.

Koppitz, E. M. (1975). *The Bender Gestalt Test for Young Children: Volume II: Research and application, 1963–1973*. New York: Grune & Stratton.

Kovacs, M. (1992). *Children's Depression Inventory*. San Antonio: The Psychological Corporation.

Krathwohl, D. R. (1988). *How to prepare a research proposal: Guidelines for funding and dissertations in the social and behavioral sciences* (3rd ed.). Syracuse: NY: Syracuse University Press.

Kuder, F. (1960). *Kuder Occupational Interest Survey—Form DD*. Chicago: Science Research Associates DD .

Kuzma, J. W. (1984). *Basic statistics for the health sciences*. Palo Alto, CA: Mayfield.

Lachar, D. (1982). *Personality Inventory for Children—Revised*. Los Angeles: Western Psychological Services.

Lane, H. (1976). *The wild boy of Aveyron*. Cambridge, MA: Harvard University Press.

Larson, R. J. (1975). *Statistics for the allied health sciences*. Columbus, OH: Merrill.

Lawton, E.B. (1956). *Activities of daily living*. New York: New York Institute of Physical Medicine and Rehabilitation, NYU-Bellevue Medical Center.

Lawton, M. P., Moss, M., Fulcomer, M. , & Kleban, M. H. (1982). A research and service oriented multilevel assessment instrument. *Journal of Gerontology, 37*, 91–99.

Lechner, D. E., Jackson, J. R., Roth, D. L., & Straaton, K. V. (1994). Reliability and validity of a newly developed test of physical work performance. *Journal of Occupational Medicine, 36*, 997–1004.

Lechner, D. E., Roth, D., & Straaton, K. (1991). *Functional capacity evaluation in work disability. Work, 1*, 37–47.

Leiter, R.G. (1948). *Leiter International Performance Scale*. Chicago: Stoelting.

Leonardelli, C. A. (1988). The Milwaukee Evaluation of Daily Living Skills. In B.J. Hemphill (Ed.), *Mental health assessment in occupational therapy: An integrative approach to the evaluative process*. Thorofare, NJ: Slack.

Lewin, K. (1939). Field theory and experiment in social psychology: Concepts and methods. *American Journal of Sociology, 44*, 868–897.

Lewis, O. (1965). *La vida*. New York: Random House.

Lezak, M. (1984). *Neuropsychological assessment* (2nd ed.). New York: Oxford University Press.

Liberman, I. Y. (1973). Segmentation of the spoken word and reading acquisition. *Bulletin of the Orton Dyslexia Society, 23*, 65–77.

Lincoln, Y. S., & Guba, E. G. (1985). *Naturalistic inquiry*. Beverly Hills, CA: Sage.

Liu, L., Gauthier, L., & Gauthier, S. (1991). Spatial disorientation in persons with early senile dementia of the Alzheimer type. *The American Journal of Occupational Therapy, 45*, 67–74.

Llewellyn, G. (1995). Qualitative research with people with intellectual disability. *Occupational Therapy International, 2*, 108–127.

Locke, L. F., Spirduso, W. W., & Silverman, S.J. (1987). *Proposals that work: A guide for planning dissertations and grant proposals*. Newbury Park, CA: Sage.

Lofquist, L. H. (1957). *Vocational counseling with the physically handicapped*. New York: Appleton-Century-Crofts.

Longmore, D (1970). *Machines in medicine*. New York: Doubleday.

Lorge, I., & Thorndike, R. (1966). *Lorge-Thorndike Intelligence Test*. Chicago: Riverside.

Luria, A. R. (1961). *The role of speech in the regulation of normal and abnormal behavior*. London: Pergaman.

Luria, A. R. (1980). *Higher cortical functions in man* (2nd ed.).(B. Haigh, Trans.). New York: Basic Books.

Luria, A. R., & Yudovich, F. I (1959). *Speech and the development of mental process in the child*. London: Staples Press.

Maher, B. A. (1978). A reader's, writer's, and reviewer's guide to assessing research reports in clinical psychology. *Journal of Consulting and Clinical Psychology, 46*, 835–838.

Mahoney, F. I., & Barthel, D. W. (1965). Functional evaluation: Barthel Index. *Maryland State Medical Journal, 14*, 61-65.

Mann, H. B., & Whitney, D. R. (1947). On a test of whether one of two random variables is stochastically larger than the other. *Annals of Mathematical Statistics, 18*, 52-54.

Markwardt, R. (1989). *Peabody Individual Achievement Test–Revised*. Circle Pines, MN: American Guidance Services.

Marti-Ibanez, F. (1962). *The epic of medicine*. New York: Bramhall House.

Martin, R. P., Hooper, S., & Snow, J. (1986). Behavior rating scale approaches to personality assessment in children and adolescents. In H. M. Knoff (Ed.), *The assessment of child and adolescent personality* (pp. 309–351). New York: Guilford.

Maslow, A. H. (1954). *Motivation and personality*. New York: Harper.

Matheson, L. (1988). *Work capacity evaluation (procedure manual)*. Anaheim: Employment and Rehabilitation Institute of California.

Matter, S., Weltman, A., & Stamford, B.A. (1980). Body fat content and serum lipid levels. *Journal of the American Dietetic Association, 77*, 149–152.

McCall, R. B. (1986). *Fundamental statistics for behavioral sciences* (4th ed.). San Diego: Harcourt Brace Jovanovich.

McCarthy, D. A. (1972a). *McCarthy Scales of Children's Abilities.* San Antonio, TX: The Psychological Corporation.

McCarthy, D. A. (1972b). *Manual for the McCarthy Scales of Children's Abilities.* San Antonio: The Psychological Corporation.

McFall, S. A., Deitz, J. C., & Crowe, T. K. (1993). Test-retest reliability of the test of visual perceptual skills with children with learning disabilities. *The American Journal of Occupational Therapy, 47,* 819–824.

McGowan, J. F. (Ed.). (1960). *An introduction to the vocational rehabilitation services (Series no. 555; guidance, training and placement bulletin no. 3).* Washington, DC: Office of Vocational Rehabilitation, US Government Printing Office.

Mead, M. (1928). *Coming of age in Samoa.* New York: Blue Ribbon Books.

Mercer, C. (1983). *Students with learning disabilities* (2nd ed.). Columbus, OH: Merrill.

Merriam–Webster's Collegiate Dictionary (10th ed.). (1993). Springfield, MA: Merriam–Webster.

Merrington, M., & Thompson, C. M. (1943). Tables of percentage points of the inverted beta (F) distribution. *Biometrica, 33,* 73–88.

Meyen, E. L., & Skrtic, T. M. (1988). *Exceptional children and youth* (3rd ed.). Aspen, CO: Love.

Miles, M. B., & Huberman, A. M. (1994). *Qualitative data analysis. An expanded sourcebook* (2nd ed.). Thousand Oaks, CA: Sage.

Miller, L. J. (1988). *Miller Assessment for Preschoolers.* San Antonio, TX: The Psychological Corporation.

Miller, N. E. (1969). Learning of visceral and glandular responses. *Science, 163,* 434–445.

Million, T., Green, C. J., & Meagher, R. B., Jr. (1982). *Million Adolescent Personality Inventory.* Minneapolis: NM: National Computer Services, Inc.

Minichiello, V., Aroni, R., Timewell, E., & Alexander, L. (1990). *Indepth interviewing: researching people.* Melbourne: Longman Cheshire.

Montessori, M. (1912). *The Montessori method* (A. E. George ,Trans). New York: Frederick A. Stokes.

Morse, J. M. (Ed.). (1994). *Critical issues in qualitative research methods.* Thousand Oaks, CA: Sage.

Morton,T., & Godholt, S. (Eds.). (1993). *Information sources in the medical sciences.* (4th ed.). London: Bowker-Saur.

Muhr, T. (1991). ATLAS/Ti. A prototype for the support of text interpretation. *Qualitative Sociology, 14,* 349–371.

Nadolsky, J. M. (1974). The work sample in vocational evaluation: A consistent rationale. *Vocational Evaluation and Work Adjustment Bulletin, 7,* 2–5.

Naglieri, J.A., LeBuffe, P.A., & Pfeiffer, S. I. (1992). *Devereaux behavior rating scales—School Form.* San Antonio, TX: The Psychological Corporation.

Naglieri, J. A., LeBuffe, P. A., & Pfeiffer, S. I. (1994). *Devereaux scales of mental disorders.* San Antonio, TX: The Psychological Corporation.

National Center for Health Studies, (1974). *Inpatient health facilities as reported from the 1971 MFI Survey. Data on national health resources* (Series 14, Number 12), DHEW Publication No. (HRA) 74-1807.

National Information Center on Health Services Research & Health Care Technology Fact Sheet (26Apr94). Available E-mail: nichsr@nlm.nih.gov or National Information Center on Health Services Research and Health Care Technology (NICHSR), National Library of Medicine.

Newborg, J., Stock, J. R,. & Wnek, L. (1984). *Battelle Developmental Inventory Screening Test.* Allen, TX: LINC Associates.

Nicholson, C. L, & Hibpshman, T. H. (1990). *Slosson Intelligence Test—Revised.* East Aurora, NY: Slosson Educational Publications.

Northrop, F. S. C. (1931). *Science and first principles.* New York: Macmillian.

O'Conner, P. D., Sofo, F., Kendall, L, & Olsen, G. (1990). Reading disabilities and the effects of colored filters. *Journal of Learning Disabilities, 23,* 597–603.

Olds, E. G. (1938). Distribution of the sums of squares of rank differences for small numbers of individuals. *Annals of Mathematical Statistics, 9,* 133–148.

Olds, E. G. (1949). The 5 percent significant levels of sums of squares of rank differences and a correction. *Annals of Mathematical Statistics, 20,* 117–118.

Oliver, M. (Ed.). (1991). *Social work: Disabled people and disabling environments*. London: Jessica Kingsley.

Osipow, S. H., & Spokane, A. R. (1987) *Occupational stress inventory manual: Research version*. Odessa: FL: Psychological Assessment Resources.

Otis A.S., & Lennon, R.T. (1989). *Otis–Lennon School Ability Test* (6th ed.). San Antonio, TX: The Psychological Corporation.

Ottenbacher, K. (1992). Confusion in occupational therapy research: Does the end justify the method? *American Journal of Occupational Therapy, 46*, 871–874.

Ottenbacher, K. J., & Barrett, K. A. (1990). Statistical conclusion validity in rehabilitation research. *American Journal of Physical Medicine and Rehabilitiation, 69*, 102–107.

Owen. D. B. (1962). *Handbook of statistical tables*. Reading MA: Addison-Wesley.

Palmer, M. (1989). Mobilization following lumbar discectomy: A comparison of two methods of bed transfer. *Physiotherapy Canada, 41*, 146–152.

Paracelsus (1971). Paragranum. In W.P.D. Wightman, *The emergence of scientific medicine*. Edinburgh: Oliver and Boyd. (Original work published 1528)

Parsons, T. (Ed.). (1964). *Max Weber: The theory of social and economic organization*. New York: Free Press.

Patterson, C. H. (1958). *Counseling the emotionally disturbed*. New York: Harper and Bros.

Patton, M. Q. (1990). *Qualitative evaluation and research methods* (2nd ed.). Newbury Park, CA: Sage.

Pavlov, I. P. (1927). *Conditioned reflexes*. London: Oxford University Press.

Pearson, E., & Hartley, H. (1966). *Biometricka tables for statisticians* (3rd ed.). London: Cambridge University Press.

Perls, F, (1969). *Gestalt therapy verbatim*. Lafayette, CA: Real People Press.

Piaget, J. (1926). *The language and thought of the child* (M. Gabain & R. Gabain, Trans.). London: K. Paul, Trench, Trubner.

Piers, E. V., & Harris, D. B. (1984). *The Piers–Harris Children's Self-Concept Scale: Revised manual*. Los Angeles: Western Psychological Services.

Power, P. (1991). *A guide to vocational assessment* (2nd ed.). Austin, TX: PRO–ED

Poynter, N. (1971). *Medicine and man*. Middlesex, England: Penguin Books.

Pribram, K. (1958). Comparative neurology and the evolution of behavior. In A. Roe and G. G. Simpson (Eds.), *Behavior and evolution* (pp. 140–164). New Haven: Yale University Press.

Psychological Corporation, (1990). *Stanford Achievement Test series, eighth edition: Measuring progress toward America's educational goals*. San Antonio, TX: Harcourt Brace Jovanovich.

Psychological Corporation, (1992). *Stanford Achievement Test* (8th ed.). San Antonio, TX: Harcourt Brace Jovanovich.

Psychological Corporation. (1992). *Wechsler Individual Achievement Test*. San Antonio, TX: Harcourt Brace Jovanovich.

Raven, J.C. (1963). *The Progressive Matrices*. Los Angeles: Western Psychological Services.

Raven, J.C. (1992). *The Standard Progressive Matrices*. San Antonio, TX.: The Psychological Corporation.

Raven, J. C., Court, J. H., & Raven, J. C. (1977). *The Coloured Progressive Matrices Test*. London: Lewis.

Raven, J.C., Court, J.H., & Raven, J. C. (1993). *The Advanced Progressive Matrices*. San Antonio: TX: The Psychological Corporation.

Reason, P. (Ed.). (1988). *Human inquiry in action: Developments in new paradigm research*. London: Sage.

Reish, W. T. (Ed.). (1995). *Encyclopedia of bioethics*. New York: Macmillian Library Reference, Simon and Schuester.

Reynolds, M., & Walberg, H. J. (Eds.). (1987). *Handbook of special education: Research and practice, Volume I: Learning characteristics and adaptive education* (pp. 213–248). Oxford: Pergamon.

Reynolds, W. M. (1987). *Auditory discrimination test* (2nd ed.). Los Angeles: Western Psychological Services.

Richards, T., & Richards, L. (1990). *NUD.IST 2.1 Manual*. Melbourne: Replee.

Roach, E. F., & Kephart, N. C. (1966). *The Purdue Perceptual-Motor Survey*. Columbus, OH: Merrill.

Roget's Thesaurus (1994). Miami, FL: Paradise Press.

Roper, F.W., & Boorkman, J. A. (1994). *Introduction to reference sources in the health sciences* (3rd ed.). Metuchen, NJ: Scarecrow.

Rosenthal, R., & Rosnow, R. (1991). *Essentials of behavioral research: Methods and data analysis* (2nd ed.). New York: McGraw-Hill.

Rousseau, J. J. (1883). *Emile: Or, concerning education.* (J. Steeg, Ed.; E. Worthington, Trans.) Boston: D.C. Heath. (Original published 1762)

Runyon, R. P. (1977). *Nonparametric statistics.* Reading, Mass: Addison-Wesley.

Runyon, R. P., & Haber, A. (1967). *Fundamentals of behavior statistics.* Reading, MA: Addison-Wesley.

Rushmer, R. F. (1972). *Medical engineering: Projections for health care delivery.* New York: Academic Press.

Rusk, H. A. (1971). *Rehabilitation medicine.* St. Louis: C. V. Mosby.

Russell, B. (1928). *Sceptical essays.* London: Allen and Unwin.

Sailor, W. (1991). Special education in the restructured school. *Remedial and Special Education, 12* (6), 8–22.

Saint–John, L. M., & White, M. A. (1988). The effect of coloured transparencies on the reading performance of reading disabled children. *Australian Journal of Psychology, 40,* 403–411.

Salvia, J. & Ysseldyke, J. E. (1995). *Assessment* (6th ed.). Boston: Houghton-Mifflin.

Sand, R (1952). *The advance to social medicine.* London: Staples Press.

Sanford, A.R., & Zelman, J. G. (1981). *Learning Accomplishment Profile* (rev. ed.). Winston- Salem, NC: Kaplan Press.

Santa Cruz County Superintendent of Schools (1973). *Behavioral Characteristics Progression Checklist.* Palo Alto, CA: VORT Corporation.

Sarno, J. E., Sarno, M. R., & Levita, E. (1973). Functional Life Scale. *Archives of Physical Medicine and Rehabilitation, 54,* 214–220.

Sattler, J. M. (1988). *Assessment of children* (3rd ed.). San Diego: Sattler.

Schatzman, L., & Strauss, A. L. (1973). *Field research. Strategies for a natural sociology.* Englewood Cliffs, NJ: Prentice-Hall.

Schoening, H., & Iversen, I. (1968). Numerical scoring of self-care status: A study of the Kenny Self-care Evaluation. *Archives of Physical Medicine and Rehabilitation, 49,* 221–229.

Schwandt, T. A., & Halpern, E. S. (1988). *Linking auditing and metaevaluation: Enhancing quality in applied research.* Newbury Park, CA: Sage.

Schwartz, C. A., & Turner, R. L. (1995). *Encyclopedia of associations* (3rd ed.). Detroit: Gale.

Schwartz, H., & Jacobs, J. (1979). Qualitative sociology. *A method to the madness.* New York: Free Press.

Seidel, J. (1989). *The ethnograph.* Littleton: Qualis Research Associates.

Selye, H. (1956). *Stress of life.* New York: McGraw-Hill.

Semel, E., Wiig, E. H., & Secord, W. (1987). *Clinical Evaluation of Language Fundamentals—Revised.* San Antonio, TX: The Psychological Corporation.

Shaffir, W. B., & Stebbins, R. A. (Eds.). (1991). Experiencing fieldwork. *An inside view of qualitative research.* Newbury Park, CA: Sage.

Shalik, L. D. (1990). The level 1 field work process. *American Journal of Occupational Therapy, 44,* 700–707.

Shaw, G. B. (1919). Annajanska, The Bolshevik princess. In G. B. Shaw, *Collection of plays, heartbreak house, Great Catherine and playets of war.* London: Comfortable.

Shea, T. M., & Bauer, A. M. (1994). *Learners with disabilities: A social systems perspective of special education.* Madison, WI: Brown and Benchmark.

Sigmon, S. B. (1987). *Radical analysis of special education: Focus on historical development and learning disabilities.* London: Falmer Press.

Simmons, L., & Wolff, H. G. (1954). *Social science in medicine.* New York: Russell Sage Foundation.

Skinner, B.F. (1953). *Science and human behavior.* New York: Macmillan.

Slade, C., Campbell, W. G., & Ballou, S. V. (1994). *Form and style.* Boston: Houghton Mifflin.

Smith, S. L., Cunningham, S., & Weinberg, R. (1986). The predictive validity of the functional capacities evaluation. *American Journal of Occupational Therapy, 40,* 564–567.

Snow, C.P. (1964). *The two cultures and a second look.* Cambridge, England: Cambridge University Press.

Sparrow, S., Balla, D., & Ciocchetti, D. (1984). *Vineland Adaptive Behavior Scales.* Circle Pines, MN: American Guidance Service.

Spatz. C., & Johnston, J. O. (1981). *Basic statistics: Tales of distribution* (2nd ed.). Monterey, CA: Brooks/Cole.

Spearman, C. E. (1927). *The abilities of man.* New York: Macmillan.

Spence, K. V. (1948) The postulates and methods of "behaviorism". *Psychological Review, 55,* 67–68.

Spradley, J. P. (1979). *The ethnographic interview.* Fort Worth, TX: Holt, Rinehart and Winston.

Stainback, S., & Stainback, W. (Eds.). (1992). *Controversial issues confronting special education.* Boston: Allyn & Bacon.

Stanton, A. H., & Schwartz, M. S. (1954). *The mental hospital: A study of institutional participation in psychiatric illness and treatment.* New York: Basic Books.

Stein, F. (1989). *Anatomy of clinical research: An introduction to scientific inquiry in medicine, rehabilitation, and related health professions* (rev. ed.). Thorofare, NJ: Slack.

Stein, F. (1988). Research analysis of O.T. assessments used in mental health. In B.J. Hemphill (Ed.),*The mental health assessment in occupational therapy: An integrative approach to the evaluative process* (pp. 225–247). Thorofare, NJ: Slack.

Stein, F., & Nikolic, S. (1989). Teaching stress management techniques to a schizophrenic patient. *American Journal of Occupational Therapy, 43,* 162–169.

Stevens, S. (1951). *Measurement and psychophysics.* New York: Wiley.

Strauss, A. A., & Kephart, N. C. (1940). Behavior differences in mentally retarded children measured by a new behavior rating scale. *American Journal of Psychiatry, 96,* 1117–1123.

Strauss, A. A., & Lehtinen, L. L. (1947). *Psychopathology of the brain-injured child.* New York: Grune & Stratton.

Strauss, A. A., & Werner, H. (1941). The mental organization of the brain-injured mentally defective child. *American Journal of Psychiatry, 97,* 1194–1202.

Strauss, A. A., & Werner, H. (1943). Comparative psychopathology of the brain-injured child and the traumatic brain-injured adult. *American Journal of Psychiatry, 99,* 835.

Strauss, A. L., & Corbin, J. (1990). *Basics of qualitative research: Grounded theory procedures and techniques.* Newbury Park, CA: Sage.

Strong, K. E., Campbell, D. P., & Hansen, J. (1985). *The Strong–Campbell Interest Inventory.* Minneapolis, MI: National Computer Systems.

Strunk, W. Jr., & White, E. B. (1979). *The elements of style.* New York: Macmillian.

Suchman, E. A. (1967). *Evaluative research: Principles and practice in public service and social action programs.* New York: Russell Sage Foundation.

Swanson, H. L,. & Watson, B. L. (1989). *Educational and psychological assessment of exceptional children: Theories, strategies, and applications* (2nd ed.). Columbus: Merrill.

Tarlov, A. R., Ware, J.E., Greenfield, S., Nelson, E. C., Perrin, E., & Zubkoff, M. (1989). The medical outcomes study: An application of methods for monitoring the results of medical care. *Journal of the American Medical Association, 262,* 925–930

Taylor, M. L., & Marks, M. (1955). *Aphasic rehabilitation: Manual and workbook.* New York: Rehabilitation, NYU-Bellevue Medical Center.

Terman, L. (1916). *The measument of intelligence.* Boston: Houghton Mifflin.

Terman, L., & Merrill, M. (1937). *Measuring intelligence.* Boston: Houghton Mifflin.

Terman, L., & Merrill, M. (1973). *Stanford–Binet Intelligence Scale.* Boston: Houghton Mifflin.

Tesch, R. (1990). Qualitative research: Analysis types and software tools. New York: Falmer Press.

Thomas, C. L. (Ed.). (1993). *Taber's Cyclopedic Medical Dictionary* (17th ed.). Philadelphia: F.A. Davis.

Thomson, L. K. (1992). *The Kohlman Evaluation of Living Skills.* Rockland, MD: American Occupational Therapy Association.

Thorndike, R., Hagen, E. & Sattler, J. (1985). *Stanford-Binet Intelligence Scale: Fourth Edition.* Chicago: Riverside.

Thornwald, J. (1963). *Science and secrets of early medicine.* New York: Harcourt, Brace and World.

Thurstone, L. L. (1938). Primary mental abilities. *Psychometric Monographs, No. 1.*

Tukey, J.W. (1977). *Exploratory data analysis.* Reading, Mass.: Addison-Wesley.

Turabian, K. L. (1987). *A manual for writers of term papers, theses, and dissertations* (6th ed.). Chicago: University of Chicago Press.

Turnbull, H. R., III (1986). *Free appropriate public education: The law and children with disabilities.* Aspen, CO: Love.

Underwood, R. J., Duncan, C. P., Taylor, J. A., & Cotton, J. W. (1954). *Elementary statistics.* New York: Appleton-Centurn-Crofts.

United Nations (1958). *Population studies* (Number 29). New York: Author.

United States Department of Defense, Joint Service Steering Committee (1963). *Human engineering guide to equipment design.* (Morgan, C. T. et al., Eds.). New York: McGraw-Hill.

United States Department Health and Human Services, National Center for Health Statistics, (1992). United States Department of Defense, Joint Service Steering Committee (1963). *Human engineering guide to equipment design.* (Morgan, C. T. et al., eds.). New York: McGraw-Hill.

United States Department of Labor (1972–73, 1988–89, 1992–93). *Occupational outlook handbook.*

University of Chicago (1993). *Chicago manual of style* (14th ed.). Chicago: Author.

Vergason, G. A., & Anderegg, M. L. (1992). Preserving the least restrictive environment. In S. Stainback and W. Stainback (Eds.), *Controversial issues confronting special education* (pp. 45–54). Boston: Allyn & Bacon.

Vygotsky, L. S. (1962). *Thought and language.* (E.Hanfmann and G. Vaka, Eds. & Trans.). Cambridge, MA: MIT Press. (Original published 1934)

Walker, J. E., & Howland, J. (1991). Falls and fear of falling among elderly persons living in the community. *American Journal of Occupational Therapy, 45,* 119–122.

Wallas, G. (1926). *The art of thought.* New York: Harcourt Brace.

Wallis, W. A., & Roberts, H. V. (1962). *The nature of statistics.* New York: Free Press.

Walters, L., & Kahn, T. J. (Eds.). (1990). *Bibliography of bioethics* (Vol. 16). Washington, DC: Georgetown University, Kennedy Institute.

Watson, J. D. (1968). *The double helix.* New York: Atheneum.

Weaver, W. (1947). *The scientists speak.* New York: Boni and Gaar.

Webster's Intermediate Dictionary (1986). Springfield, MA: Merriam.

Wechsler, D. (1981). *Manual for the Wechsler Adult Intelligence Scale—Revised.* New York: The Psychological Corporation.

Wechsler, D. (1989). *Wechsler Preschool and Primary Scale of Intelligence—Revised.* San Antonio, TX: The Psychological Corporation.

Wechsler, D. (1991). *Wechsler Intelligence Scale for Children—III.* San Antonio, TX: The Psychological Corporation.

Weiss, C. H. (1972). *Evaluation research: Methods for assessing program effectiveness.* Englewood Cliffs, NJ: Prentice-Hall.

Weiss-Lambrou, R. (1989). *The health professional's guide to writing for publication.* Springfield, IL: Charles C. Thomas

Weitzmann, E. A., & Miles, M. B. (1995). *Computer programs for qualitative analysis.* Thousand Oaks, CA: Sage.

Welch, J., & King, T. A. (1985). *Searching the medical literature: A guide to printed and online sources.* London: Chapman and Hall.

Welkowitz, J., Ewen, R. B., & Cohen, J. (1971). *Introductory statistics for the behavioral sciences.* New York: Academic Press.

White, R. W. (1952). *Lives in progress.* New York: Reinhart and Winston.

Wiener, N. (1948). *Cybernetics.* New York: Wiley.

Wightman, W. P. D. (1971). *The emergence of scientific medicine.* Edinburgh: Oliver and Boyd.

Wilkinson, G. (1993). *Wide Range Achievement Test—3.* Wilmington, DE: Jastak Associates.

Will, M. (1986). Educating children with learning problems: A shared responsibility. *Exceptional Children, 52,* 411–415.

Willard, H. S., & Spackman, C. S. (1971). *Occupational therapy* (4th ed.). Philadelphia: J.B. Lippincott.

Willer, B., Ottenbacher, K. J., & Coad, M. L. (1994). The community integration questionnaire: A comparative examination. *American Journal of Physical Medicine & Rehabiliation, 73,* 103–111.

Winkler, A. C., & McCuen, J. R. (1979). *Writing the research paper: A handbook.* New York: Harcourt Brace Jovanovich.

Winnie, A. J. (1912). *History and handbook of day schools for the deaf and blind.* Madison, WI: State Department of Education.

Winter, S. (1987). Irlen lenses: An appraisal. *Australian Educational and Developmental Psychologist, 4,* 1–5.

Wirt, R. D., Lachar, D., Klinedinst, J. K., & Seat, P. D. (1984). *Multidimensional description of child personality: A manual for the Personality Inventory for Children* (1984 revision by D. Lachar). Los Angeles, CA: Western Psychological Services.

Wolfensberger, W. (1972). *The principle of normalization in human services.* Toronto: National Institution on Mental Retardation.

Wolpe, J. (1969). *The practice of behavior therapy.* New York: Pergamon Press.

Woodcock, R. (1987). *Woodcock Reading Mastery Tests—Revised.* Circle Pines, MN: American Guidance Service.

Woodcock, R., & Johnson, M. B. (1989). *Woodcock–Johnson—Revised.* Chicago: Riverside.

World Medical Association (1993). *Handbook of declarations.* Ferney-Voltaire, France: Author.

Zimmerman, I. L., Steiner, V. G., & Pond, R. E. (1992). *Preschool Language Scale—3.* San Antonio, TX: The Psychological Corporation.

Zinsser, W. (1990). *On writing well: An informal guide to writing nonfiction* (4th ed.) New York: Harper Collins.

Index